Obstetric and Gynecologic Anesthesia

THE REQUISITES IN ANESTHESIOLOGY

SERIES EDITOR **Roberta L. Hines, MD**
Chair and Professor of Anesthesiology
Yale University School of Medicine
New Haven, Connecticut

Obstetric and Gynecologic Anesthesia

THE REQUISITES IN ANESTHESIOLOGY

Ferne R. Braveman, MD
Professor of Anesthesiology
Adjunct Professor of Obstetrics and Gynecology
Director
Section of Obstetric Anesthesiology
Yale University School of Medicine
New Haven, Connecticut

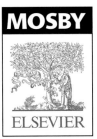

MOSBY

ELSEVIER

**ELSEVIER
MOSBY**

1600 John F. Kennedy Boulevard
Suite 1800
Philadelphia, PA 19103-2899

THE REQUISITES ™
THE REQUISITES
THE REQUISITES
THE REQUISITES
THE REQUISITES

THE REQUISITES is a proprietary trademark
of Mosby, Inc.

OBSTETRIC AND GYNECOLOGIC ANESTHESIA:
THE REQUISITES IN ANESTHESIOLOGY
Copyright © 2006 Mosby, Inc. All rights reserved.

ISBN-13: 978-0-323-02420-4
ISBN-10: 0-323-02420-3

Notice

Knowledge and best practice in this field are constantly changing. As new research and experience broaden our knowledge, changes in practice, treatment and drug therapy may become necessary or appropriate. Readers are advised to check the most current information provided (i) on procedures featured or (ii) by the manufacturer of each product to be administered, to verify the recommended dose or formula, the method and duration of administration, and contraindications. It is the responsibility of the practitioner, relying on his or her own experience and knowledge of the patient, to make diagnoses, to determine dosages and the best treatment for each individual patient, and to take all appropriate safety precautions. To the fullest extent of the law, neither the Publisher nor the Editor assumes any liability for any injury and/or damage to persons or property arising out or related to any use of the material contained in this book.

First Edition 2006.

Library of Congress Cataloging-in-Publication Data
Obstetric and gynecologic anesthesia: the requisites in anesthesiology / [edited by]
  Ferne R. Braveman.
      p. ; cm. – (Requisites in anesthesiology series)
  ISBN 0-323-02420-3
    1. Anesthesia in obstetrics. I. Braveman, Ferne R. II. Series.
    [DNLM: 1. Anesthesia, Obstetrical. WO 450 O14231 2006]
  RG732.O275 2006
  617.9'682–dc22   2005053001

Developmental Editor: Anne Snyder
Senior Project Manager: Mary Stermel
Marketing Manager: Emily Christie

Printed in the United States of America.

Last digit is the print number: 9 8 7 6 5 4 3 2 1

Working together to grow
libraries in developing countries
www.elsevier.com | www.bookaid.org | www.sabre.org

ELSEVIER   BOOK AID
            International   Sabre Foundation

I would like to dedicate this book to my family,
whose support is unwavering.

Contributors

Ferne R. Braveman, MD
Professor of Anesthesiology
Adjunct Professor of Obstetrics and Gynecology
Director
Section of Obstetric Anesthesiology
Yale University School of Medicine
New Haven, Connecticut

Pamela Flood, MD
Assistant Professor of Anesthesiology
Columbia University;
Assistant Attending
Columbia University Medical Center
New York, New York

Regina Y. Fragneto, MD
Associate Professor of Anesthesiology
Director
Section of Obstetric Anesthesia
University of Kentucky College of Medicine
Lexington, Kentucky

Stephanie Goodman, MD
Associate Clinical Professor of Anesthesiology
Columbia University;
Associate Attending
Columbia University Medical Center
New York, New York

Ana M. Lobo, MD, MPH
Assistant Professor of Anesthesiology
Section of Obstetric Anesthesia
Yale University School of Medicine
New Haven, Connecticut

Mirjana Lovrincevic, MD
Clinical Assistant Professor of Anesthesiology
School of Medicine and Biomedical Sciences
The State University of New York, University at Buffalo;
Director
Regional Anesthesia/Postoperative Analgesia
Buffalo, New York

Julio E. Marenco, MD
Assistant Professor of Clinical Anesthesiology
Columbia University College of Physicians and Surgeons;
Attending Anesthesiologist
St. Luke's Roosevelt Hospital
New York, New York

Imre Redai, MD, FRCA
Assistant Professor of Anesthesiology
Columbia University School of Medicine
New York, New York

Alan C. Santos, MD, MPH
Chairman of Anesthesiology
Ochsner Clinic Foundation
New Orleans, Louisiana

Jason Scott, FRCA
Consultant Anaesthetist
Department of Anaesthesia
St. Thomas' Hospital
London, United Kingdom

Nalini Vadivelu, MD
Assistant Professor of Anesthesiology
Yale University School of Medicine;
Attending
Yale-New Haven Hospital
New Haven, Connecticut

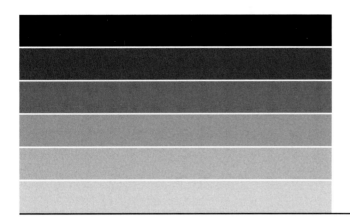

Preface

Obstetric and Gynecologic Anesthesia: The Requisites in Anesthesiology provides a thorough and concise presentation of the anesthetic considerations and management of the female patient. The book includes a discussion of the care of the pregnant patient, and it also provides information for the care and management of the female patient with unique pain management concerns as well as for her care related to gynecologic surgery.

This book is intended for a wide audience, including the anesthesiologist needing a quick review, the resident rotating in obstetrics and gynecology, and those preparing for board examinations and recertification. *Obstetric and Gynecologic Anesthesia* is presented in two major sections. The first section reviews the physiology of pregnancy and discusses care of the pregnant patient

throughout her pregnancy and into the postpartum period. The second section discusses care of the female patient for gynecologic surgery, care of the female oncology patient, and care of the patient with chronic pelvic pain. The use of illustrations, tables, summaries, and case studies should serve to make this a user-friendly text for quick reference as well as a review of the subject. In total, this volume should provide a concise reference for the care of our female patients.

I would like to acknowledge my many mentors, both past and present, without whom this book would not have been possible. Among them are Sanjay Datta, Gerry Ostheimer, Paul Barash, and Roberta Hines. The lessons I learned from them will never be forgotten.

Contents

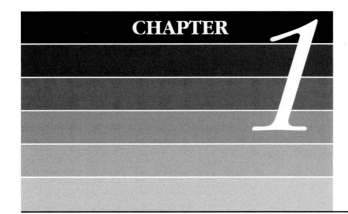

CHAPTER 1

Maternal Physiology and Pharmacology

STEPHANIE GOODMAN

PAMELA FLOOD

Physiologic changes occur during pregnancy that allow maternal adaptation to the demands of the growing fetus, supporting placental unit, and ultimately to facilitate labor and delivery. These modifications affect almost every organ system and influence the anesthetic and perioperative management of the pregnant woman. The physiologic changes of pregnancy, especially in the gastrointestinal and cardiovascular systems, directly influence the absorption, distribution, and elimination of drugs. Profound changes in the hormonal milieu, the mechanical effects of an enlarging uterus, the increased metabolic demand of the fetal-placental unit, and the presence of the low-resistance placental circulation each cause specific alterations that come together in the unique physiology of pregnancy.

The adaptations that allow for the protection and nurturing of the growing fetus are generally well tolerated by a healthy parturient. In this chapter, we will discuss the physiologic changes that occur in pregnancy in a review of systems for the parturient. We will then discuss the pharmacologic changes of pregnancy with emphasis on the physiologic changes that underlie them. These alterations should not be thought of as due to disease, but rather as normal values during pregnancy. It is easy to imagine, however, that these physiologic changes combined with the increased metabolic demand of the growing fetus can worsen pre-existing maternal health problems and can even cause subclinical illness to become manifest.

PHYSIOLOGY OF THE OBSTETRIC PATIENT

Cardiovascular

From the moment of conception, the embryo produces substances that profoundly alter the mother's physiology. These substances prevent rejection of the embryo's foreign proteins by the maternal immune system and favor transport to and implantation into the uterus. The effects of these embryonic-derived substances are largely local until implantation when there is access to the maternal vasculature. At the time of implantation (approximately 5 weeks after the last menstrual period) changes in maternal osmoregulation begin with increased maternal thirst and body water accumulation. Embryonic human chorionic gonadotropin has been implicated in these early maternal physiologic changes. Osmotic thresholds for thirst and antidiuretic hormone secretion are reset to lower levels that allow for the volume expansion of pregnancy. At term, total body water is increased by 6.5 to 8.5 liters. This enormous volume expansion results in the hemodilution of pregnancy and elevation of maternal cardiac output (Fig. 1-1).

The early volume changes of pregnancy lead to an increased left ventricular end diastolic volume by the end of the first trimester. Mild left ventricular hypertrophy is similar to that achieved with athletic training. Both left and right atrial dimensions increase as a result of the increased preload to a maximum at 30 weeks gestation. There is no increase in central venous, right ventricular, pulmonary arterial, or pulmonary capillary wedge pressures under normal circumstances because of coincident dilation of peripheral and pulmonary veins. Systemic vascular resistance starts to decrease as early as 8 weeks of gestation. Several factors, including elevated progesterone, nitric oxide, prostaglandins, and/or atrial natriuretic peptide, may play a role.

During pregnancy, cardiac output rises gradually, beginning by 8 to 10 weeks gestation. By the end of the second trimester, cardiac output is elevated by 50% of nonpregnant values, and in the immediate postpartum period, the cardiac output can be increased by as much as 100%. The elevation in cardiac output is a result of both an increase in heart rate and stroke volume. Heart rate begins to increase by 5 weeks gestation to a maximum of about 20% at term. Stroke volume reaches a maximum of a 25% increase by 20 weeks gestation. This 2 L/min increase in cardiac output mainly supplies the uterus, kidneys, and extremities. At term, the uterine artery blood flow can be as high as 500 mL/min, which explains why an obstetric hemorrhage can so quickly become life threatening.

It used to be thought that cardiac output declines around the 28th week of gestation, but it is now known that these findings were the result of positional aortocaval compression. Maternal cardiac output is dependent on position because after 24 weeks gestation, the gravid uterus can completely obstruct venous return from the inferior vena cava in the supine position. This aortocaval compression is also called the supine hypotension syndrome. At this point in gestation, women are instructed to avoid the supine position for this reason. If the parturient needs to be supine for cesarean delivery, effective prevention of aortocaval compression includes placing the patient in a modified lateral decubitus position by elevating the right hip (with a pillow or "wedge"), or by tilting the entire table or bed to the left. Cardiac output is highest when measured in the left lateral decubitus position and the knee-chest position. When fetal heart rate decelerations occur in labor, the parturient is placed in one of these positions to maximize placental blood flow and thus fetal oxygenation (Table 1-1).

During labor, cardiac output increases even more from term values. In the absence of epidural anesthesia, cardiac output can be increased from 7 to 10.5 L/m, again because of increased heart rate and stroke volume. During a uterine contraction, autotransfusion

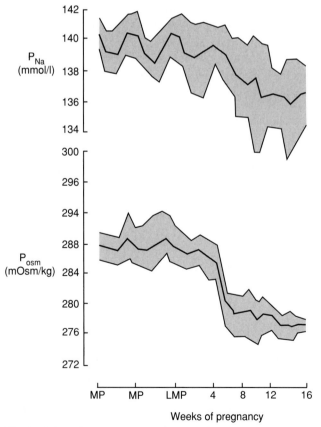

Figure 1-1   Change in maternal osmotic threshold. One of the first physiologic changes in pregnancy is a change in maternal osmotic set point that occurs approximately 4 weeks after the LMP at the time of implantation.

Table 1-1   Normal Hemodynamic Values in Pregnancy

	Normal Values	Change at Term
Systolic blood pressure	115	No change
Diastolic blood pressure	55	20% decrease
Heart rate	90 bpm	20% increase
Cardiac output	7 L/min	40% to 50% increase
Central venous pressure	4	No change
Pulmonary capillary wedge pressure	7	No change
Systemic vascular resistance	1200 dyne/cm/sec	20% decrease
Pulmonary vascular resistance	78 dyne/cm/sec	30% decrease

occurs as the blood in the uterus is expelled into the systemic circulation. This causes an acute increase in maternal stroke volume and cardiac output. Epidural analgesia prevents the baseline increase in cardiac output, which is likely due to relief of pain and a resulting decrease in heart rate, as well as vasodilatation caused by sympathectomy. The acute increase in cardiac output that occurs with uterine contractions does persist even after epidural analgesia. Approximately 10 to 30 minutes after the delivery of the baby, the parturient experiences a further 20% increase in cardiac output that is associated with sustained uterine contraction after placental expulsion. This transient phenomenon resolves within the first hour, and is counterbalanced by the normal loss of approximately 500 mL blood at vaginal delivery and 1L at cesarean delivery. All of the hemodynamic changes of pregnancy resolve within 2 to 4 weeks after delivery.

Maternal blood pressure decreases in normal pregnancy. Blood pressure is the product of cardiac output and systemic vascular resistance. Despite increases in cardiac output just described, the decrease in maternal blood pressure parallels the decrease in systemic vascular resistance. The diastolic blood pressure decreases more than the systolic blood pressure and nadirs at 15 to 20 mm Hg lower than prepregnancy values by 20 weeks gestation. This is primarily due to vasodilatation caused by progesterone as well as the presence of the low-resistance placental circuit. After 20 weeks gestation, blood pressure increases toward prepregnancy levels under the influence of increasing cardiac output and consistently reduced systemic vascular resistance. Under normal conditions, blood pressure should never exceed prepregnancy values. In addition, despite elevated angiotensin levels, pregnant women are resistant to angiotensin's hypertensive effects in the absence of pre-eclampsia.

Some pregnant women appear to have signs and symptoms of cardiovascular pathology, but these can be normal findings. Mild dyspnea on exertion, systolic heart murmurs, a prominent third heart sound, peripheral edema, and cardiomegaly can all be observed during normal pregnancy. Electrocardiographic changes such as left axis deviation and nonspecific ST-segment and T-wave changes can occur due to the heart's shifted position in the chest. Characteristic pregnancy-induced echocardiographic alterations have also been described that reflect the changes discussed. In the third trimester of pregnancy, a mild left ventricular hypertrophy reflects increased myocardial contractility and left atrial enlargement and is a result of elevated intravascular volume.

Respiratory

Early in pregnancy the shape of the thoracic cage becomes rounder and has a greater anterior-posterior

---

CASE REPORT

A 23-year-old G1P0 woman is at 24 weeks gestation with a singleton pregnancy. She presents to the labor room with acute shortness of breath and weakness. She is previously healthy except for a remote history of Rheumatic Fever at 6 years of age without known sequelae. Her blood gas analysis shows a pH of 7.50, pCO_2 is 28, and pO_2 is 76. Her cardiac exam is significant for normal S1 and S2 heart sounds with a S3 gallop, an opening snap, and a II/IV low pitched rumbling diastolic murmur. An urgent transthoracic echocardiogram shows moderate mitral stenosis and suggests elevated left atrial pressure.

QUESTIONS

1. Why would a previously asymptomatic woman with mitral stenosis become acutely ill in pregnancy?
2. Is the patient's cardiac rhythm potentially important?
3. How would you stabilize this patient?

---

diameter (Fig. 1-2). This is likely due to ligamentous relaxation. As the uterus expands and increases intra-abdominal pressure, the diaphragm elevates. These mechanical changes result in decreased static lung volumes. Total lung capacity decreases by 5%, which is mostly attributable to a 20% reduction in functional residual capacity (FRC) (Fig. 1-3). Residual volume also decreases by about 20% in late pregnancy. Vital capacity does not change. At term, the FRC has decreased to 80% of the nonpregnant level, and when the pregnant patient assumes the supine position, the FRC falls even further.

Maternal oxygen consumption increases approximately 20%, much of which is attributable to the oxygen consumption of the fetus, placenta, and uterus. The combination of reduced FRC and increased oxygen consumption puts the pregnant patient at risk for hypoxemia during periods of apnea. Decreased oxygen supply with increased demand results in a shorter period of apnea that can be tolerated before desaturation of the mother's blood occurs. One minute of apnea in the pregnant patient can result in a 150 torr decrease in P_aO_2. Adequate denitrogenation prior to the induction of general anesthesia is very important. This can be achieved by having the patient breathe 100% oxygen for a period of time before induction, to maximize the oxygen tension within the FRC. This allows more time for tracheal intubation prior to hemoglobin desaturation during induction of general anesthesia or during emergency resuscitation. Speed in establishing control of the airway and ventilation in a pregnant woman is critical.

There is no change in the strength or utilization of respiratory muscles, and thus maximum inspiratory and expiratory pressures do not change in pregnancy. By about 8 weeks of pregnancy there is an increase in tidal

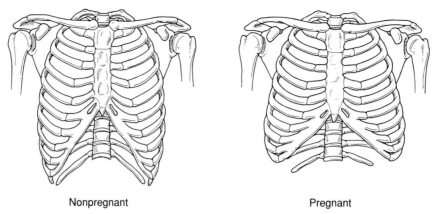

Nonpregnant   Pregnant

Figure 1-2   Maternal skeletal changes. The maternal rib cage is widened in anterior-posterior diameter and fore shortened.

volume that is centrally driven and under the control of progesterone. No significant change occurs in respiratory rate. Minute ventilation is thus increased in term pregnancy, to a level almost 50% higher than in nonpregnant women. The increased minute ventilation results in a decrease in P_aCO_2 to approximately 30 mm Hg and a small increase in P_aO_2 to 105 mm Hg. Arterial blood pH remains essentially normal (around 7.44) because of metabolic compensation. The kidneys increase excretion of bicarbonate ions resulting in reduced plasma bicarbonate levels of approximately 20 mEq/L (Table 1-2).

Central Nervous System

Neurologic changes in pregnancy are more subtle than the cardiovascular and respiratory changes, but deserve consideration nonetheless. Many people believe that the pain threshold is elevated in pregnancy. From a teleologic standpoint, an elevated pain threshold would help the mother tolerate an impending, painful delivery. In the third trimester of pregnancy, sensitivity to pain is reduced when tested with pressure or electricity. This change in pain sensitivity is thought to be due to increases in spinal dynorphin (an intrinsic κ-opioid) and upregulation of descending inhibition from noradrenergic neurons. However, sensitivity to traditional μ-opioid agonists is not changed. Changes in maternal pain sensitivity are thought to be due to increases in progesterone and estrogen. More subtle changes may occur with the hormonal changes of menstruation. These differences brought about by pregnancy are currently being evaluated as targets for pain relief modalities specific to pregnancy and delivery. An example would be utilizing α_2-adrenergic agonists as adjuvants for epidural analgesia.

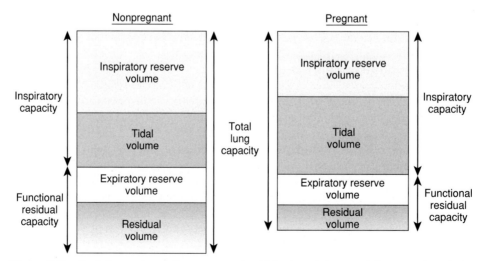

Figure 1-3   Static lung volumes. In pregnancy the tidal volume is increased. Functional residual capacity is reduced largely as a result of decreased residual volume. A smaller functional residual capacity leads to less oxygen reserve for the parturient in periods of apnea.

Table 1-2 Normal Arterial Blood Gas Values in Pregnancy

		Trimester		
	Nonpregnant	First	Second	Third
$PaCO_2$(mm Hg)	40	30	30	30
PaO_2(mm Hg)	100	107	105	103
pH	7.40	7.44	7.44	7.44
HCO_3^- (mEq/L)	24	21	20	20

CURRENT CONTROVERSIES: DOES PREGNANCY CREATE RESISTANCE TO PAIN?

- Is decreased pain sensitivity clinically relevant?
- Does the parturient have different responses to analgesic treatments than nonpregnant women? Than men?

Head, Ears, Eyes, Nose, and Throat

Pregnancy also causes anatomic changes in the airway, which can make endotracheal intubation more difficult. The maternal airway has received considerable attention due to the realization that approximately 90% of maternal deaths that are attributable to anesthetic causes occur under general anesthesia. The risk of failed intubation in a pregnant patient is approximately 1:500, which is considerably higher than in the general population. The vocal cords, arytenoids, and other glottic structures can be edematous due to fluid accumulation, and visualization of the airway and passage of the endotracheal tube may be more difficult. Mask ventilation may be hindered by airway obstruction due to weight gain and enlarged breast tissue of pregnancy. Difficult ventilation can substantially increase maternal morbidity and mortality in the event of difficulty with tracheal intubation. The increased incidence of difficult intubation in pregnancy is also correlated with higher Mallampati scores in pregnancy. Mallampati scores may actually worsen during the progress of labor, perhaps as a result of changes in fluid distribution and airway edema. For this reason, anesthesiologists must examine a patient's airway immediately prior to urgent cesarean delivery requiring general anesthesia, even if it has been assessed previously. Regional anesthesia is recommended when possible for surgical delivery, particularly for an obese parturient or one with an apparently difficult airway.

During pregnancy the oropharyngeal and nasal mucosal capillaries are engorged, which predisposes to bleeding with manipulation. Bleeding in this area can sometimes make a difficult intubation impossible. As a result, nasal intubation and nasal airways are not recommended for use in the pregnant patient. Due to increased circulating estrogen, nasal congestion frequently occurs during pregnancy and is associated with increased mucus production (Table 1-3).

CURRENT CONTROVERSIES: ENDOTRACHEAL INTUBATION IN PREGNANCY

- 90% of anesthesia-related maternal deaths occur under general anesthesia.
- Is general anesthesia more dangerous, or do sicker women get general anesthesia for more emergent situations?

Gastrointestinal

Under the influence of progesterone, gastrointestinal tone is reduced. The tone of the gastroesophageal sphincter is also reduced, increasing the incidence of gastroesophageal reflux, reflux esophagitis, and heartburn. This phenomenon affects between 50% and 80% of all pregnant women. As a result, from the first trimester of pregnancy, women have an increased risk of gastric acid aspiration when their protective airway reflexes are reduced with sedation or anesthesia. Classically, the pregnant patient has been considered to have delayed gastric emptying and prolonged intestinal transit time. This was thought to be caused by both endocrine and mechanical factors: progesterone and the enlarging uterus. More recent data suggest that pregnancy itself does not delay gastric emptying. Studies of acetaminophen absorption are used as an indirect measure of gastric emptying because it can only be absorbed when it passes into the more basic environment of the duodenum. These studies show that there is actually no reduction in gastric transit time during pregnancy. Residual gastric volume and acidity are also unchanged in pregnancy. However, gastric motility does decrease during active labor, which has been demonstrated by gastric

Table 1-3 Mallampati Classification in Pregnancy*

	First Trimester (%)	Third Trimester (%)
Class 4	42	56
Class 3	36	29
Class 2	14	10
Class 1	8	5

*The Mallampati score was obtained in 242 women during the first and third trimesters of pregnancy. The incidence of Class 4 airways was significantly increased in the third trimester ($P < 0.001$). Increased body weight was positively associated with an increase in Mallampati score ($P < 0.005$). Modified from Pilkington S, Carli F, Dakin MJ, et al: Increase in Mallampati score during pregnancy. Br J Anaesthesia 74:638–642, 1995.

ultrasound and impedance measurements, and this reduction continues into the postpartum period. Systemic and neuraxial opioids may slow gastric emptying even further. Small intestinal transit time is reduced in pregnancy. As a result, there is an increased incidence of constipation and bloating.

CURRENT CONTROVERSIES: SHOULD PARTURIENTS BE NPO IN LABOR?

● Gastric emptying is decreased in labor.
● Labor can last for over 24 hours, and starvation ketosis can occur.
● Should apparent risk for cesarean section be considered?

Because the parturient is at increased risk for gastric acid aspiration due to the relaxed barrier of the gastroesophageal junction, several strategies have been used to reduce gastric acidity (nonparticulate antacids, histamine H_2-receptor antagonists, and proton pump inhibitors) and to reduce gastric volume (metoclopramide). If surgery is elected, it is recommended to withhold oral intake for at least 6 hours before induction of anesthesia. This increased risk of aspiration again makes regional anesthesia preferable to general anesthesia because it allows the protective upper airway reflexes to remain intact. When general anesthesia is required, steps may be taken to reduce this increased risk. They include performing a rapid sequence induction of anesthesia after adequate preoxygenation while applying pressure to the cricoid cartilage in order to decrease the incidence of passive regurgitation of gastric acid into the oropharynx (a Sellick maneuver). An endotracheal tube is the device of choice for maintenance of an unobstructed airway in parturients having general anesthesia because other devices such as laryngeal mask airways do not adequately protect against aspiration.

Liver blood flow is unchanged in pregnancy, but because of increased blood volume, portal pressure is increased. Pressure in vasculature that drains to the portal system is also elevated. As such, there is an increased incidence of perianal hemorrhoids in pregnancy. Like other parts of the gastrointestinal system, the gall bladder has reduced tone. Decreased muscular activity leads to biliary sludging. In the face of increased cholesterol in pregnancy, there is an increased incidence of cholesterol-containing gallstones.

Renal

One of the earliest changes after conception is a resetting of the osmotic threshold, which results in consis-

tently increasing fluid retention throughout pregnancy. Because antidiuretic hormone is not suppressed at the new lower tonicity, body water is retained. Despite greater antidiuretic hormone production in pregnancy, there is a 3- to 4-fold increase in its metabolism due to vasopressinase, an enzyme that is synthesized by the placenta. Sodium retention increases in pregnancy because of increased renal tubular reabsorption. Renin, angiotensin, and aldosterone are all elevated during pregnancy and also contribute to sodium reabsorption. Sodium excretion, however, remains normal.

Renal blood flow and glomerular filtration rate (GFR) increase during pregnancy. Within the first trimester, renal blood flow is increased by 50% to 80%, and GFR is increased by 50%. As a result, creatinine clearance increases by 50%. Thus, serum concentrations of creatinine, urea, and uric acid are decreased by almost one third. If a pregnant patient has a "normal" creatinine concentration, then she has markedly reduced renal function. Clearance of drugs that are excreted by the kidney and unchanged by the liver is therefore also increased by 50%. Dosages of these drugs and administration schedules should be adjusted to compensate for these changes. During pregnancy the renal glucose threshold decreases, which can result in glucosuria (Table 1-4).

Hematologic

The so-called "anemia of pregnancy" is a direct result of the retention of body water and dilution that begins in early pregnancy and increases progressively to approximately 50% at 32 weeks gestation. There is increased hematopoesis during pregnancy, but the increase in red cell mass is not as great as the increase in plasma volume; thus, there is a decrease in hematocrit. By 34 weeks gestation, the normal hematocrit can be as low as 31%. The increase in blood volume provides a reserve to allow a woman to tolerate the moderate blood loss anticipated at delivery. The hematopoesis that does occur during pregnancy often outstrips the iron supply in diet and maternal stores. Thus anemia is partially responsive to iron treatment during pregnancy (Fig. 1-4).

Dilution by plasma also causes a reduction in antibody titers, although no evidence exists that this decrease

---

Table 1-4   Normal Renal Function in Pregnancy

	Pregnant	Nonpregnant
Creatinine clearance	140 to 160 mL/min	90 to 110 mL/min
Urea	2.0 to 4.5 mmol/L	6 to 7 mmol/L
Creatinine	25 to 75 μmol/L	100 μmol/L
Uric acid	0.2	0.35

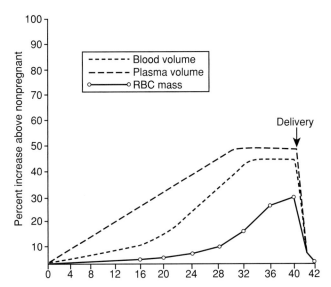

Figure 1-4 Changes in maternal blood volume and red cell mass. Both plasma volume and red cell mass increase during pregnancy. There is a greater increase in plasma volume, leading to the dilutional anemia of pregnancy. (Redrawn from Scott DE: Anemia during pregnancy. Obstet Gynecol Ann 1: 219–244, 1972.)

causes an increased susceptibility to infection. There is a reduction in leukocyte chemotaxis beginning in the second trimester that might explain the clinical improvement of some autoimmune diseases in pregnancy. The white blood cell count is normal throughout pregnancy before the onset of labor, but is often elevated during the stress of labor and remains elevated postpartum.

The platelet count is normal, but platelets often appear immature in a peripheral blood smear. Pregnancy may be a state of chronic low-grade disseminated intravascular coagulation, which causes increased platelet consumption and earlier release of immature platelets from the bone marrow in compensation. There is evidence of increased inflammatory processes in pregnancy as well. Both the erythrocyte sedimentation rate and c-reactive protein are elevated in normal pregnancy and therefore are less helpful diagnostically.

Despite decreased concentrations of total protein levels secondary to dilution, coagulation factors are increased. Normal pregnancy is a hypercoagulable state due to increases in coagulation factors made by the liver including factors VII, VIII, IX, X, and fibrinogen. The incidence of thromboembolic complications is at least five times greater during pregnancy, which places postoperative pregnant patients at higher risk for venous thrombosis and possible pulmonary embolism. Even though clotting factors and fibrinogen concentrations are increased, clotting time is not changed in pregnancy. Increases in the production of coagulation factors are thought to be due to the combination of estrogen and progesterone, as they are also seen in

women who take oral contraceptives. There is no evidence that prothrombotic factors such as protein-s, protein-c, and antithrombin III are changed in pregnancy. However, women with a pre-existing tendency to clot based on abnormalities in prothrombotic factors are at even greater risk for thromboembolic phenomenon when they become pregnant.

Endocrine

Pregnancy is a diabetogenic state and is associated with insulin resistance. Basal levels of insulin are increased, and there is an increased response to a glucose challenge. As a result, the changes in blood glucose are exaggerated, with lower preprandial and higher postprandial glucose levels. Also, higher levels of free fatty acids, lipids, and cholesterol are seen. Pregnant women are more prone to the production of ketones when fasting compared to nonpregnant women (Fig. 1-5).

The pituitary gland markedly increases in size during pregnancy such that it can be compressed by the optic chiasm. In midpregnancy, growth hormone increases, but then declines slowly until delivery. Prolactin markedly increases in pregnancy, but then sharply decreases after delivery, even in women who are breast-feeding.

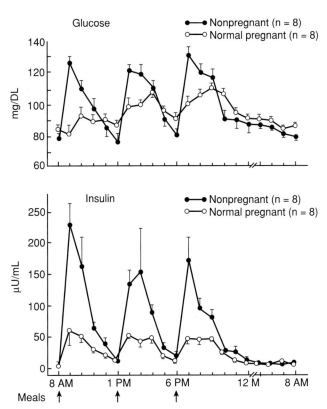

Figure 1-5 Maternal insulin and glucose homeostasis. In pregnancy changes in glucose and insulin concentrations are exaggerated.

During breast-feeding, prolactin is secreted in a pulsatile fashion in response to infant feeding. Thyroid-releasing hormone in pregnancy can act nonspecifically to favor the release of prolactin as well.

Thyroid-related proteins also undergo significant changes during pregnancy. High estrogen levels cause elevations in thyroid-binding globulin, the main carrier protein for thyroxin. Placental substances, thyrotropin and chorionic gonadotropin, stimulate the production of free thyroxin by the thyroid gland. As a result, there are changes in the normal values of thyroid function tests during pregnancy. The production of T4 can outstrip the maternal availability of iodine, like iron, and iodine-responsive goiter can result. Because only free T4 (and to a lesser extent T3) is metabolically active, the balanced increase in thyroid-binding protein and T4 results in normal values of free T4 and unchanged metabolic activity. The thyroid gland itself may be slightly hypertrophied because of increased vascularity; however, the increase is small, so a goiter in pregnancy is considered abnormal.

Parathyroid hormone decreases slightly in the first trimester of pregnancy but then increases progressively in the latter two trimesters in response to dilutional decreases in calcium concentration. In addition, estrogen makes the bones less responsive to parathyroid hormone for calcium release, providing another mechanism for decreased total maternal plasma calcium and increased parathyroid concentration. Although pregnancy and lactation significantly increase demand for maternal calcium and can deplete stores, ionized calcium is not reduced.

Circulating cortisol is increased in pregnancy, but the elevation is likely due to an elevation in the major cortisol-binding protein, transcortin. Although cortisol secretion is not increased, its metabolism is reduced. These changes are thought to be due to elevated estrogen levels. Adrenocortico-stimulating hormone, a pituitary hormone, is reduced early in pregnancy, before the rise in cortisol. This change is thought to be due to a change in set-point for feedback inhibition.

Musculoskeletal

The enlarging uterus results in exaggeration of normal lumbar lordosis. Hormonal changes, including the hormone relaxin, lead to increased mobility of joints. Under the control of progesterone and relaxin, the anterior posterior dimension of the rib cage increases, and the diaphragm is elevated. These physical changes contribute to the changes in static respiratory dynamics discussed previously. Increased mobility and changed posture can result in maternal back and leg pain in late pregnancy and exacerbation of pre-existing spinal disc disease.

PHARMACOLOGY IN THE OBSTETRIC PATIENT

The pharmacodynamics and pharmacokinetics of many drugs change during pregnancy. As a result of the enormous increase in plasma volume that begins in early pregnancy, plasma protein concentrations, especially albumin, decrease dramatically. This increased apparent volume of distribution results in lower peak plasma concentrations and an increased elimination half-life for many drugs. These changes are greatest for drugs that are highly protein bound and have low lipid solubility such as benzodiazepines. Pregnancy also changes excretion of drugs more than metabolism because of the greatly increased glomerular filtration rate. Clearance of drugs excreted by the kidney and not changed by the liver is therefore also increased by 50%.

Placental Transfer

The placenta, an organ unique to the parturient, is complex and dynamic. It brings together the maternal and fetal circulations for exchange of both nutrients and waste products. For the fetus to gain exposure to or excrete these substances, they must pass through the placenta. Because it is an incomplete barrier, the placenta also serves as a conduit to the fetus for drugs administered to the parturient. Almost all maternal drugs cross the placenta and reach the fetus to some extent. As a biological tissue, the placenta follows the same rules that determine drug transfer and distribution in the rest of the body.

The major mechanism for drug transfer across the placenta is passive diffusion, especially for anesthetic compounds and gases. Passive diffusion does not require energy use, occurs through a membrane, and net transfer depends on the concentration or pressure gradient across the membrane. These principles are described by the Fick equation:

$$dq/dt = ka(Cm{-}Cf)/d,$$

where dq/dt is the drug transfer rate; k is the diffusion constant which is specific for each drug; a is the surface area of the membrane; Cm is the maternal drug concentration; Cf is the fetal drug concentration; and d is the membrane thickness.

Several drug factors influence passive diffusion. For each drug, the diffusion constant, k, depends on the drug's molecular weight, lipid solubility, degree of ionization, and amount of protein binding. In terms of molecular weight, drugs less than 500 Daltons (D) readily diffuse across the placenta, while drugs greater than 500D are limited by their size. Size is rarely a significant constraint because the majority of drugs used in clinical practice weigh less than 500D. Lipid solubility plays a role because highly lipid-soluble drugs cross through the placenta more easily than water-soluble drugs. The degree of ionization depends on whether the drug is acidic or basic, its pKa, and the pH of the solution. Only unionized drugs diffuse across the placenta. The extent of plasma protein binding also influences diffusion because only the free or unbound drug crosses the placenta. Similar considerations apply to transfer of drugs across the blood-brain barrier. Most anesthetic drugs have the central nervous system as an effect site, and as such, readily cross the placenta as well.

The degree of passive diffusion is determined in part by the surface area and membrane thickness of the placenta. Through gestation, the number of placental villi increases and provides a growing surface area for drug transfer. While this occurs, the placental thickness decreases. Thus, as pregnancy progresses, the placenta gains a greater capacity for passive drug diffusion. This results in greater drug transfer from the parturient to the fetus in late compared to early pregnancy. However, these considerations probably only relate to the transfer rate. The total drug dose that reaches the fetus depends more on the drug factors than the placental factors (Fig. 1-6).

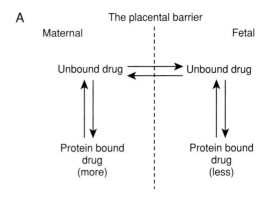

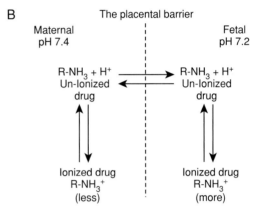

Figure 1-6 Placental transfer of drugs. **A,** Protein binding: equilibrium between bound and unbound "free" drug affects amount available for transfer. **B,** pH: maternal pH affects amount of "free" or unionized drug available for transfer.

Local Anesthetics

Local anesthetics are the most commonly used drugs by anesthesiologists caring for the parturient. Used almost exclusively for regional techniques, they provide not only analgesia for labor and delivery, but also anesthesia for instrumental deliveries and cesarean delivery. Local anesthetics act as sodium channel blockers in the neuraxis. They reduce the conduction of action potentials and decrease the information that reaches the brain for processing from the primary nociceptors or pain fibers. This section focuses on the agents in current obstetric anesthetic use, bupivacaine, ropivicaine, lidocaine, and 2-chloroprocaine and the most common routes of administration, spinal and epidural.

Pregnancy changes both the pharmacodynamics and pharmacokinetics of local anesthetic drugs. The parturient is more sensitive to local anesthetic blockade. Put another way, a smaller spinal or epidural dose of local anesthetic given to a parturient provides the same level as a greater dose would in the nonpregnant adult. This effect is short lived after delivery. One study showed that a 30% increased dose of bupivacaine was necessary for postpartum tubal ligation performed within 2 days after delivery when compared to the dose required for cesarean delivery. Several mechanisms, both mechanical and hormonal, have been proposed to explain this phenomenon. Changes in intra-abdominal pressure and inferior vena cava compression from the gravid uterus as

well as increased epidural venous pressure and distension have been proposed; however, a hormonal etiology is also likely, because a reduction in required local anesthetic dose has been demonstrated as early as the first trimester, when changes in abdominal pressure are relatively insignificant.

More likely, biochemical and hormonal changes influence the increased potency and spread of local anesthetics in pregnancy. Several studies have suggested that maternal nerve fibers are more sensitive to local anesthetic effects. Bupivacaine in vitro blocks pregnant rabbit vagus nerves faster than those from nonpregnant animals, and treatment of animals with exogenous progesterone is associated with an increased susceptibility to blockade. Lidocaine inhibits sensory nerve action potentials in the median nerves of pregnant women to a greater extent than in nonpregnant women. The cerebrospinal fluid (CSF) of pregnant women contains a higher progesterone concentration than in nonpregnant women, which may directly augment the effect of local anesthetics in pregnancy. Another mechanism may be associated with the pH of CSF. In pregnancy, women have increased minute ventilation, creating a mild respiratory alkalosis. The higher pH of the CSF causes more local anesthetic to remain unionized and able to penetrate membranes, and may thus increase its potency.

Bupivacaine is the most commonly used local anesthetic in epidurals for labor in the United States, mostly because it produces significant sensory and pain blockade while relatively sparing motor effects. This property is considered especially useful in obstetrics for maintaining maternal muscle tone during the descent of the fetus and the second stage of labor. Epidural bupivacaine administered for cesarean delivery has a similar serum absorption rate and elimination half-life compared to nonpregnant women. With a dose of 1.78mg/kg, the maximum serum concentration of 1.39mg/L was reached in 26 minutes. The elimination half-life was 12 to 15 hours, which is much longer than with an intravenous injection because of the prolonged absorption from the epidural space. One study demonstrated a maternal arterial peak concentration of 0.78 µg/mL after epidural dose for cesarean delivery. None of the patients had concentrations in the toxic range. It has been thought that the significantly smaller doses of bupivacaine used for spinal anesthesia would not reach any significant level in the maternal plasma. Detectable plasma levels of bupivacaine after spinal for cesarean delivery have been shown to be only 5% of those found after epidural.

Bupivacaine is extensively bound to plasma proteins, so as the α_1-acid glycoprotein levels decrease with pregnancy, an increased percentage of the drug remains unbound in the maternal serum compared to nonpregnant women. The liver metabolizes bupivacaine mainly to 2,6-pipecolylxylidine (PPX), and PPX can be detected in maternal plasma 5 minutes after epidural administration for cesarean delivery and continues to be detectable 24 hours later. There does not appear to be a difference in the urinary excretion of bupivacaine with pregnancy.

Ropivacaine, a newer local anesthetic, is still being evaluated in pregnant humans. Potential advantages of ropivacaine compared to bupivicaine in obstetric use include decreased cardiac toxicity and decreased depth of motor blockade. Pregnant sheep had significantly lower total clearance of intravenously administered ropivacaine, slightly decreased volume of distribution, and no significant change in elimination half-life compared to nonpregnant sheep. The pregnant sheep also had lower urinary excretion of unchanged ropivacaine. Although it is quite similar in structure to bupivacaine, some pharmacokinetic differences have become apparent. When compared for epidural use in cesarean delivery, the free maternal plasma concentration of ropivacaine was almost twice as high as bupivacaine at delivery, while the elimination half-life of ropivacaine was significantly shorter than bupivacaine by almost 3 hours.

For lidocaine, an increased volume of distribution and total clearance have been demonstrated after intravenous injection in pregnant sheep compared to non-pregnant sheep. However, these changes did not cause a difference in the elimination half-life, and no difference was detected in the urinary excretion of lidocaine. When compared to sheep at an earlier time in gestation, these pharmacokinetic changes appear stable. Lidocaine is primarily bound to α_1-acid glycoprotein, and as the protein level decreases in pregnancy, the free concentration of lidocaine increases. Peak maternal blood levels of 6.39 µg/mL were found at 31 minutes in women given epidural lidocaine for cesarean delivery. The liver metabolizes lidocaine to monoethylglycinexylidine (MEGX) and glycinexylidine (GX). MEGX can be detected in maternal blood within 15 minutes after spinal lidocaine given for cesarean delivery, although the mean maternal levels are one tenth those after epidural doses.

One ester local anesthetic, 2-chloroprocaine, has particular advantages as well as disadvantages when used in obstetric anesthesia. As an ester, 2-chloroprocaine undergoes rapid plasma metabolism by pseudocholinesterase to 2-chloroaminobenzoic acid (CABA). Its *in vitro* half-life is less than 15 seconds. Although pseudocholinesterase activity decreases approximately 30% with pregnancy, the *in vitro* half-life of 2-chloroprocaine in maternal plasma is 11 seconds. With an epidural dosage *in vivo*, the half-life increases to about 3 minutes because of continuous uptake. This rapid metabolism accounts for a short duration of action, making 2-chloroprocaine a relatively safe drug to use because, even if a toxic plasma level were inadvertently achieved, the ill effects would be short lived. However, the extremely short half-life also makes its use for labor analgesia impractical.

The main disadvantage to using 2-chloroprocaine in obstetric anesthesia for cesarean delivery is that it may decrease the quality and duration of analgesia from epidural morphine or fentanyl. Several investigators have reported this apparent antagonism of prior 2-chloroprocaine administration which inhibits the subsequent action of epidural opioids. The mechanism of this interaction remains to be elucidated. Epidural fentanyl produces less efficacious sensory analgesia of shorter duration compared to butorphanol given after epidural 2-chloroprocaine. It is hypothesized that the etiology is µ-receptor based, given that the analgesic action of the κ agonist, butorphanol, is not antagonized by prior use of 2-chlorprocaine. Even a 2-chloroprocaine test dose of 7 mL can inhibit the duration of action of epidural morphine. 2-Chloroprocaine does bind the µ-opioid receptor; however, it has not been proven to act as a receptor antagonist. Interestingly, 2-chloroprocaine has also been shown to interfere with the efficacy and duration of action of bupivacaine. Although the pH of the 2-chloroprocaine solution was shown not to be the cause, a metabolite of 2-chloroprocaine has been implicated in the bupivicaine interaction. In isolated rat sciatic nerves, the inactive metabolite remains bound to the receptor, interfering with bupivacaine's subsequent effect.

Epinephrine is frequently added to epidural local
anesthetic solutions used for regional anesthesia to
intensify and prolong the duration of local anesthetic
action and to decrease the peak local anesthetic blood
levels. The efficacy depends upon the drug used, its
concentration, and the site of administration. With
epidural bupivacaine and lidocaine for labor, epinephrine speeds the onset, and increases the duration and
intensity of analgesia without causing a significant
increase in hypotension.

Local anesthetic toxicity, both central nervous and
cardiovascular, can become apparent after an inadvertent intravascular dose of a drug intended for the
epidural space. Compared to other local anesthetics,
bupivacaine is known to have a narrower range
between the serum concentration that causes convulsions and cardiovascular collapse. After several case
reports of cardiovascular collapse in pregnant women
given bupivacaine, a decreased threshold for local
anesthetic toxicity in pregnancy was investigated and
initially confirmed.

Pregnant sheep given intravenous bupivacaine manifested cardiovascular collapse at lower doses and mean
serum concentrations compared to nonpregnant sheep.
When studied in a similar fashion, there were no differences between pregnant and nonpregnant animals for
lidocaine or mepivacaine toxicity. The increased toxicity
of bupivacaine in pregnancy was thought to be due to
the increased unbound bupivacaine present in this
hypoproteinemic state or to the selective cardiac depressant effects of progesterone combined with bupivacaine.
A more recent random and blinded study in sheep suggested that there is no enhancement in the toxicity of
ropivacaine or bupivacaine in pregnancy. The applicabil-
ity of these animal studies to humans remains uncertain
as does the issue of enhanced bupivacaine toxicity in
pregnancy.

With enough uterine blood flow for delivery of local
anesthetics to the membrane, the transfer of local anesthetics across the placenta is influenced predominantly
by two factors: the extent of protein binding and the
degree of ionization. Placental transfer·is often measured
at delivery and expressed as the ratio of umbilical venous
to maternal venous drug concentration, or the UV/M
ratio.

Because only unbound drug can freely diffuse across
the placenta, protein binding limits the degree of drug
transfer to the fetus. Because bupivicaine is highly protein bound, it has a lower UV/M ratio than other local
anesthetics, which implies less fetal transfer. However,
the ratios usually refer to total concentrations, not free or
unbound concentrations. Equilibrium occurs between
the unbound species, which is the active drug form,
so a low UV/M ratio does not necessarily mean low
fetal exposure or risk. Similarly, the UV/M ratio is often
quoted as proportional to the amount of placental transfer, a low ratio reflecting less total transfer. Because the
umbilical samples are measured at delivery and are not
necessarily at equilibrium, the ratio is not always an accurate measure of placental transfer.

Of equal importance to placental transfer of local
anesthetics is the pH gradient between the parturient
and the fetus. Most local anesthetics are weak bases and
have pKa's ranging from 7.6 to 8.9. The local anesthetics
with higher pKa's (or further from maternal pH) have
smaller amounts of unionized drug and therefore less placental transfer. Because the fetus exists in an acidotic
environment compared to the parturient, unionized
local anesthetic becomes ionized upon transferring from
the parturient to the fetus and is "trapped" because it cannot then transfer back. With fetal acidosis, this becomes
more significant. Also, the higher the pKa, the more ion
trapping can occur, so bupivicaine (pKa 8.1) is more susceptible than mepivicaine (pKa 7.7) on the basis of pKa.
However, the more protein bound, the less impact pH
has on the local anesthetic, so bupivacaine is actually
least affected by pH.

The maternal blood concentration of local anesthetics
also contributes to their transfer across the placenta.
A larger dose of drug will lead to a higher plasma concentration and more placental transfer. This occurs with
higher local anesthetic concentrations and more frequent epidural dosing causing drug accumulation. This
effect can be minimized with dilute concentrations of
local anesthetics or with the use of 2-chloroprocaine, as
it is rapidly hydrolyzed.

Opioids

Opioids have diverse uses in obstetric anesthesia.
They can be used systemically for labor analgesia and for
postoperative pain control after cesarean delivery.
Opioids are also used neuraxially for labor analgesia,
both in the epidural and spinal spaces, either alone or in
combination with local anesthetics. This section will
focus on the most commonly used systemic opioids:
meperidine, morphine, butorphanol, and nalbuphine; as
well as those used commonly in the neuraxis: fentanyl,

sufentanil, and morphine. Despite this focus, crossover exists between locations of drug use. All opioid agonists have efficacy in the CNS for the treatment of labor pain. Currently, the role of κ- and δ-opioid agonists is under investigation because of specific upregulation of these systems in the maternal spinal cord.

Systemic opioids can be given to the parturient by several routes: intravenously, intramuscularly, or subcutaneously; and their pharmacokinetic profile depends to some extent on the route and method of administration. Often they are given by bolus injection, but also can be provided as patient-controlled analgesia (PCA). Continuous infusions are not recommended because of the intermittent intensity of the pain and the risk of overdose. Typically for labor pain, systemic opioids do not provide adequate efficacy of analgesia, but allow the parturient to better tolerate labor pain by providing sedation. Numerous studies have documented the poor quality of pain relief after systemic opioids. The choice of which drugs to use often depends more on institutional tradition and physician preference than on scientific evidence that one opioid is better than another. Maternal dosing of systemic opioids is largely limited by placental transfer and by the risk of sedation and respiratory depression in the newborn (Table 1-5).

Meperidine is probably the most commonly used systemic opioid for labor because of long experience and tradition. When 25 to 50 mg is given intravenously, the onset is within 5 minutes, and when 50 to 100 mg is given intramuscularly, the onset is within 45 min-

utes. It is 63% bound to protein in the maternal plasma mostly to α_1-acid glycoprotein. The pharmacokinetics of meperidine are not changed in pregnancy. After a single 50-mg intravenous dose, maternal peak plasma concentration of 1.5 to 3 μg/mL occurred within the first 5 to 10 minutes, and maternal elimination half-life was 2.5 to 3 hours. Volume of distribution and clearance were similar between pregnant and nonpregnant subjects.

Normeperidine, an active and potentially epileptogenic metabolite of meperidine, is produced readily by the pregnant patient within 10 minutes of meperidine injection. The maternal plasma concentration of normeperidine increases rapidly during the next 20 minutes and continues to rise slowly throughout labor. No differences in metabolism or urinary excretion of meperidine or normeperidine were found in pregnancy. When several doses of meperidine are given during labor, normeperidine accumulation occurs with an elimination half-life of over 20 hours.

Morphine, in contrast to meperidine, does have altered pharmacokinetics in pregnancy. It can be given in 2- to 5-mg doses intravenously with an onset of 3 to 5 minutes or 5 to 10 mg intramuscularly with an onset of 20 to 40 minutes. It is metabolized to morphine-3-glucuronide (M3G), which is inactive. In pregnancy, morphine has a faster clearance, shorter elimination half-life, and a faster peak M3G level, which suggests increased morphine metabolism.

Nalbuphine, a mixed opioid agonist and antagonist, has a maternal elimination half-life of 2.5 hours when given intravenously. Another mixed agonist and antagonist is butorphanol, which also has the benefit of a short half-life, inactive metabolites, and provides better labor analgesia than meperidine. Because of their antagonistic properties that overtake their agonist properties at increased doses, these drugs have a ceiling effect and thus theoretically carry less risk of respiratory depression and other adverse events.

Epidural and intrathecal opioids are useful for both labor and postoperative analgesia, especially during the first stage of labor, which involves dilation of the cervix and lower uterine segment. They can be used by bolus technique or continuous infusion, in combined spinal-epidurals (CSE) and patient-controlled epidural analgesia (PCEA). In general, the analgesia from neuraxial opioids is superior to systemic opioids, and much lower doses are required to achieve adequate efficacy. As lower doses are required, lower maternal plasma levels occur, and there is less danger of fetal effects. However, neuraxial opioids alone are not usually sufficient analgesia for labor and delivery. The addition of at least a low concentration of local anesthetic is usually required to provide adequate pain relief throughout labor and delivery. Intrathecal and epidural fentanyl and sufentanil are commonly used for

Table 1-5   Placental Transfer of Opioids*

	Transfer	Equilibrium
Morphine	30%	225 min
Meperidine	100%	NM
Fentanyl	25%	NM
Sufentanil	12%	45 min
Buprenorphine	29%	90 min

*The extent of transfer of narcotic from maternal plasma to fetus. Morphine, sufentanil, and buprenorphine were studied in isolated human placentas. Meperidine and fentanyl were studied in rabbit placentas *in vivo*. Time to equilibrium was not measured for meperidine and fentanyl. (Data from Gaylard DG, Carson RJ, Reynolds F: Effect of umbilical perfusate pH and controlled maternal hypotension on placental drug transfer in the rabbit. Anesth Analg 71(1):42–48, 1990; Kopecky EA, Simone C, Knie B, Koren G: Transfer of morphine across the human placenta and its interaction with naloxone. Life Sci 65(22):2359–2371, 1999; Krishna BR, Zakowski MI, Grant GJ: Sufentanil transfer in the human placenta during in vitro perfusion. Can J Anaesth 44(9):996–1001, 1997; Nanovskaya T, Deshmukh S, Brooks M, Ahmed MS: Transplacental transfer and metabolism of buprenorphine. J Pharmacol Exp Ther 300(1):26–33, 2002; Vella LM, Knott C, Reynolds F: Transfer of fentanyl across the rabbit placenta. Effect of umbilical flow and concurrent drug administration. Br J Anaesth 58(1):49–54, 1986) labor analgesia. The advantage of intrathecal fentanyl and sufentanil is rapid onset of pain relief in labor, little sympathetic block, and no motor block. Morphine is less lipid soluble, has a slower onset, but a much longer duration of action, which makes it useful for the treatment of postoperative pain. A mixture of both fentanyl and morphine or sufentanil and morphine can be used during cesarean delivery to take advantage of the beneficial aspects of both types of opioid.

Early studies of epidural morphine showed that it alone did not provide adequate analgesia for labor and resulted in significant maternal blood levels of morphine. Sufentanil, in contrast, does provide adequate epidural analgesia for the first stage of labor, with a single dose lasting for 80 to 140 minutes. With doses between 5 and 50 µg of epidural sufentanil, maternal serum levels were undetectable.

For the treatment of postoperative pain after cesarean delivery, 2 to 5 mg of epidural morphine provides analgesia for a mean duration of 23 hours. The optimal dose is thought to be 3 mg because side effects increase with increased dose, and the analgesic effect is maximal at 3 mg. Epidural morphine has been shown to provide better analgesia than morphine given intramuscularly or by PCA. Intrathecal morphine has similar duration and side effects compared to epidural morphine, but a smaller dose is required. With an intrathecal dose of 0.6-mg morphine, maternal plasma levels peaked at 3 hours at a concentration of 0.61 ng/mL. Doses as low as 0.1 to 0.25 mg of intrathecal morphine have been used effectively for pain after cesarean delivery and provide analgesia for 18 to 28 hours.

In general, because opioids alone do not provide complete analgesia for labor and delivery, they are most often used in combination with local anesthetics. Very dilute local anesthetic solutions that would alone be ineffective can be used because the local anesthetic and the opioid have a synergistic interaction. This strategy helps reduce side effects from each drug. In obstetric anesthesia, this is particularly useful because reduced local anesthetic doses cause less motor blockade. As the epidural dose of fentanyl increases, the minimum local analgesic concentration (MLAC) of epidural bupivacaine for labor significantly decreases. This effect is true for epidural 2-chloroprocaine as well. Local anesthetics, combined with opioids, can be useful for anesthesia for cesarean deliveries, and continuous infusions of PCEA treatment provide effective postoperative pain relief and enhanced mobility after surgery.

All opioids are readily transferred across the placenta because they have molecular weights less than 500. Meperidine can be detected in the fetal plasma 2 minutes after maternal drug administration. The ratio between umbilical to maternal venous meperidine concentrations increases with time from 1 to 4 hours, and ratios of one or higher can be found after 2 hours. After 5 minutes of

intravenously administered morphine to parturients and up to 1 hour, the fetal to maternal ratio of morphine is close to one. The ratio for nalbuphine is 0.78 and for butorphanol is 0.9.

When fentanyl was given intravenously to pregnant women, an umbilical to maternal ratio of 0.31 was found. This low value is thought to result from high fentanyl protein binding because it is a very lipid-soluble drug. One hundred µg of epidural fentanyl has a similar umbilical artery to maternal vein ratio of 0.32. An in vitro study of sufentanil showed that its placental transfer is increased with increased maternal dose and increased fetal acidemia but decreased with increased maternal protein binding. After epidural sufentanil of a mean dosage of 24 µg, the UV/MV ratio was 0.81.

General Anesthetics

Intravenous induction agents are used most frequently to induce general anesthesia for patients who require emergency cesarean delivery or have contraindications to regional anesthesia. Smaller doses of these drugs, however, are useful in cases in which some pain relief and sedation are necessary, such as during removal of a retained placenta. In obstetric anesthesia, thiopental and ketamine are used much more than propofol and etomidate. Although the choice of agent does depend on the specifics of each clinical situation, maintaining maternal hemodynamic stability and uterine blood flow and minimizing neonatal sedation are important considerations.

In the first trimester of pregnancy, a reduced dose of thiopental (by as much as 18%) is required to anesthetize a pregnant woman when compared to a nonpregnant woman. After an average induction dose of 261 mg, the mean venous thiopental concentration was 17 µg/mL in pregnant women. Although there is no change with pregnancy in the percentage of thiopental bound to plasma proteins, thiopental does have a relatively larger volume of distribution and longer elimination half-life in pregnant patients.

The pharmacokinetics of ketamine in pregnancy have not been studied as extensively as barbiturates. The useful properties of ketamine in general, its sympathomimetic effects on the cardiovascular and pulmonary systems, make it similarly useful in obstetric anesthesia, especially for hypovolemic or asthmatic patients. A unique side effect of ketamine, increased uterine contraction frequency and intensity, has important consequences for the parturient. Ketamine-induced uterine hypertonicity and uterine artery vasoconstriction could worsen a placental abruption or decrease the uteroplacental blood flow to the fetus. This increased uterine tone is dose related and not generally seen with doses less than 1 mg/kg. Ketamine causes hallucinations in the parturient, as it does in nonpregnant women. When ketamine is used to induce anesthesia for emergency cesarean delivery, consideration should be given to the coadministration of an anesthetic or sedative that provides amnesia, such as a benzodiazepine or barbiturate.

Etomidate is not routinely used for parturients unless there is particular concern for maintaining hemodynamic stability because it has the benefit of causing minimal cardiovascular depression. Its pharmacokinetics in pregnancy have not been well studied. After 0.3 mg/kg of etomidate for induction of general anesthesia for cesarean delivery, the mean maternal plasma etomidate concentration was 1242 ng/ml, which decreased quickly and was undetectable at 2 hours after injection. In one study, APGAR scores were not different when the mother was induced for cesarean delivery with etomidate compared to methohexital. Cortisol levels initially dropped in the newborns born after etomidate induction, but there was no difference after 6 hours. Etomidate is initially found in the colostrum but is undetectable at 4 hours after injection.

Propofol has similar pharmacokinetic properties in pregnant women compared to nonpregnant women. No difference exists in volume of distribution or elimination half-life, but pregnant women do have a more rapid clearance of propofol. It is not known whether this represents increased hepatic metabolism or simply removal of the drug through the delivery of the placenta and loss of blood. Propofol does not seem to have significant advantages over other induction agents for the parturient.

Inhalation Agents

A mixture of 50% nitrous oxide and 50% oxygen used to be intermittently self-administered by a laboring woman with each contraction for labor analgesia. Now, with the effective pain relief provided by spinal and epidural analgesia, this less efficacious treatment is no longer routinely available in the United States. If general anesthesia is used for cesarean delivery, then the inhalation agents are frequently used for maintenance of anesthesia but not for induction because the parturient requires a rapid sequence induction and rapid airway control to prevent regurgitation and aspiration. In emergency situations in which profound uterine relaxation is needed, such as for delivery of a second twin or removal of a retained placenta, these agents are particularly useful. Most commonly, nitrous oxide is used in combination with isoflurane, but the newer agents, desflurane and sevoflurane, can also be used. The combination of gasses decreases maternal awareness and increases the inspired concentration of oxygen.

It is well known that pregnancy is associated with lower general anesthetic requirements. While the mechanism remains uncertain, it has been attributed to higher maternal progesterone concentrations because the change occurs as early as the first trimester of pregnancy. The minimum alveolar concentration (MAC) in animals was demonstrated to be lower with pregnancy, by as much as 40% for isoflurane. More recently, similar reductions have been shown in humans. MAC for isoflurane in humans is reduced by 28% as early as 8 to 12 weeks gestation and returns to normal by 12 to 24 hours postpartum. Other inhalation agents, such as halothane and enflurane, have equal pregnancy-induced decreased MAC.

The volatile anesthetics all produce uterine relaxation. In experiments with human uterine muscle strips there is an equal depression of contractility caused by enflurane, halothane, and isoflurane, and this decrease is dose dependent. Although a statistically significant reduction in contractility exists even at 0.5 MAC, these doses of isoflurane and halothane used with nitrous oxide in oxygen for maintenance of general anesthesia for cesarean delivery have not been associated with increased maternal blood loss. Similarly, the newer inhalation agents, desflurane and sevoflurane, do not increase postpartum blood loss.

If used for labor analgesia, isoflurane administered in subanesthetic doses ranging from 0.2% to 0.7% during the second stage of labor can provide satisfactory analgesia in approximately 80% of mothers. This was not associated with significant maternal amnesia or blood loss. In contrast, desflurane, which has a very low blood–gas partition coefficient of 0.41 and is similar to nitrous oxide in this respect, was associated with a significant rate of maternal amnesia for the delivery of the baby.

Benzodiazepines

As sedatives and anticonvulsants, the benzodiazepines have limited use in obstetric anesthesia. In large doses, they can be used for a hemodynamically stable induction of general anesthesia but cause significant neonatal side effects, often described as "floppy infant syndrome." While diazepam can be used to prevent eclamptic seizures, magnesium is more commonly used for this purpose in the United States. In addition, the amnesia caused by benzodiazepines, which is beneficial in many nonobstetric situations, is not desirable in labor and delivery because most women want to remember the experience of childbirth. For some women, however, a small dose of a short-acting benzodiazepine such as midazolam can be useful to decrease severe anxiety when receiving a neuraxial anesthetic for cesarean delivery and should not be sufficient to impair memory of the birth.

After a 5-mg intravenous bolus dose of midazolam, the mean plasma midazolam concentration is lower in pregnant than in nonpregnant women due to the larger apparent volume of distribution. The elimination half-life of midazolam, approximately 50 minutes, is not affected by pregnancy. When used for induction, midazolam has a slower induction time compared to thiopental, which could put the parturient at risk for aspiration. Unlike midazolam, the elimination half-life of diazepam is greatly prolonged, 65 hours compared to 29 hours in nonpregnant women.

Muscle Relaxants

When general anesthesia is used for cesarean delivery or other obstetric surgical procedures, muscle relaxants are often necessary to facilitate intubation of the trachea and to provide abdominal muscle relaxation to improve the surgical conditions. Obstetric patients require rapid sequence induction of general anesthesia, and succinylcholine is the drug of choice because of its rapid onset and rapid degradation by plasma cholinesterases. The nondepolarizing muscle relaxants are used most frequently for maintenance of muscle relaxation and for induction if the use of succinylcholine is contraindicated, such as in pseudo-cholinesterase deficiency. Long-acting nondepolarizers such as pancuronium, curare, and metocurine are rarely used in obstetrics because the intermediate-acting drugs like vecuronium, atracurium, and rocuronium are available and have a more appropriate duration of action for the average cesarean delivery.

Succinylcholine is rapidly metabolized by plasma cholinesterase, and its limited time of effect is what makes it so useful. In patients with decreased enzyme activity, succinylcholine has a longer duration of action. It is well established that plasma cholinesterase activity is 30% less with pregnancy, but the recovery from succinylcholine is not significantly prolonged in pregnant women. This apparent contradiction is best explained by an increased volume of distribution of succinylcholine in pregnancy, which causes a decreased apparent dose. However, in the postpartum period, when enzyme activity remains decreased, but the volume of distribution begins to normalize, the recovery from succinylcholine is prolonged by 3 minutes compared to control patients. The common side effects of succinylcholine, fasciculations and myalgias, are significantly decreased in pregnant compared to nonpregnant patients, and pretreatment with d-tubocurarine does not further decrease the incidence of these side effects in pregnancy.

Several muscle relaxants have prolonged action in pregnancy. Vecuronium, when administered in a dose according to body weight, has a significantly faster onset in pregnant women, 80 seconds compared to 144 seconds in nonpregnant females, and a longer duration of action, 46 minutes compared to 28 minutes. As such, to maintain stable muscle relaxation, pregnant patients require smaller doses of vecuronium than controls.

Pregnant patients also have a more rapid clearance of vecuronium than nonpregnant patients. In pregnant patients, rocuronium has a very similar onset of action, 79 seconds, and duration of action, 33 minutes after 0.6 mg/kg, compared to vecuronium. The duration of rocuronium is also prolonged in postpartum patients compared to nonpregnant patients. Recovery from mivacurium is slightly prolonged (from 16 to 19 minutes) in pregnancy, perhaps because of reduced plasma cholinesterase available for its metabolism. In contrast to vecuronium, rocuronium, and mivicurium, atracurium does not have a prolonged duration of action in peripartum patients. Magnesium, used in the treatment of pre-eclampsia, will prolong the duration of all nondepolorizing neuromuscular blocking drugs, but the duration of action of succinylcholine is not affected.

DRUG INTERACTION: MAGNESIUM AND MUSCLE RELAXANTS

- Magnesium enhances the neuromuscular blockade produced by nondepolarizing neuromuscular blocking drugs.
- Magnesium is used frequently in obstetrics for both the treatment of preterm labor and seizure prophylaxis in pre-eclampsia.
- Neuromuscular blocking drugs must be dosed carefully in these patients.

Vasopressors

It is very common after placement of a spinal anesthetic for cesarean delivery or even after the spinal dose of a CSE analgesic to require a vasopressor to support the blood pressure. In this case, rapid resolution of hypotension is important because neonatal acidemia will otherwise result. Vascular tone is tonically modulated by activation of both α_1- and β_2-adrenergic receptors in blood vessels. Because maternal sensitivity to catecholamines is reduced, more agonist drug is required to activate both receptor subtypes in pregnancy. There is a larger reduction in α_1-adrenergic sensitivity compared to β_2, which might contribute to the vasodilatory state of pregnancy. Ephedrine has traditionally been the drug of choice for the treatment of hypotension in pregnancy due to its α and β receptor-stimulating properties and because it does not decrease uterine blood flow in moderate doses. Other drugs have previously been considered contraindicated in obstetric anesthesia because of a fear of placental vasoconstriction leading to fetal asphyxia. More recent work has shown that treating the hypotension effectively is much more important than which agent is chosen. Increasing the pressure head to the placenta is more important than any vascular constriction that might be caused by an α-adrenergic agonist. In this regard, phenylephrine had always been thought to decrease uterine blood flow, but when used to treat hypotension after spinal anesthesia for cesarean delivery, it has been shown to result in less maternal hypotension and neonatal acidemia than ephedrine. Because phenylephrine has primarily α-receptor agonist effects, it can be used to avoid or decrease the tachycardia associated with excessive ephedrine use.

DRUG INTERACTION: ERGOT ALKALOIDS AND VASOPRESSORS

- Ergot alkaloids effect uterine contractions and are useful in the treatment of postpartum hemorrhage.
- Their mechanism of action is probably via α-adrenergic receptors.
- The combination of an ergot alkaloid and a vasopressor may lead to extreme hypertension.

Vagolytic Drugs

After a single 0.01-mg/kg dose of intravenous atropine given during cesarean delivery, the distribution half-life is 1 minute while the elimination half life is 3 hours. Intramuscular glycopyrrolate is rapidly absorbed prior to cesarean delivery and has an elimination half-life of 33 minutes, which is shorter than in nonpregnant females. Approximately half of the drug is excreted in the urine within 3 hours. Intravenous glycopyrrolate (0.005 mg/kg) and intravenous atropine (0.01 mg/kg) administered to laboring parturients have equal effects on maternal heart rate and blood pressure. Scopolamine, used in the past for "twilight sleep" in labor, has a similarly rapid intramuscular absorption rate with an elimination half-life during pregnancy of 1 hour.

Antihypertensive Drugs

Several different classes of drugs can be used for the treatment of hypertension in pregnancy. Angiotensin-converting enzyme (ACE) inhibitors are the only class contraindicated due to its association with fetal renal failure and intrauterine death. These drugs would not be very effective in pregnancy anyway because the normal pregnant woman is resistant to the action of angiotensin-II. For acute treatment of hypertension, especially in preeclampsia, hydralazine is used most frequently because of its long safety history and rapid pharmacokinetics. After intravenous bolus, it has an onset of action of 20 to 30 minutes. Sodium nitroprusside lowers blood pressure much more quickly, but this drug is used only as a last

resort because of the risk of rapid fluctuations in maternal pressure and the increased risk of cyanide toxicity to the fetus. β-Blockers are becoming more commonly used in pregnancy. The pharmacokinetics of propranolol are similar during pregnancy and the postnatal period. Labetolol has theoretical advantages over pure β-receptor antagonists due to its ability to antagonize α receptors as well. When administered orally, it has an elimination half-life ranging from 4 to 7 hours. The calcium channel antagonists have not been well studied in pregnancy but have specific utility for treatment of both maternal and fetal arrhythmias in addition to maternal hypertension.

Antacids

Most studies involving antacids traditionally assess efficacy by using a gastric volume of greater than 25 mL and a pH of less than 2.5 as indicators of increased risk of aspiration. More recently, though, these cutoffs have been challenged because no outcome data has suggested that obtaining these values reduces the risk of acid aspiration syndrome. Still, most drug therapy is used to increase gastric pH because altering gastric volume is much more difficult to accomplish. Both H2 antagonists and proton-pump inhibitors, particularly in combination with nonparticulate antacids, are effective at reducing gastric pH.

Because the aspiration of particulate matter can be as damaging to the lung as acid aspiration, nonparticulate antacids are recommended. One effective oral antacid is the administration of 30 mL of 0.3-molar sodium citrate given no more than 60 minutes in advance of cesarean delivery. When more time is available between drug administration and surgery, such as for an elective cesarean delivery, 400 mg of cimetidine, the prototypic histamine H_2-receptor antagonist, can be given orally 90 to 150 minutes in advance. Ranitidine has several advantages over cimetidine. It does not have as many interactions with other drugs; it raises gastric pH within an hour of intravenous administration, and it lasts longer. Several studies have shown its improved efficacy when given in conjunction with sodium citrate. Omeprazole, a proton pump inhibitor, is also useful in reducing gastric pH in pregnant patients. It has a long duration of action and binds directly to the pump. Its plasma half-life, on the other hand, is only 0.5 to 1.5 hours. This results in relatively low maternal plasma concentrations. Omeprazole has also been shown to be efficacious when used with metaclopramide and sodium citrate.

Antiemetics

There are many causes of nausea and vomiting in the parturient. Some of these include pregnancy itself, labor, opioids administered systemically, intrathecally, or epidurally, as well as spinally mediated hypotension during cesarean delivery. If treatment is required, options include ondansetron, dolasetron, droperidol, and metoclopramide. Depending on the situation, each has advantages and disadvantages. Most studies involving the use of these drugs in pregnancy assess efficacy and not pharmacology. Ondansetron and dolasetron, the newest and most expensive of the four, are less studied during pregnancy.

Metoclopramide has been shown to decrease the volume of stomach contents in early pregnancy, in established labor, and before elective cesarean delivery. There is also evidence that metoclopramide can be used prophylactically in women having spinal or epidural anesthesia for elective cesarean delivery to decrease the incidence of nausea and vomiting throughout the perioperative period. In sheep, the maternal elimination half-life of metoclopramide is 71 minutes, which is only slightly prolonged compared to the nonpregnant value of 67 minutes. Total body clearance and volume of distribution are lower in the pregnant ewe compared to the nonpregnant ewe, but dose reduction is not necessary. Ondansetron and droperidol have each been shown to be effective prophylaxis against nausea and vomiting after elective cesarean delivery compared to placebo, but there was no statistical difference in prophylaxis between treatments. Ondansetron has been shown to be more effective at preventing nausea than metoclopramide and placebo in a randomized trial during cesarean delivery. Because the FDA has placed a "black box" warning on droperidol packaging indicating its possible implication in cardiac arrhythmias, metoclopramide, dolasatron, and ondansetron remain the best alternatives for prophylaxis and treatment of nausea and vomiting after cesarean delivery.

Pregnancy represents a "new normal" state with markedly increased body fluid volume, increased cardiac output, and lung and kidney function. These changes are easily accommodated in the healthy parturient, and some are beneficial, for instance in preparation for blood loss at the time of birth. It is easy to imagine, however, how these changes could overcome physiologic compensation in a patient with subclinical disease of any organ system. It is thus the role of the anesthesiologist, along with our obstetric colleagues, to ensure that the new normal values of pregnancy are maintained and well tolerated by the parturient, to ensure successful delivery of the newborn.

SUGGESTED READING

Chadwick HS, Posner K, Caplan RA, et al: A comparison of obstetric and nonobstetric anesthesia malpractice claims. Anesthesiology 74(2):242–249, 1991.

Gintzler AR, Liu NJ: The maternal spinal cord: Biochemical and physiological correlates of steroid-activated antinociceptive processes. Prog Brain Res 133:83–97, 2001.

Gordon MC: Maternal physiology in pregnancy. In Gabbe SG, Niebyl JR, Simpson JL (eds): Obstetrics: Normal and Problem Pregnancies. 4th edition, Philadelphia, Churchill Livingstone, 2002, pp 63–92.

Kanto J: Obstetric analgesia: Clinical pharmacokinetic considerations. Clin Pharmacokinet 11(4):283–298, 1986.

Krauer B, Krauer F, Hytten FE: Drug disposition and pharmacokinetics in the maternal-placental-fetal unit. Pharmacol Ther 10(2):301–328, 1980.

Maternal adaptation to pregnancy. In Cunningham FG, Gant NF, Leveno KJ, et al (eds): Williams Obstetrics, 21st edition. New York, McGraw-Hill, 2001, pp 167–200.

Mucklow JC: The fate of drugs in pregnancy. Clin Obstet Gynaecol 13(2):161–175, 1986.

Pacifici GM, Nottoli R: Placental transfer of drugs administered to the mother. Clin Pharmacokinet 28(3):235–269, 1995.

Pilkington S, Carli F, Dakin MJ, et al: Increase in Mallampati score during pregnancy. Br J Anaesth 74(6):638–642, 1995.

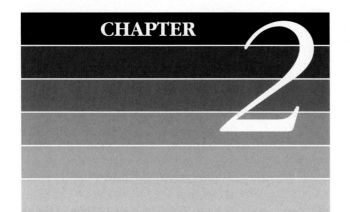

CHAPTER

2

Anesthesia for Nonobstetric Surgery During Pregnancy

JULIO E. MARENCO

ALAN C. SANTOS

INTRODUCTION

The need for surgery during pregnancy is not uncommon. It is estimated to occur in approximately 2% of all pregnancies and, in the United States alone, accounts for 50,000 cases per year. Surgery during pregnancy may be related to obstetric causes, such as cervical incompetence, or may be due to trauma and other abdominal emergencies. Anesthetic management must consider both maternal and fetal well-being. However, in contrast to obstetric anesthesia at term of pregnancy, prevention of labor is of paramount importance in women having surgery while pregnant. Also, whereas avoiding fetal depression due to placental transfer of anesthetic agents is a primary concern in obstetric anesthesia, it is less important when surgery is performed during pregnancy because the fetus is able to excrete anesthetics back to the mother for biotransformation and elimination. Finally, in contrast to obstetric anesthesia, teratogenicity and spontaneous abortion are immediate concerns when surgery is required during early pregnancy.

MATERNAL SAFETY

Pregnancy is associated with changes in maternal physiology that affect anesthetic management. Whereas these changes are well described at the end of pregnancy, there are few systematic studies on how altered physiology due to pregnancy can affect anesthetic management in the first or second trimester. Generally speaking, physiologic alterations in the first half of pregnancy are under hormonal control; whereas in the latter half of pregnancy, the mechanical effects of a growing uterus supervene.

Cardiovascular Changes

During pregnancy, the cardiovascular system becomes progressively more hyperdynamic to meet increasing fetal metabolic demands. This is both a result of changes in blood volume and constituents, as well as hemodynamics, which occur as early as the first trimester. There is an increase in plasma volume that, by term of pregnancy, is 50% greater than in the nonpregnant state. The most rapid increase in plasma volume occurs toward the middle of gestation, between 24 and 28 weeks. Concomitantly, an increase in red blood cell volume occurs, which is disproportionately lower than the increase in plasma volume. Accordingly, even in early pregnancy, the hematocrit of pregnant women is lower (33% to 35%) as compared to nonpregnant women. The increase in plasma volume also results in hemodilution of other blood constituents. For instance, although the total amount of plasma protein is increased during pregnancy, the concentration of protein per milliliter of plasma is decreased relative to nonpregnant women. As a result, there may be enhanced anesthetic effect because the free fraction of protein-bound anesthetic agents, such as diazepam and bupivacaine, may be increased during pregnancy.

Cardiac output increases progressively during pregnancy, in part, related to the aforementioned increase in total blood volume. However, there is also a redistribution of cardiac output resulting in an increase in blood flow to the uterus and mammary glands. Concomitantly, systemic vascular resistance is decreased due to the smooth muscle-relaxing effects of progesterone and prostacyclin, which are elevated during pregnancy, and also due to the growth of the placenta, which acts as a low-resistance vascular bed. The net result is that arterial blood pressure tends to be normal or slightly decreased in pregnant as compared to nonpregnant women.

A decrease in cardiac output may occur in the supine position during the second half of pregnancy due to compression of the aorta and inferior vena cava by a growing uterus. Compression of the vena cava may result in reduced venous return to the heart and a decrease in cardiac output whereas aortic compression results in reduced blood flow (and pressure) below the level of obstruction. In its most severe form, compression of the great vessels in the supine position results in the "Supine Hypotension Syndrome," which affects 10% to 15% of mothers and is manifested by lightheadedness, hypotension, tachycardia, diaphoresis, and even syncope. Thus, it is critical to ensure that the uterus be adequately displaced during anesthesia and surgery from the fifth month of gestation onward.

Respiratory System

Pregnancy increases the risk of hypoxemia during periods of apnea and hypoventilation, particularly after the fifth month of gestation. This is mostly related to two factors: a 15% to 20% decrease in functional residual capacity and an almost equal increase in the rate of oxygen consumption. Therefore, supplemental oxygen should be administered routinely to pregnant women during the immediate perioperative period. Indeed, the rate of decline in maternal PaO_2 is greater in pregnant (139 mm Hg/min) as compared to nonpregnant women (58 mm Hg/min) during periods of apnea. Thus it is imperative that denitrogenation (preoxygenation) precede induction of general anesthesia. This can be accomplished by the mother breathing 100% oxygen for 5 minutes or by taking four vital capacity breaths. Supplemental oxygen should also be administered routinely to women having regional anesthesia.

Minute ventilation increases during pregnancy, and, as a result, $PaCO_2$ lower (32 to 34 mm Hg) mostly due to an increase in tidal volume. It is ironic that pregnant women are more vulnerable to developing hypoxemia, considering that the resting PaO_2 is actually higher (PaO_2 104 to 106 mm Hg) than that of nonpregnant women due to the aforementioned alveolar hyperventilation. Alveolar hyperventilation may also result in faster induction with an inhalational agent due to a greater rate of rise in the alveolar partial pressure of the gas.

Vascular engorgement of the oropharynx and respiratory tract may render laryngoscopy and tracheal intubation difficult due to edema and bleeding, particularly if repeated attempts are required. Indeed, studies in pregnant women have shown that the use of general anesthesia is associated with a case fatality rate that is 16.7 times greater, almost exclusively due to difficulties with airway management, than for regional anesthesia. There are other reasons why a pregnant woman may be more difficult to intubate. During pregnancy, the mammary glands enlarge, making it technically difficult to perform laryngoscopy. Also, the anterior–posterior diameter of the thorax increases, which may make it difficult to place the woman in an optimum "sniff position." Consequently, the likelihood of a pregnant woman being unable to be intubated is almost 10 times more common than for surgical patients.

Gastrointestinal Changes

It's well accepted that the pregnant woman at term, particularly if in labor or having received systemically administered opioids, is at risk for aspiration pneumonitis. Unfortunately, it is less clear at what point in gestation individual women become at risk for aspiration. During pregnancy, increasing progesterone levels inhibit gastric emptying and intestinal motility. The competency of the gastroesophageal sphincter is compromised by the relaxant effects of progesterone and due to the mechanical effects of the uterus pushing the stomach upwards. Indeed, a delay in gastric emptying has been observed as early as 8 to 11 weeks of gestation and becomes significant at 12 to 14 weeks of pregnancy. Women who complain of frequent heartburn may be at greatest risk of aspiration. Finally, the pH of gastric secretions is lower as early as the first trimester in pregnancy due to placental secretion of gastrin.

Prevention of aspiration is of the utmost importance (Box 2-1). Preoperative administration of histamine H_2-receptor antagonists may be used to decrease the volume and acidity of gastric secretions. However, these require time to be effective and will not increase the pH of gastric secretions that are present in the stomach prior to drug administration. In this regard, nonparticulate antacids, such as sodium citrate, are very effective in neutralizing gastric secretions and should be routinely administered prior to induction of anesthesia. Particulate antacids, on the other hand, should be avoided because aspiration of colloidal suspensions may result in a severe form of aspiration pneumonitis having long-term consequences. Advance administration of metoclopramide promotes

---

Box 2-1 Measures to Avoid Aspiration

Follow strict NPO guidelines
Histamine H2-receptor antagonist
Metoclopramide
Sodium citrate
Avoid undue sedation during regional anesthesia
Rapid sequence induction with cricoid pressure and
    intubation if general anesthesia is chosen

---

gastric emptying and increases esophageal sphincter tone, but this requires 20 to 40 minutes for maximal effect.

Unfortunately, it is difficult to assess at what point in gestation individual women become at risk for aspiration. It would seem logical that women with comorbid diseases, such as morbid obesity and severe diabetes, may be vulnerable earlier. It is our practice to consider women by the end of the first trimester at increased risk of aspiration and to administer sodium citrate antacid routinely prior to anesthesia and surgery to decrease the risk for the syndrome of acid aspiration (Mendelson's syndrome). Avoiding general anesthesia and administering regional anesthesia, when possible, may theoretically decrease the risk of aspiration. However, the inappropriate use of sedatives and opioids may obtund airway reflexes during regional anesthesia and result in vomiting and aspiration. If general anesthesia is selected, rapid sequence induction with cricoid pressure and tracheal intubation with a cuffed endotracheal tube are required to reduce the risk of inhalation of gastric contents. If active vomiting occurs during induction, the oropharynx should be suctioned, and the woman should be placed in Trendelenburg position to prevent secretions from tracking down the trachea. With active vomiting, depending on the intensity, consideration should be given to releasing the cricoid pressure to prevent esophageal rupture.

If intubation is difficult, arterial oxygen desaturation must be prevented between attempts at intubation by intermittent positive pressure mask ventilation through cricoid pressure. If mask ventilation proves difficult, alternative techniques such as the laryngeal mask airway or Combitube may be required to maintain oxygen saturation. Once ventilation is assured, intubation using other equipment, such as intubating a laryngeal mask airway (LMA) or a fiber-optic bronchoscope, may be attempted. If ventilation is difficult, consideration should also be given to awakening the patient and using a different anesthetic technique.

Changes in Anesthetic Requirement

Pregnancy has been shown to be associated with a decrease in anesthetic drug requirement for both regional and general anesthesia. The decrease in local anesthetic requirement has been demonstrated as early as the first trimester of pregnancy and is mediated by a specific effect of progesterone (or a metabolite) on the sodium channel that makes it more receptive to local anesthetic blockade. As pregnancy progresses, epidural venous engorgement decreases the cerebrospinal fluid volume and the epidural space. As a consequence, lower doses of spinal and epidural drug are required to achieve a sensory level comparable to nonpregnant women. Vascular engorgement may also increase the risk of inadvertent intravascular injection of local anesthetic.

In animals, the minimum alveolar concentration (MAC) of inhalational agents has been shown to be 25% to 40% lower in pregnant as compared to nonpregnant ewes. Similar findings have been reported with nitrous oxide (NO_2) in humans. These effects have been attributed to the sedative effects of progesterone elaborated during pregnancy.

FETAL OUTCOME

The potential risks to the fetus from maternal anesthesia and surgery during pregnancy include the potential for congenital abnormalities, spontaneous abortion, intrauterine fetal death, and preterm delivery (see Box 2-2). Fetal exposure to anesthetic agents may be acute, as occurs during surgical anesthesia or subacute as may happen with exposure of one or both parents to sub-anesthetic concentrations of inhalational agents in the workplace. This chapter will focus only on acute exposure such as may occur during anesthesia for surgery during pregnancy.

TERATOGENICITY

It is well accepted that anesthetic agents may slow cell growth and division, and their cytotoxic and teratogenic effects have been demonstrated in many *in vitro* and animal models. However, extending these findings to women undergoing anesthesia for surgery during pregnancy is difficult for several reasons (Box 2-3). First, a drug may be a teratogen in one species but not in others. For instance,

---

Box 2-2 Adverse Fetal Outcomes

Congenital anomalies
Spontaneous abortion
Intrauterine fetal death
Premature labor

Box 2-3   Factors Affecting Teratogenicity

Species differences
Genetic predisposition
Timing of exposure
Magnitude of exposure
Effect on specific organ system

studies of the drug thalidomide in animals failed to identify the drug's potential for causing congenital anomalies in humans. Also, the timing of exposure is crucial because each organ system has its own critical period of vulnerability when it is most susceptible to teratogenic effects of specific drugs. In humans, the critical period of organogenesis is between the 15th and 56th day of gestation. In addition to the timing of exposure, consideration should be given to the magnitude and duration of the exposure. For instance, 12 to 24 hours of drug exposure in a rat having gestational period of 21 days is probably not comparable to 1 to 2 hours of surgical anesthesia in a woman whose gestation is 40 weeks.

The only anesthetic drug that has been shown conclusively to be a teratogenic in humans is cocaine. This effect is most likely mediated through the drug's sympathomimetic actions that reduce uteroplacental perfusion rather than to its direct local anesthetic effect. Some retrospective studies have also demonstrated a link between sustained maternal diazepam use and cleft lip/palate in the children of women using the drug during pregnancy, while other studies have not.

Perhaps the best-studied and most commonly administered anesthetic drug is nitrous oxide (N_2O). For a long time, N_2O was thought to be inert and devoid of metabolic effects. However, more recent evidence suggests that N_2O may interfere with important biochemical pathways leading to the synthesis of thymidine, a DNA component (Fig. 2-1). Indeed, nonpregnant patients exposed to N_2O for prolonged periods (greater than 5 days) have developed a megaloblastic anemia and peripheral neuropathy reminiscent of vitamin B_{12} and folate deficiency. The relationship between N_2O and vitamin B_{12} (cobalamin) is illustrated in Figure 2-1. Cobalamin is a cofactor to methionine synthetase, which is the enzyme catalyzing the transfer of a methyl group from methyltetrahydrofolate to homocysteine, thereby generating methionine, the precursor of the major methyl donor S-adenosyl methionine. Through intermediate steps, S-adenosyl methionine is converted to formyl-tetrahydrofolate that ultimately is involved in the synthesis of thymidine from uridine. N_2O exerts its adverse metabolic effects by oxidizing cobalamin I (the active form of vitamin B_{12}) to cobalamin III (inactive form) and thus prevents methionine from being formed. Studies have demonstrated that the inhibition of the methionine synthetase–cobalamin complex is irreversible and requires *de novo* synthesis of a new enzyme complex.

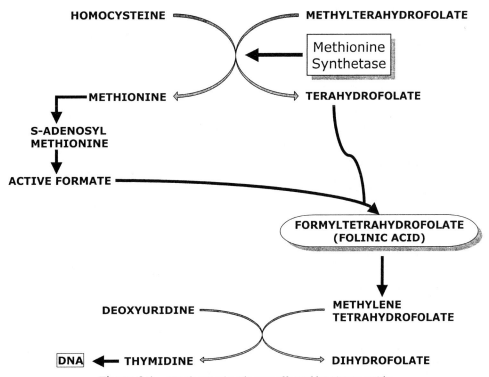

Figure 2-1   Biochemical pathways affected by nitrous oxide.

Similar metabolic effects of N_2O may also occur in the fetus during maternal exposure. This would be particularly important during periods when rapid fetal growth and development occur. Indeed, methionine synthetase activity is greater in the brains of midtrimester human abortuses than neonates or adults. Maternal exposure to N_2O results in decreased methionine synthetase activity in the fetal rat.

The results of fetal outcome studies in animals exposed to N_2O are conflicting. The effect of N_2O appears to be dose related, with studies using inhaled concentrations of less than 50% reporting no adverse effect of the drug, whereas inhaled concentrations greater than 50% may result in increased fetal wastage and impaired growth and skeletal development.

Although it would be tempting to assume that the adverse reproductive effects of N_2O are due to impairment of DNA synthesis, pretreatment with folinic acid, the missing intermediate, fails to prevent the teratogenic effects of N_2O in pregnant rats. In fact, adverse reproductive outcome in animals exposed to N_2O may not be at all related to its metabolic effects but a consequence of decreased uterine blood flow due to the drug's sympathomimetic effects. This is supported by data showing that administration of the α-receptor antagonist, phenoxybenzamine, or a potent inhalational agent, such as halothane or isoflurane, reduces adverse reproductive outcome in animals exposed to N_2O.

Whether N_2O should be used during human pregnancy has been a source of controversy (Box 2-4). In contrast to animal studies, no adverse reproductive outcome has been detected in women briefly exposed to N_2O for short periods of time during cervical cerclage. A Swedish registry study[1] involving 5405 women having anesthesia and surgery during pregnancy failed to implicate the use of N_2O in adverse perinatal outcome. Considering the results of animal studies, it would seem prudent to use inhaled concentrations of N_2O that are 50% or lower and to limit the duration of exposure to reasonable intervals associated with routine surgery (see Box 2-4). Furthermore, a potent inhalational agent may be useful in preventing decreases in uterine blood flow related to N_2O-mediated sympathomimetic effects or light anesthesia (see Box 2-4). The animal studies do not support routine maternal pretreatment with folinic acid prior to N_2O exposure.

Reproductive Outcome Studies

Studies have demonstrated that routine clinical anesthesia administration during pregnancy does not increase the risk of congenital anomalies. However, there is an increased risk of spontaneous abortion with anesthesia and surgery, particularly when procedures are performed during the first trimester of pregnancy or involve placement of a cervical cerclage or if surgery is performed on the pelvic organs. Two major reproductive outcome studies after anesthesia and surgery during pregnancy have been published.

Box 2-4   Avoiding N_2O Teratogenicity

Avoid prolonged exposure.
Use inhaled concentrations <50%.
Use in combination with a potent halogenated agent.

In one study, the health insurance codes for the population of Manitoba, Canada from 1971 to 1978[2] were surveyed. Each of 2565 women having surgery while pregnant was paired with a pregnant woman of similar characteristics who did not undergo surgery. For both groups of mothers, the rate of spontaneous abortion was similar: 7.1% in the surgery group and 6.5% in the nonsurgery group. In contrast to earlier studies, the site of surgery did not affect the incidence of spontaneous abortion. Also different from earlier studies, there was an increased incidence of spontaneous abortion with surgery on the pelvic organs or cervical cerclage; particularly when general anesthesia was used. This finding has been questioned for two reasons. First, general anesthesia was preferentially chosen for gynecologic and cervical cerclage; regional anesthesia was rarely used. Secondly, it is possible that more seriously ill mothers were given general anesthesia more frequently than regional anesthesia and that the maternal underlying disease alone could be sufficient to account for the higher incidence of fetal wastage had it been studied.

The other large study was also a registry study of 880,000 women delivering in Sweden between 1973 and 1981.[1] During that time period, 5405 women underwent surgery while pregnant. The incidence of spontaneous abortion and congenital anomalies was no different in woman having surgery during pregnancy as compared to those who did not. However, the likelihood of delivering an infant with intrauterine growth retardation was greater in women having surgery during pregnancy as was the risk of neonatal death in the first 7 days following birth. These risks were not related to prematurity because infants born to women having surgery earlier in their pregnancy and carrying to term had similar adverse outcome. The authors suggested that perhaps the disease that necessitated surgery played an important role in adverse perinatal outcome in women having surgery. In contrast to the aforementioned study, the use of general anesthesia was not associated with adverse reproduction outcome.

LAPAROSCOPY

Laparoscopic surgery has gained in popularity because it is less invasive than other approaches. It requires minimal hospitalization time and more comfortable recovery. Laparoscopic procedures have been performed for chole-

Box 2-5   Safeguards During Laparoscopy

DVT prophylaxis (pneumatic stockings)
Ultrasound rather than cholangiogram during chole-
    cystectomy
Pneumoperitoneum with N_2O rather than CO_2
Intra-abdominal pressure <15 mm Hg
Prevent maternal (fetal) respiratory acidosis by adjusting
    ventilation

cystitis, appendicitis, and other abdominal emergencies during pregnancy. In a retrospective review, there was no significant difference in obstetric outcome with laparoscopy compared to laparotomy. However, if laparoscopy is performed during pregnancy, there need to be some safeguards (Box 2-5).

Preventing maternal hypercarbia during insufflation should be a primary objective because respiratory acidosis alone may result in adverse fetal effects. In this regard, some have suggested insufflating the abdomen with N_2O rather than carbon dioxide. The intra-abdominal pressure during pneumoperitoneum should be adjusted so as not to exceed 15 mm Hg. Caution should be taken if the patient is to be placed in reverse Trendelenburg position for two reasons: venous pooling in the lower extremity may increase the incidence of thromboembolism (DVT), and it may also augment the effects of aortocaval compression.

PRESERVING UTERINE BLOOD FLOW

The foremost goal of the anesthesiologist should be to ensure maternal safety and preserve uteroplacental perfusion. Adequate oxygenation and ventilation must be preserved particularly because both hypoxia and hypercarbia have been shown to increase the risk of congenital anomalies in animals. Maternal hypotension may be due to aortocaval compression or anesthesia. Aortocaval compression is particularly hazardous to the fetus because it may reduce uteroplacental perfusion. From the fifth month of pregnancy on, uterine displacement should be a routine practice. Hypotension should be treated with increasing uterine displacement, increasing the rate of crystalloid infusion, and if needed, administering a small dose of an indirect-acting vasopressor, such as ephedrine. Vigorous controlled ventilation under general anesthesia may increase intrathoracic pressure and reduce uteroplacental perfusion in animals as a result of decreased venous return and cardiac output. Hypocarbia may further exacerbate the problem by causing umbilical cord constriction and a leftward shift of the maternal oxyhemoglobin dissociation curve.

CLINICAL RECOMMENDATIONS

1. Purely elective surgery should be postponed until after delivery (Fig. 2-2). If necessary, it is prudent to

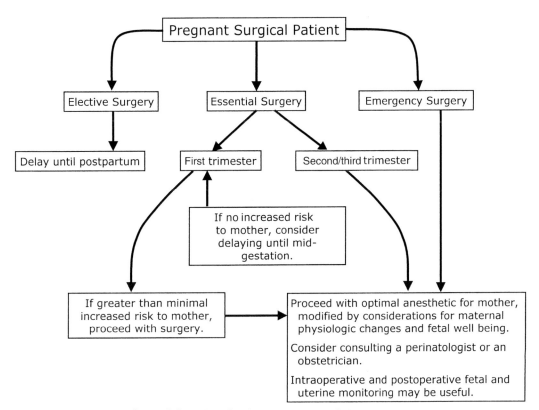

Figure 2-2   Algorithm for timing surgery during pregnancy.

wait until after the first trimester (where the theoretic risk of teratogenicity is lower), as long as the mother's condition allows. The optimum period for surgery during pregnancy may be from the 20th to 24th week of gestation when there is the lowest risk of teratogenicity and premature labor.

2. Pain and anxiety should be treated with the appropriate medication. Considering the available evidence and the many alternatives at hand, it would seem prudent to avoid the use of diazepam in the first trimester.

3. Prophylaxis for aspiration (see Box 2-1) may include preoperative administration of an H_2-receptor antagonist and metoclopramide. Sodium citrate should be routinely administered to neutralize existing gastric secretions.

4. From the fifth month of pregnancy on, uterine displacement should be routine.

5. Supplemental oxygen should be administered perioperatively, particularly when maternal illness, anesthesia, or postoperative pain medications may result in hypoventilation.

6. No one anesthetic technique has emerged as preferable. Rather, the choice of anesthetic should be based on maternal condition, the proposed surgery, and anticipated duration. Procedures involving the pelvic organs or for obstetric indications carry an additional risk of adverse reproductive outcome.

7. If general anesthesia is chosen, it is critical to prevent arterial oxygen desaturation during the period if induction by meticulous preoxygenation. Currently, there is no evidence preventing the use of N_2O as long as the inhaled concentration is less than 50% and exposure is not prolonged (see Box 2-4). Regional anesthesia, although theoretically decreasing the risk of aspiration, has its own complications, such as hypotension.

8. Maternal surveillance should at least include all of the basic monitors recommended by the American Society of Anesthesiology. Depending on the severity of maternal disease and the extent of the proposed surgery, additional invasive monitors may be required.

9. Fetal monitoring remains controversial. Most would agree that it is sufficient to confirm a fetal heart rate prior to and at the conclusion of the procedure if the fetus is previable. If the fetus is viable, decisions regarding continuous fetal monitoring during anesthesia and surgery should be made on an individual case-by-case basis, taking into consideration the mother's condition, the site of surgery, and the potential jeopardy to the fetus. To date, there is no known study suggesting that continuous fetal monitoring results in better fetal outcome if the mother has anesthesia and surgery while pregnant. However, if the fetus is viable, it would seem prudent that an obstetrician be available to manage obstetric complications related to the surgical procedure.

10. Surgical pain may mask premature labor, and for that reason, it may be necessary to monitor uterine activity in the immediate postoperative period.

11. Maternal pain relief should be a priority. The patient should receive postoperative supplemental oxygen for as long as required. Uterine displacement should be routinely practiced intraoperatively and immediately postoperatively.

REFERENCES

1. Mazze RI, Kallen B: Reproductive outcome after anesthesia and operation during pregnancy: A registry study of 5405 cases. Am J Obstet Gynecol 161:1178-1185, 1989.

2. Duncan PG, Pope WDB, Cohen MM, Greer N: Fetal risk of anesthesia and surgery during pregnancy. Anesthesiology 64:790-794, 1986.

SUGGESTED READING

Archer GW, Marx GF: Arterial oxygenation during apnoea in parturient women. Br J Anaesth 46:358-360, 1974.

Baden JM: Mutagenicity, carcinogenicity, and teratogenicity of nitrous oxide. In Eger EI II, (ed): Nitrous Oxide/N_2O. New York, Elsevier, Inc., 1985.

Hawkins JL, Koonin LM, Palmer SK, Gibbs CP: Anesthesia-related deaths during obstetric delivery in the United States, 1979-1990. Anesthesiology 86:277-284, 1997.

Heinonen OP, Slone D, Shapiro S: Birth Defects and Drugs in Pregnancy. Littleton, MA, Publishing Sciences Group, 1977.

Mazze RI, Kallen B: Appendectomy during pregnancy. A Swedish registry study of 778 cases. Obstet Gynecol 77: 835-840, 1991.

Reedy MB, Kallen B, Kuehl TJ: Laparoscopy during pregnancy: A study of five fetal outcome parameters with the use of the Swedish Health Registry. Am J Obstet Gynecol 177:673-679, 1997.

Rosen MA. Management of anesthesia for the pregnant surgical patient. Anesthesiology 91:1159-1163, 1999.

Samsoon GLT, Young JRB: Difficult intubation. Anaesthesia 42:487-490, 1987.

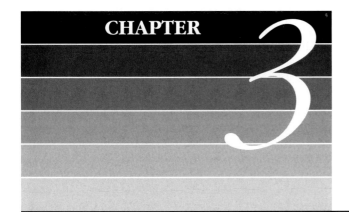

CHAPTER 3

Anesthetic Considerations for Fetal Surgery

FERNE R. BRAVEMAN

INTRODUCTION

Improved prenatal diagnosis has allowed for the recognition of fetal abnormalities much earlier in gestation. Whereas fetal surgeries 5 years ago were primarily EXIT (*ex utero* intrapartum therapy) procedures to treat the fetus just prior to delivery, earlier diagnosis, coupled with the availability and application of minimally invasive surgical procedures, has allowed for early treatment of abnormalities with the continuation of the gestation.

As a result, the anesthetic care of the mother for fetal surgery will be to provide anesthesia for either minimally invasive surgery during pregnancy, anesthesia for hysterotomy in early pregnancy, or anesthesia for cesarean delivery following a fetal EXIT procedure.

MATERNAL–FETAL SURGERIES: FETAL INDICATIONS

Surgical intervention directed at improved fetal outcome must be carefully considered with respect to "acceptable" maternal risk. One must remember that the mother's involvement in the fetal surgery, unlike emergent maternal surgery during pregnancy, entails only risk to the mother, without specific maternal benefit. The mother and fetus are considered appropriate for surgery only when the risk

of death or severe disability to the fetus is greater than with no intervention AND the risk to the mother is low.

Ex utero intrapartum therapy (EXIT) procedures are beneficial to the fetus and occur at or near term, as part of a cesarean delivery. The EXIT procedure entails delivering the fetal head through a controlled hysterotomy. Intubation using direct or indirect laryngoscopy or tracheostomy may be performed. This allows for fetal airway management while gas exchange is maintained via the placenta. Also, thoracentesis and pericardiocentesis can be done as EXIT procedures when indicated. Indications for EXIT procedures are listed in Table 3-1.

Other open procedures—those procedures requiring hysterotomy—include thoracic, cardiovascular, and neurologic procedures on the fetus in the first or second trimester. Table 3-2 lists procedures performed via hysteroscopy. Not all of these procedures have been shown to definitively decrease fetal morbidity or improve fetal outcome. Anomalies requiring an open procedure must be followed by cesarean delivery in this and all subsequent pregnancies, as the hysterotomy incision precludes trial of labor.

Thoracic procedures on the fetus usually take place between 18 and 25 weeks gestation. The goals of these operations are to correct problems which obstruct heart and lung development. These corrective procedures will result in better lung growth and improve postnatal viability.

Repair of meningomyelocele *in utero* is to prevent shunt-dependent hydrocephalus and loss of spinal cord function. Currently, closure of the meningomyelocele is done between 22 and 25 weeks gestation and results in a lower incidence of shunt-dependent hydrocephalus. Sacrococcygeal teratomas have also been removed from fetuses *in utero*. Resection of all or part of these highly vascular tumors restores cardiovascular stability.

Minimally invasive fetal procedures (fetoscopy) include insertion of stents or shunts, occlusion of fetoplacental structures, and the transfusion of medications

	Table 3-1 Indications for EXIT Procedures	
Disease	**Complicating Factors**	**Treatment**
CHAOS (Congenital High Airway Obstruction Syndrome)	Hydrops fetalis 2 degrees to *in utero* airway obstruction	Bronchoscopy and intubation *or* tracheostomy
Neck Mass	Polyhydramnios High output state	Tracheostomy followed by delivery and excision of the mass
Tracheal Atresia	—	Intubation
Pleural effusion	—	Drainage of effusion
Pericardial effusion	—	Drainage of effusion

or blood products into the fetus (Table 3-3). These procedures do not require hysterotomy and thus may be followed by vaginal delivery.

ANESTHETIC CONSIDERATIONS FOR FETAL SURGERY

Maternal considerations for fetal surgery occurring in the first or second trimester are those of any pregnant patient undergoing surgery (see Chapter 2).

	Table 3-2 Fetal Defects That May Be Indications for Open Fetal Surgery	
Fetal Defect	**Rationale for Treatment**	**Therapy**
Urethral valves	Prevention of renal failure and pulmonary hypoplasia	Vesicostomy
Congenital cystic adenoma	Prevention of pulmonary hypoplasia, hydrops fetalis, demise	Pulmonary lobectomy
Congenital diaphragmatic hernia	Prevention of pulmonary hypoplacia and pulmonary failure	Reduction and repair Temporary tracheal occlusion
Sacrococcygeal teratomas	Prevention of high output cardiac failure/hydrops fetalis	Resection of tumor, vascular occlusion
Meningomyelocele	Prevention of shunt-dependent hydrocephalus and further loss of spinal cord function	Closure of the defect

Unlike nonobstetric procedures undertaken in pregnancy, uteroplacental factors must be considered for fetal surgery. These include the location of the placenta and umbilical cord, maintenance of uteroplacental blood flow, and uterine relaxation for fetal exposure.

Fetal considerations for fetal surgery include the impact of anesthesia on a fetus with an immature cardiovascular system, fetal blood loss during surgery (total fetal blood volume may be less than 50 mL), and the significant evaporative fluid and heat losses from the fetus, as the thin, immature fetal skin provides little barrier to these losses. The risk for fetal demise intraoperatively is significant due to this combination of decreased myocardial contractility, hypovolemia, and hypothermia.

Nociceptive sensory pathways are present by midgestation, thus requiring administration of anesthesia to the fetus to prevent pain perception.

ANESTHESIA FOR OPEN FETAL SURGERY, EXCLUDING EXIT PROCEDURES

General anesthesia is usually selected for open fetal surgery because both mother and fetus must be anesthetized, and the uterus must be atonic. Maternal regional anesthesia may be used, and the fetus must then be anesthetized with neuromuscular paralysis for the procedure, independent of maternal anesthesia. As always, the decision between regional versus general anesthetic is determined by maternal comorbid diseases, such as an asthma history, or physical concerns, such as the potential for airway difficulties. Anesthetist and patient preference must also always be considered.

Prior to the day of surgery, a preanesthetic visit should be undertaken. At that time any confounding medical history should be reviewed, the anesthetic care of the mother and fetus discussed with the mother, and a plan of care clearly outlined for the mother.

On the operative day, the obstetrician will examine the mother and assess fetal status to confirm fetal well-being. Also, ultrasound assessment of placental location is essential because surgical access to the fetus is easier if the placenta is located on the posterior uterine wall. Type and cross-matched packed red blood cells should be available for the mother and O-negative blood available for the fetus. The mother should be premedicated for acid aspiration prophylaxis and administered a tocolytic.

As previously mentioned, preparation for care of the fetus includes having O-negative blood readily available. Also, drugs for fetal anesthesia care and resuscitation should be prepared, labeled, and available on the surgical table for administration by the surgeons in consultation with the anesthesiologist. Table 3-4 lists the

Table 3-3   Fetal Defects That May Be Indications for Repair via Fetoscopy

Fetal Defect	Rationale for Treatment	Therapy
Chorioangioma	Prevention of cardiac failure and hydrops fetalis	Legation of major vessels to the angioma
Amniotic bands	Prevention of amniotic band syndrome	Ligation of band
Twin-to-twin transfusion syndrome (TTTS) in monochorionic twins	Prevention of cardiac failure in "recipient;" prevention of anemia, hypotrophic hypoxia growth retardation in "donor"	Laser coagulation of anastomosing vessels
TTTS in the presence of one nonviable fetus	Prevention of cardiac failure in viable time	Fetal cord ligation

Table 3-4   Drugs to Be Immediately Available for Intraoperative Fetal Administration

Atropine	0.02 mg/kg
Epinephrine	1 μg/kg
Vecuronium	0.2 mg/kg
Fentanyl	20 μg/kg
0-Negative blood	50 mL aliquots

necessary medications. Continuous fetal echocardiography will provide monitoring of intraoperative fetal hemodynamics.

Maternal preparation, in addition to the premedication just mentioned, often includes placement of an epidural catheter. This can be used for intraoperative anesthesia, with fetal anesthesia obtained by fetal intravenous or intramuscular drug administration. If maternal general anesthesia is selected, an epidural should still be considered for postoperative analgesia. In addition to routine maternal monitoring, a radial arterial catheter and urinary catheter should be placed. The arterial catheter is helpful for blood pressure control, as most medications (noted later) used to maintain uterine relaxation also decrease maternal blood pressure.

Intraoperatively, because fetal circulation is dependent on uterine tone and maternal blood pressure, maternal blood pressure should be maintained greater than 100 mm Hg systolic, and uterine relaxation should also be maintained. Volatile agents and/or nitroglycerin should be administered as needed to decrease uterine tone while appropriate vasopressors may be needed to maintain maternal blood pressure. Total maternal intravenous fluids should be limited to 500 mL, unless maternal blood loss is significant to require volume resuscitation. Postoperative maternal pulmonary edema has been reported as a complication when excessive intravenous fluid was administered in these cases.

A small uterine incision limits fetal and maternal risk. The fetal operative site will be delivered through the inci-

sion, and warm fluids will be administered continuously into the uterine cavity to prevent cord kinking, to replace amniotic fluid loss, and to maintain fetal body temperature. Medications administered to the fetus intramuscularly, prior to fetal surgery, include fentanyl 5 to 20 μg/kg and vecuronium 0.2 mg/kg. Atropine 20 μg/kg may also be administered. Fetal hemoglobin and blood gases may be checked by taking an umbilical blood sample. Blood and medications can be administered through the umbilical vein as needed. At the end of the procedure, the amniotic fluid should be replaced by normal saline.

Postoperative care should be in an obstetric high-risk setting. Tocolysis is imperative, and maternal observation for the development of pulmonary edema and premature labor is required. Maternal pain should be treated with patient-controlled epidural analgesia or intravenous patient-controlled analgesia (Table 3-5).

ANESTHESIA FOR FETOSCOPY AND ENDOSCOPIC SURGERY

Fetoscopic surgery can be performed under general or regional anesthesia. General anesthesia is the least complicated method of providing both maternal and fetal anesthesia. However, since fetoscopic procedures

Table 3-5   Tocolytic Agents

Agent	Maternal Side Effect	Maternal Anesthetic Considerations
β-Mimetic agents	Hypovolemia Palpitations Tachycardia Hypoglycemia	Prone to pulmonary edema
Magnesium sulfate	Nausea/vomiting CV collapse	Prone to pulmonary edema Sensitivity to muscle relaxants
Nitroglycerin (venodilator)	Hypotension Headache	Prone to pulmonary edema
Nifedipine (calcium channel blocking agent)	Hypotension	—

are presently only being performed on the placenta, cord, and amniotic membranes; fetal anesthesia is not essential. Future procedures may involve the fetus directly, and thus general anesthesia would be preferred. In contrast to traditional laparoscopy, visualization and working space are achieved not with carbon dioxide insufflation but with the infusion of a warm lactated Ringer's solution. Fetal body temperature and hydration are thus maintained. The fetus can be monitored with a special pulse oximetry probe. Maternal monitoring is limited to standard monitors—no additional monitoring is necessary intraoperatively.

Postoperative care should be in an obstetric high-risk setting. Tocolysis is imperative preoperatively, intraoperatively, and postoperatively. Maternal observation for the development of premature labor is required. Maternal pain will be minimal, and treatment with intravenous patient-controlled analgesia or oral analgesics should suffice.

ANESTHESIA FOR EXIT PROCEDURES

Anesthesia for EXIT procedures is either with general or epidural anesthesia. The patient does not require tocolytics except for the short period of time while the fetal procedure is performed. This can be achieved either with high concentrations of volatile anesthetics or by administering intravenous nitroglycerin. If epidural anesthesia is used for the EXIT procedure and subsequent cesarean delivery, fetal analgesia should be obtained with intravenous fentanyl if a procedure other than laryngoscopy is performed. Fetal muscle relaxation is rarely needed for these procedures. Fetal oxygenation can be monitored using a sterile pulse oximeter probe applied to the hand.

CASE PRESENTATION

You are asked to see a 27-year-old, gravida 2, para 1 female who is scheduled for a primary cesarean section and EXIT procedure to treat a fetus with a large neck mass of unclear origin. She was seen in the preadmission testing center on the day prior to surgery and requests that her procedure be done under regional anesthesia. She wishes to be aware of her newborn's status at all times. She also requests that her husband be present in the operating room for the procedure.

1. How would you proceed to counsel this patient regarding her anesthetic management?
2. What recommendation will you make to the obstetric and pediatric staff regarding management of the infant if you proceed with regional anesthesia? General anesthesia?

SUMMARY

The choice of anesthesia for fetal surgery is dependent on maternal status and preference, anesthetist's preference, and the type of fetal procedure to be performed. Maternal benefit is lacking and fetal benefit controversial for many of the procedures; thus, the procedure should be undertaken only when maternal risk is minimal.

SUGGESTED READING

Cauldwell, CB: Anesthesia for fetal surgery. Anesth Clin North Am 20(1):211–226, 2002.

Gaiser, RR, Kurth, CD: Anesthetic considerations for fetal surgery. Semin Perinatol 23(6):507–514, 1999.

Galinkin JL, Gaiser RR, Cohen DE, et al: Anesthesia for fetoscopic fetal surgery: Twin reverse arterial perfusion sequence and twin-twin transfusion syndrome. Anesth Analg 92:1394–1347, 2000.

Myers LB, Cohen D, Galinkin J, et al: Anaesthesia for fetal surgery. Paediatr Anaesth 12:569–578, 2002.

Analgesia for Labor and Delivery

IMRE REDAI

PAMELA FLOOD

For most women, childbirth is a highly anticipated, joyful experience. However, it can also be accompanied by the most severe pain a woman will ever experience. In one study, women rated labor pain as only slightly less painful than the amputation of a digit. Nulliparous women rate their pain as more severe than multiparous women, and dysfunctional labors due to fetal malposition or dystocia can also be more painful. Despite the agreement that labor can cause severe pain, there is varied opinion on how it should be addressed. Labor pain is one of the few medical issues that has a large, vocal lay audience. Arguments for and against treatment of labor pain vary from religious to philosophic to scientific. The American College of Obstetrics and Gynecology notes that parturition is the only circumstance in which it is considered acceptable to experience severe pain, amenable to safe relief, while under a physician's care. They further recommend that a laboring woman's request for pain relief be sufficient for its implementation.

CLINICAL CAVEAT

Women with dysfunctional labors or nulliparous women may request earlier epidural analgesia.

Analgesia for labor first became possible with the development of general anesthetic techniques in the 1840s. At this time, the practice of analgesia for childbirth was highly controversial, in part because of the incomplete separation of church and state in many countries. Christian theologians argued that it was God's design that women suffer pain in childbirth. They argued that according to the story of Adam and Eve, women were destined to suffer in childbirth as punishment for Eve's sin. As such, many concluded that to relieve that pain would be sinful. Medically, techniques for analgesia were unrefined and consisted of the inhalation of chloroform or ether in uncontrolled amounts. There were many incidences of maternal hypotension, hypoxia, and gastric aspiration. Obstetric analgesia gained more public acceptance in 1853 when Queen Victoria of England was given chloroform for the birth of Price Leopold.

Although physicians remained divided on the morality and safety of the use of anesthesia and analgesia for childbirth, patients demanded it. In the early twentieth century, a new technique was developed in Germany, termed "twilight sleep." This treatment was a combination of scopolamine for amnesia and an opioid for analgesia. Twilight sleep remained popular through the mid-twentieth century when effects on the newborn began to be recognized and placental transfer was better understood. Regional analgesia for childbirth also developed during the early years of the twentieth century, but developed slowly because of the difficulty of the techniques and the lack of wide availability of local anesthetic drugs.

PAIN TRANSMISSION IN PARTURITION

Pain during the first stage of labor occurs mostly during contractions and is due to contraction of the uterus and distention of the cervix and vagina. Visceral afferent pain fibers from the uterus, cervix, and upper vagina form the cervical plexus and enter the spinal cord at the T10–L1 levels. The visceral afferent fibers also enter the sympathetic chain at L2 and L3 levels.

In the second stage of labor, expulsion of the fetus activates somatic afferent pain fibers from the mid and lower vagina, vulva, and perineum. These signals are conveyed via the S2–S4 spinal nerve roots that form the pudendal nerve. The pudendal nerve projects bilaterally through the inferior sciatic foramen, where it is accessible for blockade by local anesthetics. Neuraxial representation of labor pain is not continuous, and the interceding segments represent and mediate the sensory and motor innervation of the lower extremities.

Neurophysiology of Pain Transmission

The primary afferent pain fibers are bipolar, and their cell bodies are located in the dorsal root ganglia. The proximal axons of these neurons synapse in the dorsal spinal cord, where extensive sensory integration occurs. Many studies have been conducted on the role of gender and hormonal environment on pain sensation. The results of such studies are made more difficult to interpret by the subjective nature of pain and cultural and individual differences in pain reporting. There are likely gender-related differences in pain such that women experience less pain in response to a given noxious stimulus than men but are more likely to report that pain. Women are less sensitive to analgesia from μ-opioid agonists such as morphine when compared to men, whereas men are insensitive to κ-opioid agonists. Pain sensitivity is reduced in pregnancy. This reduction is likely hormonally mediated, as it occurs as early as 8 to 12 weeks gestation.

There are intrinsic inhibitory systems that are tonically active to reduce pain transmission. Two major inhibitory pathways are mediated by the neurotransmitters norepinephrine and serotonin. Noradrenergic fibers originate in the periaqueductal gray and other noradrenergic nuclei in the brain and project caudally to the dorsal horn of the spinal cord, where they synapse on the presynaptic aspects

of the afferent nociceptive fibers and on the receptive dorsal horn neurons as well. The descending noradrenergic pathway is a tonically active modulatory system that can be thought of as a volume control for pain transmission. This system is upregulated in pregnancy and is also involved in the analgesia associated with stress and trauma. The norepinephrine released from these neurons activates α_2-adrenergic receptors just as do the synthetic analogs clonidine and dexmedetomidine to provide analgesia.

The serotonergic neurons that provide native analgesic mechanisms are located in the median raphe nuclei in the brain. They also project caudally in the spinal cord, where they synapse on the dorsal horn neurons. These serotonergic inputs can be either facilitatory or inhibitory, but overall they provide analgesia. There is also evidence for tonic activity of this system.

NONPHARMACOLOGIC TECHNIQUES FOR LABOR PAIN

During the early years of analgesia and anesthesia for labor, there were significant maternal and fetal complications. Beside maternal hypotension, fetal asphyxia, and maternal gastric aspiration, the most common complaint about early techniques for labor analgesia was the lack of maternal participation in the birth experience. Ether and chloroform provided anesthesia in addition to analgesia. "Twilight sleep" including the anticholinergic drug scopolamine produced more amnesia than analgesia. Mothers often had no memory of the birth of their babies when these techniques were used. In response to these issues, a social movement against pharmacologic analgesia for childbirth gained popularity in the 1950s. Objections to the pharmacologic treatment of labor pain have at times been embraced by the movement for women's equality on the basis that doctors (mostly male) were taking women's childbirth experience away. These issues have largely dissipated as techniques available for labor analgesia have become safer and now do not induce amnesia or depression of consciousness.

Psychoprophylaxis was popularized by obstetricians Grantly Dick-Read and Fernand Lamaze. Their theories were based on the concept that the pain of childbirth was an unnatural symptom found only in Western cultures and was induced by fear of childbirth. Accordingly, the incorporation of relaxation techniques would allow women to experience childbirth without pain. There is some evidence that anxiety can potentiate pain. In some studies, nulliparous women who had attended classes in psychoprophylaxis had slightly less pain than nulliparous women who did not. There was no difference for women who had experienced childbirth previously. These methods are useful in preparing parents for a potentially stressful event. Although there is great variety in the experience of labor pain, practitioners should help to develop reasonable expectations for the pain relief that can be expected from these methods.

Many other nonpharmacologic techniques have been used for labor analgesia. Many of these methods have not been studied adequately by Western scientists, but they have been used for analgesia in other cultures for years. Maternal ambulation, bathing, showering, massage, and labor support appear to result in temporary pain relief and can hardly be recommended against as they have few side effects. Hypnosis and acupuncture have had variable reported success in relieving labor pain, and that success may be culturally determined. Transcutaneous electric nerve stimulation is a technique in which a constant electric current is used to produce activation of sensory input to the dorsal horn. According to the "Gating Theory," continuous sensory input (perhaps like that achieved with massage) reduces the activation achieved by the noxious sensory input.

SYSTEMIC ANALGESIA

Historically, systemic analgesics were part of "twilight sleep," analgesia induced with scopolamine and morphine. Although scopolamine has fallen out of favor because of its amnestic effect, systemic opioids are still used for labor analgesia. Opioid agonists exert their effects largely in the maternal central nervous system, although there is evidence for a role for peripheral opioid receptors. All opioid analgesics cross the placenta and reduce fetal heart rate variability due to CNS depression. Babies born under the influence of opioids have decreased respirations and reduced muscle tone. These effects can be reversed by opioid antagonists. Long-acting opioid agonists such as morphine and meperidine have been used for labor analgesia. The problem with the use of these drugs for this indication is that they are not very efficacious. The concentrations required to adequately relieve labor pain may cause maternal respiratory depression, nausea and vomiting, sedation, and increase the risk of maternal aspiration. As such, they are mostly used for partial relief of labor pain in early labor or when other methods are not available and for early labor. Mixed opioid agonist antagonists have the benefit of a ceiling effect; at higher concentrations the antagonist properties of the drug overtake the agonist properties. As such, analgesic efficacy is limited, but the risk of toxicity is smaller.

Table 4-1	Parenteral Opioids for Labor Analgesia		
Drug	**Dose**	**Duration**	**PCA Administration**
Meperidine	25 to 50 mg IV	~2 hr	12.5 to 15 mg q10min 300-mg 4 hr lockout
Morphine	5 mg IV	~2 to 3 hr	1.0 to 1.3 mg q8 to 10min plus 0.2 mg/hr CI 30-mg 4 hr lockout
Remifentanil	25 to 50 μg	5 to 10 min	10 to 25 μg q + 5 min plus 0.8 to 1 μg/kg/hr CI 1-mg 4 hr lockout
Fentanyl	25 to 50 μg IV	30 to 45 min	10 to 25 μg q6 to 8min 500-μg 4 hr lockout
Nalbuphine	10 to 20 mg IV	~3 to 4 hr	-

CI, Continuous infusion.

More recently, shorter-acting synthetic opioids (fentanyl, sufentanil, alfentanil, and remifentanil) have been used by intravenous patient-controlled analgesia infusions. The drug remifentanil has a pharmacokinetic advantage in that it is metabolized very rapidly by tissue esterases. As such, it is very short acting and reaches a peak effect approximately 3 minutes after dosing. It is so rapidly metabolized that although it crosses the placenta, it is unlikely to cause ill effects in the newborn. Although several different dosing regimens have been trialed, an ideal formula that ensures good analgesia but limits respiratory depression has not been developed. Table 4-1 provides dosages of commonly used parenteral analgesics.

NEURAXIAL TECHNIQUES

Epidural Anesthesia

Anatomy and Technique

The spinal cord terminates in the majority of adult women at the level of the first lumbar vertebra. It is extremely rare for the conus terminalis to extend beyond the L2 vertebral body. The dural sac, containing the cauda equina, continues to the level of the second sacral vertebra. The segmental spinal nerve roots are enveloped in lateral extensions of the meninges, which continue in the perineurium once the nerves exit the spinal column. The inside of the bony vertebral canal is not cylindrical. The ligaments connecting the vertebral bodies and laminae, the inner aspects of the pedicles, and intervertebral foramina all provide incongruences. These incongruences, containing the peridural venous and lymphatic plexus embedded in areolar fatty tissue, are what we perceive as epidural space. The posterior border of the epidural space is formed by the ligamentum flavum. The ligamentum flavum is not one ligament, but is composed of two curvilinear ligaments fused in the middle (Fig. 4-1). In some cases, there is no midline fusion, particularly at thoracic levels.

Epidural anesthesia for labor is performed with the patient in the sitting or the lateral decubitus position. Although the most common determinant for patient positioning is the preference of the operator performing the block, we will review briefly the potential advantages and disadvantages of the two positions. Patient comfort and preference seem to divide between the two options evenly although obese patients appear to favor the sitting position somewhat more than the lateral decubitus. Fortunately, most anesthesiologists also prefer their obese patients sitting for epidural placement for better landmark identification. Flexion of the lumbar spine is adequate in most patients, regardless of whether they are sitting or on their side. Lumbar flexion may be improved by another 10 to 15 degrees in the sitting position if the patient is sitting cross-legged ("Turkish" or "Indian" style). The lateral decubitus position provides more stability and may lessen patient movement during the procedure. When the patient is sitting, an assistant is often required to provide support and minimize patient motion.

It has been suggested that concealed aortocaval compression may occur in the lateral decubitus position. This phenomenon probably occurs only in exaggerated flexion, and there is no evidence derived from fetal heart tracing that uteroplacental flow or fetal well-being is compromised in the lateral decubitus position. Some have speculated that the left lateral decubitus position may be hemodynamically more advantageous. However, the position of the patient is often determined by which side the fetal heart rate monitor is situated: the patient has to turn facing the monitor so the cables running from the monitor to the patient do not cross the sterile field. Finally,

there is a reduced incidence of intravascular catheter placement using the lateral decubitus position. This is likely due to a gravity-related increase of venous pressure and intravascular volume in the sitting position. The position of the patient has minimal, if any, effect on the spread of the anesthetic solution injected into the epidural space.

Once the patient is positioned, an intervertebral interspace is selected. Any space below the L1–L2 space is acceptable. When determining the level of the interspace to be used, the most common anatomic guide utilized is the line joining the iliac crests. It is important to remember that in the nonpregnant state, this line is at the L4–L5 level, but in most pregnant women the line actually marks the L3–L4 interspace.

Following antiseptic preparation of the insertion site and local anesthetic infiltration, the epidural needle is advanced until the tip is engaged in the ligamentum flavum. It is important to identify and engage the needle in the ligament initially, as this step reduces the possibility of false loss of resistance and catheter misplacement. Furthermore, advancing the epidural needle without a stylet through loose fat or connective tissue may result in coring and plug formation in the needle lumen. This in turn blunts the loss-of-resistance response of crossing the ligament and could result in inadvertent dural puncture. Once engagement is achieved, a loss-of-resistance technique is used to determine the entry into the epidural space. Whether it is air, saline, "hanging drop," or any other ingenious method does not affect success or complication rates: operator preference determines the technique. Loss of resistance is not always clearly felt: this is perhaps related to the incomplete fusion of the two parts of the ligamentum flavum and the resulting relative thinness of the central part of the ligament.

Opinions differ as to whether the bevel of the needle should be advanced parallel or perpendicular to the sagittal plane. Some suggest parallel advancement decreases the incidence of headache if an inadvertent dural puncture occurs. However, when the needle is inserted parallel to the sagittal plane, it should be turned 90 degrees once in the epidural space. This maneuver may increase the possibility of inadvertent dural puncture because the turning needle may act like a corkscrew.

Once the epidural space is identified, a catheter is advanced through the epidural needle. There are two types of epidural catheter designs: open-ended single orifice and closed-end multiorifice catheters. Closed-end multiorifice catheters deposit local anesthesia over a length of about 1 to 1.5 cm in two or three different directions and provide a more even spread of the injected local anesthetic and perhaps a lesser likelihood of uneven or unilateral block than a single orifice catheter. Catheter material is also varied: soft, flexible catheters have gained popularity over the earlier rigid designs. It is more difficult to pass a soft, flexible

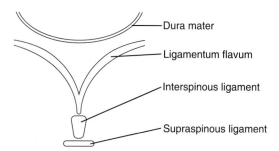

Figure 4-1 Schematic drawing of the relationship between the various ligaments encountered during epidural placement and the dura. Note that the ligamentum flavum is formed by the fusion of two curvilinear ligaments.

catheter; however, intravascular placement or migration of these catheters is less likely than with rigid catheters. True soft catheters, however, are all open-ended single orifice catheters. Soldering closed the end of the catheters results in a hard tip which will penetrate any vein situated adjacent to the orifice of the epidural needle. Thus when avoidance of vascular injury is important (e.g., patients with marginal coagulation status), use of open-ended soft catheters may have an advantage.

Once the catheter is advanced 5 to 6 cm beyond the tip of the epidural needle, the needle is carefully withdrawn and removed. Do not withdraw the catheter from the needle once the tip of the catheter is beyond the tip of the epidural needle; this may result in sheer or damage to the catheter. The catheter is secured with 3 to 6 cm left in the epidural space. The deeper the epidural space from the skin, the more of the catheter should be left in the epidural space to prevent accidental dislodgement. However, placement of the epidural catheter more than 4 cm into the epidural space increases the likelihood of a unilateral or patchy block, likely due to advancement of the catheter away from the middle. After placement, the catheter is then secured with an adhesive tape.

The catheter is then tested for inadvertent intrathecal or intravascular placement. Testing for intrathecal placement is based on the fact that the intrathecal analgesic dose of local anesthetics and narcotics is about ⅕ to ⅒ of the epidural dose. Between 30 and 45 mg of lidocaine or 7.5 to 10 mg bupivacaine is used for this purpose. Onset of profound analgesia in less than 5 minutes suggests intrathecal placement. Detecting intravascular placement is more difficult. The use of the classic approach of adding 15 to 20 µg epinephrine to the test solution and observation for heart rate (HR) changes is difficult in the laboring patient. Maternal HR variability secondary to uterine contractions and associated pain make interpretation of HR changes with epinephrine-containing test doses difficult. This may be minimized by injecting the epinephrine-containing test dose immediately at the end of a contraction. Some believe that intravenous administration of even this small dose of epinephrine may decrease uteroplacental perfusion. However, at this small dose, epinephrine would have predominantly β-adrenergic effects, and no clinical evidence exists to support this fear. The most sensitive and specific test in laboring patients for detection of intravascular placement of epidural catheters is the injection of 1 mL of air via the catheter while heart tones are continually monitored with a Doppler ultrasound probe placed over the maternal precordium. This simple test is underutilized in clinical practice.

Should a catheter be shown to be intrathecal, it can be used for continuous or intermittent subarachnoid analgesia or it can be removed and replaced with an epidural catheter. An intravascular catheter should be removed and replaced—most maneuvers recommended to salvage the catheter (e.g., gradual withdrawal of the catheter with repeat testing using boluses of local anesthetics with or without epinephrine) only delay analgesia for the patient and predispose to local anesthetic toxicity.

Continuous labor analgesia can be provided by an initial loading dose of an anesthetic (Table 4-2) followed by either a continuous infusion of a local anesthetic solution or intermittent boluses of a local anesthetic. Continuous techniques are the common clinical practice: these provide more even analgesia utilizing lower drug concentrations (0.0625% to 0.125% bupivacaine or 0.075% to 0.125% ropivacaine with 2 to 4 µg/mL fentanyl, hydromorphone 3µg/mL, sufentanil 2µg/mL, or 1 to 2 µg/ml clonidine at 8 to 12 mL/hr), producing good or excellent quality labor pain relief with minimal motor blockade of the lower extremities than with intermitted techniques. Drug administration is titrated according to patient needs, and patient-controlled epidural analgesia may be used. With this technique, the epidural infusion is administered with an epidural pump and can be programmed for patient-controlled use. With this device, a continuous infusion of one of the previously mentioned dilute analgesic solutions is administered at rates between 4 and 12 mL/hr, and a patient has access to self-administer boluses of 3 to 8 mL with lockout intervals ranging from 5 to 10 minutes. There is some increase in patient satisfaction due to this technique, although no significant improvement in analgesia.

A modification of epidural anesthesia is the combined spinal-epidural technique. After the epidural space is identified, a long pencil point spinal needle is advanced

Table 4-2 Epidural Infusions for Labor Analgesia

Loading Dose	Infusion Local Anesthetic Concentration*	Infusion Opioid Concentration
Bupivacaine 0.125% or Ropivacaine 0.075% Hydromorphone 10 µg/mL Volume: 10 mL	Bupivacaine 0.0625% to 0.125% or Ropivacaine 0.075% to 0.125%	Hydromorphone 3 µg/mL
Bupivacaine 0.125% or Ropivacaine 0.075% Fentanyl 5 µg/mL Volume: 10 mL	Bupivacaine 0.0625% to 0.125% or Ropivacaine 0.075% to 0.125%	Fentanyl 2 µg/mL
Bupivacaine 0.125% or Ropivacaine 0.075% Sufentanil 1 µg/mL Volume: 10 mL	Bupivacaine 0.0625% to 0.125% or Ropivacaine 0.075% to 0.125%	Sufentanil 2 µg/mL

*Clonidine 1 to 2 µg/mL may also be added with or without the opioid.

through the epidural needle into the subarachnoid space, and the initial analgesia is provided by administering drugs intrathecally (Table 4-3). Following the intrathecal dose, the spinal needle is withdrawn, and the epidural catheter is passed as previously described. Use of the combined spinal-epidural technique provides a rapid onset of analgesia with no or minimal lower extremity motor block. The catheter should be tested or observed for intravascular or intrathecal placement. It is not possible to reliably test the quality of analgesia provided by the epidural catheter until the initial spinal medication has worn off. This major drawback of the combined spinal-epidural technique should be noted when providing labor analgesia for patients at increased risk for operative delivery. Should the initial intrathecal dose prove to be inadequate or insufficient, the epidural loading dose should be given following testing for subarachnoid and intravascular placement.

CURRENT CONTROVERSY

Has the advent of combined spinal-epidural techniques for labor analgesia resulted in an increased failure rate in the conversion of epidural analgesia to surgical anesthesia and thus an increased rate of general anesthesia in some patient populations?

Although most epidural catheters provide good or excellent analgesia for part or all of labor, 10% to 15% of patients will experience significant pain even after receiving epidural analgesia. By understanding the concepts of troubleshooting inadequate analgesia, one can rescue patients with functional but inadequately dosed catheters and can avoid unnecessary delays in replacing catheters that are nonfunctional. Several characteristic signs indicate an inadequate epidural drug dose or level. Diffuse pain over the abdomen and/or back are commonly associated with need for additional bolus doses. However, a typical bolus dose (Table 4-4) should be effective in these cases. If the bolus dose is ineffective, it indicates that either the pain is not what it was initially interpreted to be (e.g., it is actually pain of second stage of labor) or the catheter is not in the epidural space. Unilateral or bilateral pain localized to the groin

Table 4-4   Recommended Bolus Doses for Epidural Catheters

Drug	Volume	Caveats
Lidocaine 2%	5 mL	Good to diagnose a clear level when analgesia is equivocal.
Bupivacaine 0.25%	5 mL	Useful to increase concentration in a patient with a clear epidural level, but incomplete effect. If effective, should be followed by an increase in concentration of infusion. Opioid may be added.
Ropivacaine 0.2%	5 mL	Useful to increase concentration in a patient with a clear epidural level, but incomplete effect. If effective, should be followed by an increase in concentration of infusion. Opioid may be added.
Clonidine	100 µg	Although clonidine is not approved by the FDA for epidural use, it has been used in obstetric analgesia as a second-line drug. It is particularly effective to resolve sacral sparing. It may induce hypotension approximately 20 min after use. If effective clonidine may be added to the epidural infusion at 1 to 2 µg/mL.

area is related to the L1 segment. The L1 segment is one of the thickest nerve roots in the body, and diluted concentrations of local anesthetics may be inadequate to penetrate this root. Injection of small doses of concentrated local anesthetics (3 to 5 mL 0.25% bupivacaine or 3 to 5 mL 2% lidocaine) usually provides good analgesia. Pain referred to the distribution of the lumbar or the sacral plexus along the lower extremity is caused by direct pressure and irritation by the presenting part. This pain is often severe and difficult to control until the presenting part passes the level of the plexus. Pain in the vulvoperineal area is associated with the second stage of labor. This necessitates the extension of analgesia toward the sacral segments. However, caudal spread of local anesthetics is poor: drugs injected to the epidural space preferentially spread cephalad. Epidural narcotics or α_2-receptor antagonists are useful in this context.

It is important to recognize when the catheter is not in the epidural space. Subdural placement has historically been described as an extensive neuraxial block with a delayed onset following a relatively low dose of a local anesthetic. It was hypothesized that the catheter is placed in the "virtual" space between the dura and the arachnoid, which allows for this uneven and unpredictable spread. However, a recent clinical and radiographic study has

Table 4-3   Intrathecal Opioids for Labor

Opioid	Dose
Sufentanil	2 to 5 µg in 1 mL NS
Fentanyl	10 to 25 µg in 1 mL NS
Meperidine	10 mg in 1 mL NS

NS, Normal saline.

brought attention that a poor-quality block with restricted spread and slow onset is likely to be due to a subdural catheter. These catheters should be removed and replaced.

Intravascular placement was previously discussed. However, it is important to recognize that a catheter may migrate intravascular at any time during labor, and this may result in loss of analgesia. Timely replacement is the best solution.

Unilateral analgesia occurs in 5% to 10% of patients. The most common reason is lateral migration of the catheter. Withdrawal of the catheter 1 to 2 cm may be attempted followed by administration of a bolus of an anesthetic solution. Should analgesia remain unilateral, replacement of the catheter is the best option.

Indications, Contraindications, Complications, and Caveats

Epidural anesthesia is indicated at any stage of labor when the laboring woman desires analgesia. It was shown to be the most effective way of relieving pain with the least amount of maternal and fetal side effects among the current choices for labor analgesia. The American College of Obstetricians and Gynecologists has stated that barring medical contraindication, a patient's request should be sufficient for epidural placement.

Contraindications for epidural placement include coagulopathy, local infection at the planned site of insertion, patient refusal or inability to cooperate, and inadequate training or experience of the anesthetist. Relative contraindications include mild to moderate coagulopathy, systemic infection, increased intracranial pressure, history of spina bifida, and other lumbosacral neuromeningeal malformations, and uncorrected maternal hypovolemia.

CURRENT CONTROVERSY

What is the lower limit of platelet count when epidural placement remains safe? Or rather should we monitor platelet *function* routinely or at least in select patients?

Common maternal side effects include lumbar sympathectomy-induced hypotension, narcotic-induced pruritus, nausea, and urinary retention. Hypotension following epidural or combined spinal-epidural placement is usually mild and easily treated. It is not prevented reliably by fluid loading, and excessive fluid loading may slow labor. As such, the routine infusion of more than 250 to 500 mL crystalloid prior to epidural placement is not recommended. Narcotics, whether administered epidurally or intrathecally, slow or halt gastric emptying in about 80% of laboring patients, and oral intake of food or liquids should be strongly discouraged in association with neuraxial narcotic use. Local anesthetic toxicity, even when the infusate is administered intravenously via a migrated catheter, is very rare with current low-dose epidural infusions.

CURRENT RESEARCH INTEREST

What is the underlying mechanism of maternal pyrexia associated with epidural analgesia?

Maternal temperature rises gradually during epidural analgesia. The temperature rise is usually noticed hours after placement of the epidural and is not associated with any infectious event. The etiology remains unclear. However, recognition of this phenomenon is important in preventing unnecessary diagnostic and therapeutic interventions in the mother and the newborn.

Common postpartum maternal complications include postdural puncture headache, pain at the epidural insertion side, and prolonged effects of the anesthetic agents (motor block, sensory deficit, urinary retention). Rare but serious complications include epidural hematoma, infection, granuloma, and arachnoiditis.

In experienced hands, unintended dural punctures with large epidural needles occur in approximately 1% of patients, and the incidence of postdural puncture headache is between 70% and 80%. Several maneuvers have been attempted to prevent the onset of these headaches, including prophylactic blood patch and prolonged maintenance of and saline infusion into the spinal catheter. These issues are addressed elsewhere.

Fetal/neonatal side effects are relatively uncommon with epidural anesthesia in the absence of maternal decompensation. Apgar and neurobehavioral scores, umbilical artery pH, and base deficit are no different in newborns of mothers with or without epidural anesthesia. No effect of the epidurals on postnatal bilirubin metabolism is seen.

CURRENT CONTROVERSY

Is the continued use of intrathecal fentanyl justified, given the knowledge of their potential to cause significant fetal bradycardia?

Fetal bradycardia associated with subarachnoid opioids, given as part of the combined spinal-epidural technique, was described. Rapid onset of maternal analgesia resulting in a precipitous reduction of circulating β-agonist concentrations may cause an unopposed increase in uterine tone, leading to decreased uteroplacental perfusion and fetal bradycardia. Also, reduction in maternal blood pressure, particularly when the opioid is combined with a local anesthetic, can lead to utero-placental insufficiency evidenced by fetal heart rate deceleration. Cases that do not resolve spontaneously usually respond to change in maternal position, intravenous terbutaline, or ephedrine in the setting of maternal hypotension. Intramuscular injection of 25 mg of ephedrine 10 minutes prior to the subarachnoid injection of fentanyl was found to be effective in reducing the incidence of maternal hypotension after combined spinal-epidural analgesia for labor.

Caudal Anesthesia

Anatomy and Technique

Caudal anesthesia is a variant approach for epidural anesthesia. The epidural space is accessed via the sacral hiatus. The patient is placed in the lateral decubitus position, and the sacral cornua are identified. Following local infiltration of the skin, a short beveled needle is passed between the cornua at a 45 degree angle. The crossing of the sacrococcygeal ligament is felt as a distinct loss of resistance. The needle is then redirected cephalad and advanced 1 to 2 cm farther. It is imperative not to advance the needle farther to avoid inadvertent puncture of the dural sac. Position of the needle can be confirmed using the following tests. Injection of 3 to 4 mL of air through the needle with simultaneous auscultation over the thoracic spine will result in a characteristic whoosh sound heard if the needle is correctly placed in the sacral epidural space. Rapid injection of 3 to 5 mL saline while palpating at the projected level of the tip of the needle will reveal subcutaneous placement of the needle tip. However, this test will not differentiate between a needle in the caudal epidural space and one passed deep between the sacrum and the coccyx. Once the operator is satisfied with the location of the needle, a soft catheter is passed 4 to 6 cm into the sacral epidural space. Testing and intrapartum management of the catheter are similar to that of a lumbar epidural catheter.

Indications, Contraindications, Complications, and Caveats

Indications and contraindications are similar to those for lumbar epidural anesthesia. Caudal anesthesia is superior for analgesia for the second stage of labor because of proximity of the catheter to sacral nerve roots. It may be successful in patients in whom attempts to place an epidural catheter via the lumbar route have failed (prior back surgery, kyphoscoliosis, obesity).

Side effects and complications are similar to those of lumbar epidural analgesia. An uncommon but serious potential neonatal complication is inadvertent injection into the fetal head when the needle is accidentally passed between the sacrum and the coccyx.

ALTERNATIVE REGIONAL ANESTHETIC TECHNIQUES

CURRENT CONTROVERSY

What is the role, if any, of the alternative regional anesthetic techniques in modern labor analgesia?

Paracervical Block

Anatomy and Technique

The paracervical ganglion or Frankenhäuer's ganglion is located lateral and posterior to the cervicouterine junction. Sensory nerve fibers from the uterine corpus, the cervix, and the upper vagina pass through the paracervical ganglion: these are the fibers conducting the painful sensation of the first stage of labor. Finger-guided infiltration of the posterolateral aspect of the vaginal fornix results in adequate analgesia for the first stage of labor in about 75% of patients. A further advantage of the paracervical block is the superficial position of the ganglion: it is rarely deeper than 2 to 4 mm from the vaginal mucosal surface. The patient is positioned in the lithotomy position with left uterine displacement. A needle guard is used to prevent the needle from penetrating deeper than 2 to 3 mm into the vaginal vault. This will minimize but not abolish the possibility of vaginal injury or penetration of the fetal presenting part. The ganglia are located at approximately 4 and 8 o'clock positions just under the mucosa of the vaginal vault. Care should be taken by the operator not to put undue pressure on the mucosa with the examining finger, as this may distort the anatomy and result in a failed block. After careful aspiration, 5 to 10 mL of local anesthetic solution is injected. There should be a 5 to 10 minute interval between the left- and right-sided blocks while the fetal heart rate is monitored. On occasion, fetal bradycardia may result from a paracervical block, and fetal heart rate monitoring is recommended during and after the procedure. 0.125% bupivacaine, 1% lidocaine, and 2% 2-chloroprocaine have all been used for paracervical blocks. Epinephrine-containing solutions are AVOIDED. It seems that 2% 2-chloroprocaine is associated with the least amount of fetal side effects and the lowest reported neonatal local anesthetic blood levels while the duration of action is not remarkably different from the other local anesthetics. The duration of the block is about 30 minutes to 1 hour, after which the block can be repeated as necessary.

Indications, Complications, and Caveats

The paracervical block is indicated for analgesia for the first stage of labor.

Maternal complications are rare and avoidable. Using small doses of dilute drugs can prevent systemic toxicity from inadvertent intravascular injection of the local anesthetic solution. Injury of the injection site with hematoma or abscess formation has been reported. The paracervical block has no effect on the duration or progress of labor.

Fetal complications are more common. The most common unwanted side effect of the paracervical block is transient fetal bradycardia, which occurs in up to 40% of cases. The etiology remains unclear. Fetal bradycardia occurs 2 to 20 minutes after the injection of the local anesthetic solution and resolves within 5 to 10 minutes. Fetal bradycardia is more common in patients who had a nonreassuring fetal tracing prior to the block, and most obstetricians avoid using a paracervical block in such patients. Furthermore, although fetal bradycardia is usually transient, the severity and duration of the bradycardia correlate with pre-existing fetal acidosis and neonatal depression.

Severe fetal injury may result from direct injection of the local anesthetic solution into the presenting part. This is more common when the block is performed during advanced stages of cervical dilatation.

The paracervical block is associated with a significant risk for physician for needlestick injury. The needle and the palpating fingers are in close proximity, deep in the vagina of a patient who may have difficulty staying motionless.

To summarize, the paracervical block is clearly inferior to a continuous epidural or spinal technique, as it is only effective during the first stage of labor. Sacral nerve roots that conduct pain during the second stage of labor are not affected with this technique. It has a well-recognized potential to cause fetal bradycardia and should not be used in the presence of a nonreassuring fetal heart trace. The risk of needlestick injury in the era of HIV and hepatitis C awareness has further reduced the popularity of the paracervical block. However, it is a relatively easy block to learn and to perform, and the only additional equipment needed is an adjustable needle guard. It is clearly superior to systemic analgesics and may provide improved labor analgesia to women who cannot have neuraxial blockade for a variety of reasons.

Lumbar Sympathetic Block

Anatomy and Technique

Uterine and cervical visceral afferent fibers join the sympathetic chain at L2-L3. Sympathetic blockade performed at this level will alleviate pain of the first stage of labor.

The patient is placed in the sitting position. The L2 level is identified. Following local infiltration, a 3.5-inch 22-gauge needle is inserted 6 to 8 cm lateral from the mid-line and directed at 30 to 45 degree from the sagittal toward the vertebral body. Once bony resistance is identified, the needle is redirected so it just misses the anterolateral surface of the vertebral body. 10 to 15 mL 0.375% to 0.5% bupivacaine with 1:200,000 epinephrine is injected after careful aspiration. The procedure is then repeated on the contralateral side. The onset time for the block is about 5 to 8 minutes, and the duration is approximately 3 to 6 hours. There is no associated motor block, as only the sympathetic fibers are affected. Some evidence suggests that lumbar sympathetic blockade may accelerate the first stage of labor.

Indications, Complications, and Caveats

Lumbar sympathetic block was used successfully for analgesia in the first stage of labor in patients when prior spine surgery precluded the use of epidural or spinal analgesia. Reported cases and series are from trained individuals: these practitioners have a 75% to 100 % success rate.

The most common side effect observed was maternal hypotension, which can be prevented by administering 250 to 500 mL IV crystalloid solution prior to the block and/or by treating with sympathetic agonists.

Inadvertent intravascular, epidural, or intrathecal injection of local anesthetic solution may lead to unwanted side effects of systemic toxicity, high spinal anesthesia, or postdural puncture headache.

The need for two separate injections, the unsuitability of the block for continuous techniques, and the lack of ability to extend the block for the second stage of labor have limited the use of lumbar sympathetic block in obstetric analgesia. However, familiarity with the block allows the anesthesiologist to relieve pain in patients with prior back surgery and instrumentation who otherwise would not be able to receive the benefits of conduction anesthesia.

Pudendal Nerve Block

Anatomy and Technique

The pudendal nerve provides sensory innervation to the mid to lower vagina, perineum, and vulva, and is thus responsible for conduction of pain information during the second stage of labor. The pudendal nerve originates from the S2-S4 segments of the spinal cord. In its initial course, it follows the sciatic nerve to the lesser sciatic foramen just below the ischial spine. The nerve then runs in the pudendal canal just lateral and inferior to the sacrospinous ligament. It then branches into numerous terminal branches innervating the perineum.

There are two approaches to block the pudendal nerve: the transvaginal and the transperineal. The patient is placed in the lithotomy position. The operator places a finger in the vagina or the rectum and identifies the ischial spine and the sacrospinous ligament. In the transvaginal approach, the needle is restricted by a needle guard. No more than 1 to 1.5 cm should protrude beyond the guard. The needle is inserted into the vaginal mucosa and then directed toward the sacrospinous ligament. When the ligament is passed through, there is a loss-of-resistance sensation. From 3 to 10 mL of local anesthetic solution is injected after careful aspiration. When using the transperineal approach the needle is inserted between the rectum and the ischial tuberosity and is directed just inferior and lateral to the ischial spine and sacrospinous ligament. The same amount of local anesthetic solution is deposited as with the transvaginal approach. 0.5% bupivacaine, 1% lidocaine, 1% mepivacaine, and 3% 2-chloroprocaine with or without epinephrine can all be used for pudendal nerve block in labor without any significant maternal or fetal side effects.

Indications, Complications, and Caveats

Pudendal nerve block is indicated for pain in the second stage of labor. Administration of the block requires considerable experience, and unilateral or bilateral failure of the block is common.

Loss of the bearing down reflex occurs in about a third of women following pudendal nerve block, and use of epinephrine-containing solutions accentuates this unwanted effect. Systemic toxicity may result from inadvertent intravascular injection: the close proximity of the pudendal vascular bundle predisposes to this complication. Absorption of local anesthetic from the injection site is rapid and reaches peak in maternal and fetal blood within 10 to 20 minutes. However, neonatal well-being is not or is minimally affected by a pudendal nerve block. Other maternal complications include hematomas, which are rarely significant, and deep pelvic or subgluteal abscesses, which are rare but serious. Fetal complications are mainly associated with direct needle trauma and injection into the presenting part. As the injection is performed blind and in close proximity to the palpating finger of the operator, needlestick injuries are common.

The pudendal nerve block may be useful in a patient presenting in advanced labor when neuraxial blockade is "too late." When successful, it is also an excellent supplement for the pain of the second stage in patients who have received paracervical or lumbar sympathetic blocks for analgesia in the early part of their labor. Failure of the block is perhaps its most common complication.

Although there are many options for labor analgesia, by far the most popular modalities are epidural and combined spinal-epidural analgesia. They have the benefit of excellent efficacy and a low incidence of side effects. The perfect labor analgesic, however, would also be relatively noninvasive, inexpensive, and widely available. The achievement of these objectives, combined with the enormous recent progress in the safety and efficacy of labor analgesia, would be a great boon for women's health.

CASE REPORT

A 21-year-old woman G_1P_0 in active labor requests labor analgesia. Her vaginal examination is 1 to 2 cm dilated. Contractions are occurring every 8 to 10 minutes. Discuss options for analgesia. Is it different for G_3P_2 at 8 cm?

SUGGESTED READING

Andrews PJ, Ackerman WE III, Juneja MM: Aortocaval compression in the sitting and lateral decubitus positions during extradural catheter placement in the parturient. Can J Anaesth 40(4):320–324, 1993.

Collier CB: Accidental subdural injection during attempted lumbar epidural block may present as a failed or inadequate block: Radiographic evidence. Reg Anesth Pain Med 29(1):45–51, 2004.

Friedlander JD, Fox HE, Cain CF, et al: Fetal bradycardia and uterine hyperactivity following subarachnoid administration of fentanyl during labor. Reg Anesth 22(4):378–381, Jul–Aug 1997.

Friedman EA, Sachtleben MR: Caudal anesthesia: The factors that influence its effect on labor. Obstet Gynecol 13(4): 442–450, 1959.

Fusi L, Steer PJ, Maresh MJ, Beard RW: Maternal pyrexia associated with the use of epidural analgesia in labor. Lancet 1(8649):1250–1252, 1989.

Merry AF, Cross JA, Mayadeo SV, Wild CJ: Posture and the spread of extradural analgesia in labor. Br J Anaesth 55(4):303–307, 1983.

Mulroy M, Glosten B: The epinephrine test dose in obstetrics: Note the limitations. Anesth Analg 86(5):923–925, 1998.

Palmer CM, Cork RC, Hays R, et al: The dose-response relation of intrathecal fentanyl for labor analgesia. Anesthesiology 88(2):355–361, 1998.

Rosen MA: Paracervical block for labor analgesia: A brief historic review. Am J Obstet Gynecol 186(5 Suppl Nature):S127–S130, 2002.

CHAPTER 5

Fetal Monitoring and Resuscitation

ANA M. LOBO

During pregnancy and throughout labor and delivery, both the mother and fetus are routinely evaluated, to decrease morbidity and mortality. A thorough understanding of fetal monitoring and resuscitation is essential to anesthetic practice, as the administration of anesthesia may profoundly affect maternal and fetal physiology and outcome. Information obtained through fetal monitoring suggests how a fetus will tolerate labor, delivery, and anesthetic intervention and guides anesthetic management of the parturient. With the advent of improved monitoring techniques, perinatal mortality has decreased approximately 3% per year in the United States since 1965.

Over 50% of all fetal deaths are associated with fetal asphyxia or maternal factors (i.e., pregnancy-induced hypertension, placental abruption). Intrauterine hypoxia/birth asphyxia accounts for 3% of perinatal deaths while placental or umbilical complications are responsible for 2%. Fetal monitoring is one important vehicle by which fetuses at risk may be identified and promptly treated, with the goal of reducing perinatal morbidity and mortality.

FETAL STRESS REACTIONS

Both acute fetal distress and chronic fetal stress reactions are detected through fetal monitoring. Fetal oxygen deprivation may result in various physiologic responses. These include vagal activity (bradycardia); tachycardia; a decrease in fetal breathing movements; gasping movements; redistribution of blood flow to the brain, heart, and adrenals; increased circulatory catecholamines; and systemic hypertension.

Acute fetal distress is the result of severe and/or prolonged deprivation of oxygen. Fetal hypoxia or asphyxia may occur due to the delivery of a hypoxic mixture of gases and/or a critical reduction of blood flow to the uterus. If severe, or prolonged, the preceding may result in decreased fetal oxygen tension, increased carbon dioxide tension, and respiratory and metabolic acidosis, leading to lactate accumulation. Fetal compensatory mechanisms may be inadequate, resulting in asphyxia and permanent tissue damage. Urgent delivery may be indicated.

Chronic fetal stress may lead to hypoxemia, which may or may not require immediate treatment. Factors which may cause chronic fetal stress include the following: fetal congenital anomalies, decreased hemoglobin concentration (i.e., hemolytic disease), inadequate maternal oxygenation (i.e., asthma, pulmonary disease), decreased placental oxygen delivery (i.e., maternal hypertension, heart disease, smoking, diabetes, anemia) or decreased placental oxygen transfer (i.e., placental abruption, placenta previa), and inadequate maternal nutrition (i.e., excessive narcotic, alcohol use). Some of these factors may be controlled with specific maternal interventions that minimize fetal stress, thereby decreasing the need for immediate obstetric treatment. Routine antepartum fetal assessment and evaluation, as well as intrapartum fetal monitoring techniques, are critical because they detect fetal stress, thereby preventing poor maternal and fetal outcome.

ANTEPARTUM FETAL ASSESSMENT

Antepartum fetal assessment incorporates various tools which monitor and evaluate maternal and fetal well-being. A detailed explanation of routine prenatal evaluation and care is beyond the scope of this chapter. Pregnancy dating and fetal growth evaluations are part of routine care. Additional indicators of fetal well-being include estimations of fetal movement. After 28 weeks gestation, normal fetuses have gross body movements 20 to 50 times/hr, although quiet times lasting 20 to 75 minutes occur. A change in movement pattern (appreciated by the parturient) may indicate a need for further fetal evaluation. Lack of movement may reflect fetal hypoxia or asphyxia requiring immediate intervention. Parturients at high risk for fetal compromise (i.e., postdate gestation, diabetes, pregnancy-induced hypertension, premature labor, etc.) may require fur-

ther fetal assessment to ensure fetal well-being. Tests used to further evaluate the fetus include the nonstress test, the contraction stress test, and biophysical profile scoring.

The Nonstress Test

The nonstress test (NST) is frequently used as an initial screening test in the high-risk parturient to evaluate fetal well-being. It is noninvasive and has no contraindications. Normally, fetal movement is associated with temporary accelerations in fetal heart rate (FHR) which occur at frequent intervals. Infrequent movement not associated with FHR accelerations may indicate a compromised fetus.

During a NST, the baseline heart rate and long-term variability (discussed later) of the FHR tracing are also evaluated. A normal baseline FHR is between 110 and 160 beats/min (bpm). Bradycardia may suggest fetal hypothermia, congenital heart block, exposure to a β-adrenergic receptor antagonists, and acute fetal hypoxia. Fetal tachycardia (FHR > 160) may reflect maternal fever, chorioamnionitis, fetal exposure to anticholinergics or β-adrenergic agonists, fetal anemia, or fetal hypoxia. Normal long-term variability is present when the FHR tracing demonstrates a sinusoidal wave pattern which cycles every 3 to 6 minutes (Fig. 5-1).

The parturient lies in the Semi-Fowler's position, tilted to the left, for 20 minutes. Fetal movements are detected by maternal report, and the FHR tracing is recorded using an external monitor. The tracing is evaluated for FHR accelerations immediately following fetal movement. A normal, or reactive, NST requires that the FHR be in the normal range, that two or more fetal movements occur

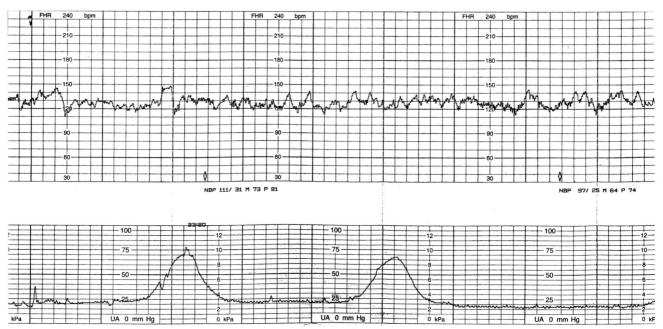

Figure 5-1   Presence of short- and long-term variability in a normal FHR tracing.

CLINICAL CAVEAT: ETIOLOGY OF FETAL BRADYCARDIA AND TACHYCARDIA

Bradycardia
Increased vagal tone
Hypoxia
Congenital heart block
Hypothermia
Drugs (narcotics, β-blockers)

Tachycardia
Maternal fever
Chorioamnionitis
Drugs (anticholinergics)
Fetal anemia
Fetal hypoxia
Tachyarrhythmias

within 20 minutes, and that these are accompanied by FHR accelerations of at least 15 bpm lasting at least 5 seconds. An abnormal, or nonreactive, NST occurs when no FHR accelerations are noted during a 40-minute period. The FHR may or may not be in the normal range. Poor or absent long-term variability is observed. This test is repeated weekly if reactive. Further evaluation in the form of a contraction stress test (CST) or biophysical profile (BPP) is necessary if the NST is nonreactive. If uncertain reactivity is present (i.e., the baseline FHR is not normal, fewer than two fetal movements are observed, or the acceleration is <15 bpm), the NST should be repeated or followed by a CST.

Contraction Stress Test

The CST, or oxytocin challenge test, is performed when uteroplacental insufficiency is suspected. Not infrequently, it follows a suspicious or nonreactive NST. This test requires the presence of uterine contractions, which normally and temporarily decrease uteroplacental perfusion and fetal oxygen delivery. This brief interruption of blood supply will not negatively affect a fetus that

has adequate reserves. A fetus that is compromised may become hypoxic and bradycardic during this period of decreased blood supply. A CST is contraindicated in patients with placenta previa, third trimester bleeding, polyhydramnios, multifetal gestation, incompetent cervix, premature rupture of membranes, and those at risk or being treated for premature labor.

An external ultrasound transducer and a tocographic unit are placed on the maternal abdomen. Uterine activity and FHR are recorded for 15 to 20 minutes. This test requires three mild to moderate contractions over 10 minutes. If spontaneous contractions are not present, pitocin can be used for augmentation. Alternatively, nipple stimulation, triggering release of oxytocin from the posterior pituitary, may be used to stimulate contractions. Possible interpretations of this test are listed in Table 5-1.

A negative CST indicates that placental reserves are most likely sufficient to maintain fetal viability for approximately 1 week. However, fetal health is not guaranteed with a negative CST, as 8% are falsely negative. The CST is not useful for predicting a compromised fetus. The false positive rate is 50%. For this reason, when the CST is indicative of fetal stress, other tests, such as a BPP, should be used to confirm an undesirable fetal state prior to any obstetric intervention.

Biophysical Profile (BPP)

Yet another tool utilized by obstetricians to evaluate the fetus at risk is the BPP. BPP scoring incorporates the evaluation of several fetal biophysical activities, which are regulated by the fetal central nervous system and reflect fetal well-being. Fetal biophysical activity is compromised by varying degrees of hypoxemia. Breathing movements and heart rate variability are most sensitive to hypoxemia, whereas fetal tone and movement are least sensitive. Ultrasound examination is useful for evaluating multiple fetal activities including breathing, tone, movement, sucking, swallowing, eye movements, heart rate, and urination. Other parameters readily evaluated by ultrasound include amniotic fluid volume, placental

Table 5-1   CST Interpretations

	Negative	Positive	Suspicious	Hyperstimulation	Unsatisfactory
Findings	Normal FHR 3 contract/10 min Contract last ≥40 sec No late decelerations	Absent FHR variability Persistent late FHR decelerations	Inconsistent late FHR decelerations Variable FHR decelerations Abnormal baseline FHR	Uterine contract >q2 min Uterine contract last >90 sec cause late FHR decelerations or fetal bradycardia	<3 uterine contract in 10 min Poor recording quality
Actions	Repeat in 1 week BPP if indicated	BPP Consider delivery	BPP Repeat in 24 hr	Repeat in 24 hr	Repeat in 24 hr

grade and structure, umbilical cord condition, and umbilical vessel blood flow.

During BPP evaluation, five fetal biophysical activities are examined. Each is given a score ranging from 0 (abnormal) to 2 (normal) as outlined in Table 5-2. The scores are added, and risk of fetal asphyxia is determined. Based on these results, management decisions are made (Table 5-3). Diminished fetal movement, absence of breathing movements, poor tone, and/or oligohydramnios may herald poor fetal outcome. The simultaneous evaluation of several biophysical parameters is necessary for accurate BPP scoring.

INTRAPARTUM FETAL ASSESSMENT

Intrapartum fetal assessment evaluates ongoing fetal well-being during the process of labor and birth. At term, a normal FHR ranges from 110 to 160 bpm. *In utero,* both the fetal sympathetic and parasympathetic nervous systems innervate the myocardium, thereby regulating the FHR. Throughout gestation, parasympathetic tone increases and becomes more predominant. In fact, the beat-to-beat variability observed in FHR tracings is the result of parasympathetic innervation.

Electronic FHR Monitoring

Continuous electronic FHR monitoring provides an ongoing tracing of the FHR from early labor through delivery. This method of FHR monitoring is the cornerstone for evaluation of fetal well-being. The continuous FHR tracing and uterine contraction pattern are recorded on the fetal monitoring strip (Fig. 5-2). The top grid is used to record FHR over time. Each small

Table 5-2 Biophysical Profile Scoring

Parameter	Findings	Normal	Abnormal
Antepartum fetal heart rate testing Nonstress test	Reactive nonstress test	2	0
Fetal breathing	One or more episodes within 30 min, lasting 30 sec or more	2	0
Fetal movements	Three or more discrete body or limb movements within 30 min	2	0
Fetal tone	One or more episodes of limb extension with return to flexion within 30 min	2	0
Amniotic fluid volume	Adequate volume defined as one or more 1 cm or larger pockets of fluid in two perpendicular planes	2	0

From Manning FA: Fetal biophysical profile scoring: A prospective study in 1,184 high-risk patients. Am J Obstet Gynecol 140:289–294, 1981.

box (*) represents 10 seconds of time in the longitudinal axis, while the bolder lines (↑) divide the grid into 1-minute time intervals. The bottom grid displays the presence and duration of contractions. When a tocodynamometer is used (i.e., internal monitoring), the vertical axis measures uterine contraction intensity (in mm Hg). Two techniques of electronic FHR monitoring are

Table 5-3 Biophysical Profile Score and Recommended Management

Score	Interpretation	Recommended Management
10	Nonasphyxiated fetus	Repeat test weekly
8 to 10 (Normal fluid)	Nonasphyxiated fetus	As above
6	Suspect chronic fetal asphyxia	Consider delivery as soon as possible 1. If amniotic fluid is abnormal—deliver 2. If amniotic fluid is normal, >36 weeks, favorable cervix—deliver 3. If <36 weeks EGA or L/S ration is <2 or cervix not favorable—repeat test in 24 hr 4. If repeat test is <6—deliver If repeat test is >6—observe and repeat test as above
4	Probable fetal asphyxia	Repeat test same day If repeat score is <6—deliver If repeat score is >6—as above
0 to 2	Fetal asphyxia	Immediate delivery

From Manning FA: Fetal assessment based on fetal biophysical profile scoring experience in 19,221 referred high-risk pregnancies. II. An analysis of false-negative fetal deaths. Am J Obstet Gynecol 157:880–886, 1987.

EGA, Estimated gestational age; L/S, lecithin/sphingomyelin.

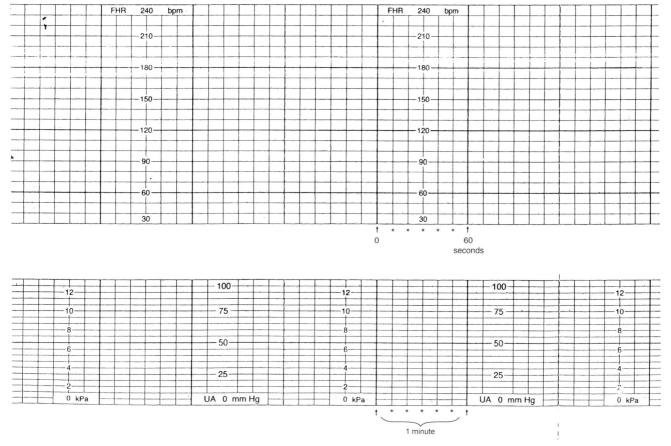

Figure 5-2   Fetal heart rate/uterine contraction monitoring strip.

currently in use: external (or noninvasive) and internal (or invasive).

External FHR monitoring involves placement of both a Doppler ultrasound transducer (measuring FHR) and a tocodynamometer (identifying uterine contractions and their duration) over the gravid uterus. The Doppler ultrasound transducer identifies fetal cardiac events over time, but does not accurately reflect beat-to-beat variability (described later). Both FHR and uterine contraction presence and duration are simultaneously recorded over time on the FHR/uterine contraction strip. External monitors are easy to use and noninvasive in design but are less sensitive than internal monitors.

Internal FHR monitoring is more invasive but most sensitive in evaluating FHR patterns, FHR variability, and intensity of uterine contractions. A small electrode is inserted via the cervix onto the fetal presenting part. Placement requires that the cervix be at least 1 cm dilated, the presenting part be vertex or breech, the fetal head be well applied, and membranes be ruptured. Internal monitors are more accurate, have fewer artifacts, and are sensitive in recording fetal heart rate beat-to-beat variability (see later). They are indicated if the external monitor tracing is of poor quality and/or

demonstrates a nonreassuring FHR pattern. Use is limited by a maternal history of herpes, hepatitis C, and/or HIV disease, as fetal transmission may occur. Internal uterine contraction monitors are used to evaluate the duration, intensity, and quality of uterine contractions. An open-ended, fluid-filled, plastic catheter is placed in the uterine cavity, and the pressure generated by each contraction is converted to and electric signal and recorded on the strip. Contractions which generate 60 mm Hg of pressure and last 60 seconds are generally considered adequate to dilate the cervix.

Internal monitoring is useful in the diagnosis of delayed labor progression, secondary to inadequate contractions, and uterine hyperstimulation (which may lead to fetal distress, placental abruption, and/or uterine rupture). It can also be utilized as an adjunct to pitocin administration for labor augmentation or induction.

FHR Patterns

There are two types of FHR patterns: the baseline FHR (i.e., FHR in the absence of a contraction) and the periodic FHR (i.e., FHR changes associated with uterine contractions).

At term, the baseline FHR may be normal (110 to 160 bpm), elevated, or depressed. Fetal tachycardia is present when the FHR exceeds 160 bpm. Tachycardia may be mild (160 to 180 bpm) or severe (>180 bpm). Both maternal issues (e.g., fever, chorioamnionitis, or thyrotoxicosis) and/or fetal conditions (e.g., extreme prematurity or tachyarrhythmias) may contribute to fetal tachycardia. A persistent baseline FHR of <110 bpm is considered fetal bradycardia. Persistently severe bradycardia (FHR 60 to 100 bpm) may suggest fetal compromise. Maternal hypotension, fetal hypoxemia, and/or congenital heart block may be present. A FHR that persists at <60 bpm requires prompt treatment, and emergent delivery may be indicated.

At term, a normal, reassuring baseline FHR tracing also exhibits both short- and long-term variability. Short-term variability refers to the presence of differing time intervals, between the same points in the cardiac cycle, of successive beats. Irregularity in a FHR baseline tracing reflects an intact nervous system pathway between the fetal cerebral cortex and its cardiac conduction system (see Fig. 5-1). Short-term variability is most accurately assessed by a fetal electrocardiogram. When a fetus becomes hypoxic, cerebral function may become impaired and cause a loss of short-term variability, or a "flat" tracing (Fig. 5-3). Maternal narcotic administration or fetal sleep may temporarily cause a paucity of beat-to-beat variability.

Long-term variability refers to changes in the FHR over a period of 3 to 6 minutes. An irregular sinusoidal oscillation of FHR (6 to 10 bpm) occurring at 3 to 6 cycles per minute is considered normal long-term variability (see Fig. 5-1). It is described as normal, decreased, absent, or

> ### CLINICAL CAVEAT: SHORT- AND LONG-TERM FHR VARIABILITY
>
> - The presence of short- and long-term variability suggests fetal well-being.
> - In practice, short- and long-term FHR variability are interpreted together.
> - A "flat" FHR tracing is nonreassuring and requires further evaluation.

salutatory, based on the amplitude range of the FHR tracing. Fetal asphyxia, vagal blockade, cardiac conduction delays/heart block, and drug effects can all reduce long-term variability (see Fig. 5-3).

Periodic FHR changes may occur in association with uterine contractions. They are categorized as accelerations, early decelerations, variable decelerations, and late decelerations.

Accelerations in FHR, occurring with contractions, are associated with good fetal outcome. An acceleration is observed when the FHR increases at least 15 bpm above baseline and lasts at least 15 seconds (Fig. 5-4). These accelerations are the result of fetal sympathetic activity outweighing parasympathetic activity and suggest a reactive, healthy fetus.

Early decelerations are typically recognized as being the mirror image of the uterine contraction curve. They occur with contraction onset, and the nadir in FHR occurs as the contraction reaches its peak. FHR recovery occurs as the contraction subsides (Fig. 5-5). Early decelerations are uniform in shape, and the FHR nadir is usually <20 bpm

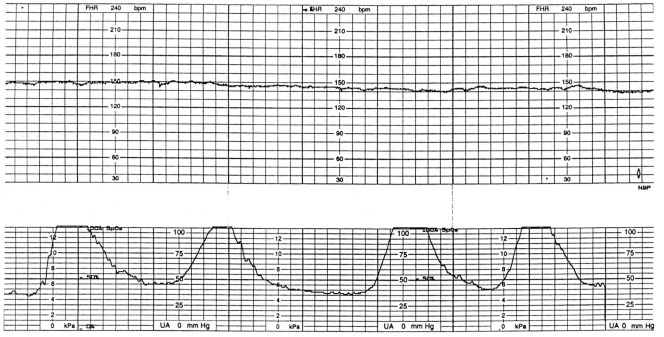

Figure 5-3   A "flat" FHR tracing. Minimal/absent short- and long-term variability.

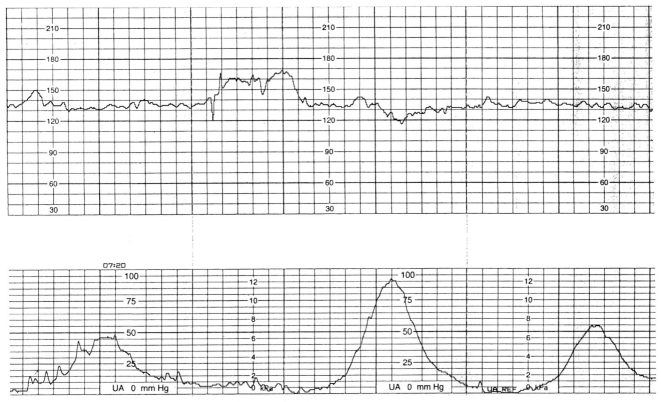

Figure 5-4   Fetal heart rate acceleration.

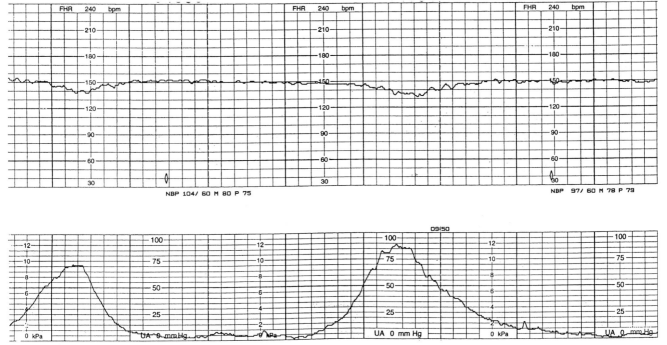

Figure 5-5   Early FHR decelerations.

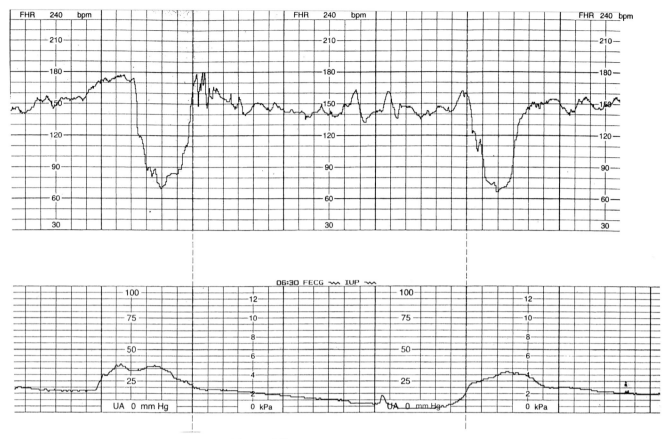

Figure 5-6   Deep variable decelerations.

below baseline. These decelerations are the result of mild fetal hypoxia or head compression (temporary increase in intracranial pressure) leading to reflex vagal stimulation. If mild, they are usually benign and well tolerated. Early decelerations are rarely severe in nature, and further evaluation of fetal status is usually not indicated.

Variable decelerations in FHR are the result of umbilical cord compression leading to vagal stimulation and bradycardia. Typically, they are irregular in intensity and duration and nonuniform in shape (Fig. 5-6). They are variable in onset, severity, and duration. Not infrequently, the FHR drops dramatically with the onset of a contraction (as the umbilical cord is compressed), and recovery is variable. If severe, meaning a FHR drop of 60 bpm below baseline and/or lasting >60 seconds, these variables may progress to late decelerations. Often, variables will improve by changing the parturient's position (i.e., left uterine displacement) and administering oxygen. A normal fetus is usually able to tolerate mild to moderate variable decelerations for a period of time without being compromised.

Late decelerations, caused by uteroplacental insufficiency, contour and mirror the uterine contraction curve. Characteristically, the FHR begins to decelerate approximately 10 to 20 seconds after the onset of the uterine contraction. The nadir of the FHR is observed after the contraction peak and recovery of the FHR is observed following the end of the uterine contraction (Fig. 5-7). Late decelerations are classified as either reflex- or nonreflex-based upon their etiology. Reflex late decelerations typically occur secondary to maternal hypotension (causing decreased uterine blood flow, cerebral hypoxia, increased fetal vagal tone, and FHR deceleration). Typically, the FHR maintains good short-term variability throughout the deceleration, and the FHR returns to baseline with resolution of the contraction. Correction of maternal hypotension normalizes the FHR pattern. Conditions such as pre-eclampsia, intrauterine growth retardation, and repetitive late decelerations may result in prolonged fetal hypoxia and lead to fetal myocardial depression, causing nonreflex late decelerations. Progressive decompensation of fetal cardiac function is the result of inadequate fetal oxygen supply during contractions. Poor or absent short-term FHR variability is present.

Terminal fetal bradycardia refers to a severe, prolonged decrease in FHR (Fig. 5-8). FHR typically falls below 60 bpm without prompt recovery. Not infrequently, beat-to-beat variability is diminished or absent. This type of deceleration may suggest a hypoxic insult to

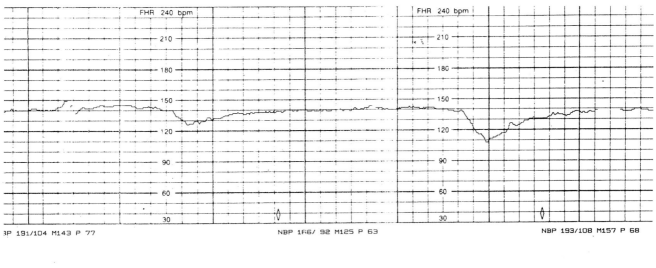

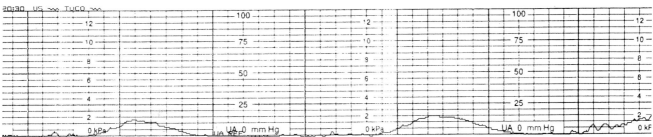

Figure 5-7   Late decelerations.

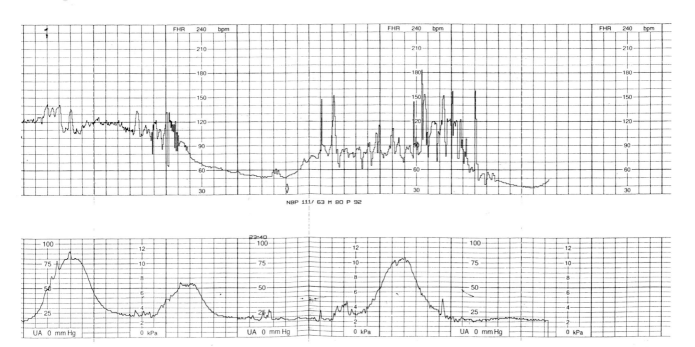

Figure 5-8   Terminal fetal bradycardia.

the fetus. Emergent delivery may be necessary to prevent severe permanent fetal damage and/or intrauterine fetal demise.

Treatment of FHR Decelerations

Once FHR decelerations are detected, it is important to identify the type of deceleration and its most probable cause. If possible, correcting the cause of the decelerations, in an expeditious manner, will return the FHR to normal. Improving fetal oxygenation and relieving fetal stress are the treatment goals.

Early decelerations caused by fetal head compression are generally mild in nature and infrequently result in poor fetal outcome. Changing maternal position and/or maternal oxygen administration may benefit the fetus. Fetal scalp stimulation, if possible, may result in FHR acceleration. In the presence of fetal meconium or severe early decelerations, further fetal evaluation may be necessary (i.e., fetal scalp sampling, see following section).

Variable decelerations, caused by umbilical cord compression, are generally well tolerated by the healthy fetus. If severe, however, fetal compromise may occur. Treatment includes changing maternal position, administering oxygen, administering intravenous fluids, and/or amnioinfusion. Further fetal evaluation and/or delivery may become necessary if variables persist or worsen.

Late decelerations are caused by uteroplacental insufficiency. Treatment involves left uterine displacement, oxygen administration, intravenous fluids, and ephedrine, if maternal hypotension is present. Fetal evaluation (i.e., scalp sampling, fetal pulse oximetry) as well as delivery may become necessary.

Terminal fetal bradycardias are ominous in nature and require immediate intervention. Treatment involves all of the aforementioned modalities and emergent delivery if no improvement in the FHR is observed.

Table 5-4 Fetal Scalp Blood Values and Acidosis

Scalp Blood Value	Normal	Metabolic Acidosis	Respiratory Acidosis
pH	≥7.25	<7.25	<7.25
PO_2 (torr)	≥20	Variable	<20
PCO_2 (torr)	≤50	>50	>50
HCO_3 (mMol/L)	≥20	<20	<20
BE (mMol/L)	<−6	>−6	<−6

BE, Base excess.
From Kryc JJ: Evaluation of the Pregnant Patient: Preoperative Concerns. In Dewan DM, Hood DD (eds): Practical Obstetric Anesthesia, Philadelphia, W.B. Saunders, 1997, pp 19–47.

CURRENT CONTROVERSIES: ELECTRONIC FHR MONITORING

Does electronic FHR monitoring improve fetal neurologic outcome?

Electronic FHR monitoring is currently the cornerstone of fetal assessment throughout the antepartum period. It is routinely used to diagnose acute and chronic fetal stress in an effort to reduce fetal morbidity. Rosen and Diskensen (1993) reviewed a decade of literature and found that electronic FHR monitoring had limited sensitivity in identifying and predicting the absence of fetal neurologic morbidity. No monitoring abnormalities were found in a significant number of neonates with poor neurologic outcome, and fetal monitoring did not lead to treatment that significantly impacted neonatal morbidity. Despite these findings, obstetricians routinely use FHR monitoring in conjunction with other modalities to evaluate fetal well-being.

Fetal Scalp Sampling

Fetal scalp sampling may be indicated to further evaluate a fetus with an abnormal FHR tracing. Based on its results, the diagnosis of suspected fetal hypoxia may be confirmed, establishing the need for urgent delivery.

A small sample of fetal blood is obtained and analyzed for pH, PO_2, PCO_2, HCO_3, and base excess. Fetal membranes must be ruptured to allow the obstetrician to make a small incision in the fetal presenting part (i.e., scalp or buttock) and collect fetal blood in a small capillary tube. The values obtained will vary, depending upon the stage of labor, sampling during a contraction, and the presence of maternal acidosis. During contractions, placental blood flow is compromised. The fetus is periodically exposed to episodes of relative hypoxia and impaired placental gas exchange. As labor progresses, fetal pH and PO_2 normally decrease, and PCO_2 normally increases. Decreased fetal pH occurs as a late sign of hypoxia.

Normal values for fetal blood scalp sampling may be found in Table 5-4. If acidosis is present, it is important to determine whether the acidosis is respiratory or metabolic in nature. Respiratory acidosis should improve with standard resuscitation. Fetal metabolic acidosis requires immediate delivery. Good fetal outcomes are associated with a pH >7.20, while a pH <7.20 suggests fetal compromise necessitating immediate delivery. A fetal pH in the 7.20 to 7.25 range may require re-evaluation within 30 minutes to confirm fetal well-being.

Umbilical Cord pH

Umbilical cord blood pH and gas measurements are routinely performed at birth throughout the United

States. For the most part, the values obtained correlate with fetal scalp samples obtained shortly before birth. Umbilical cord blood pH values may be used to evaluate whether low Apgar scores were the result of fetal hypoxia or if poor outcome was caused by another factor.

Fetal Pulse Oximetry

Fetal pulse oximetry has emerged as a newer technique to evaluate intrapartum fetal oxygenation. Currently, it remains an adjunct to electronic FHR monitoring. The fetal pulse oximeter (FPO) is currently being used when the electronic FHR monitor shows a nonreassuring tracing or if the tracing is unreliable (i.e., fetal arrhythmia).

Basically, the obstetrician places the FPO sensor through the cervix so that it lies alongside the fetal cheek or temple. Operator placement skill is important to ensure an accurate saturation reading. Membranes must be ruptured for adequate placement. The FPO provides continuous fetal arterial oxygen saturation readings on a beat-to-beat basis.

When compared with the adult, the fetus has fetal hemoglobin and lower oxygen saturation. Fetal O_2 saturation between 30% and 70% is considered normal. Saturation readings consistently <30% for a prolonged period of time (10 to 15 min) are suggestive of fetal acidemia. Fetal blood scalp sampling and/or prompt obstetric intervention may be indicated.

Fetal pulse oximetry was introduced with the hope that it would complement electronic fetal monitoring (given its limitations in predicting fetal compromise) with the goal of preventing unnecessary cesarean deliveries. A randomized study performed over 2 years involving 1011 laboring women with nonreassuring EFM tracings found >50% reduction in cesarean deliveries performed (on patients monitored by EFM and FPO) because of nonreassuring fetal status. However, the overall cesarean delivery rate (secondary to all causes) was not reduced because of an increase in the amount of cesarean deliveries performed because of dystocia. Overall section rate, therefore, was not changed by use of the FPO.

As of September 2001, the American College of Obstetrics and Gynecology failed to endorse the use of the FPO in clinical practice. Concerns regarding escalation in medical care costs outweighing improvement in clinical outcome were expressed. Currently, studies that address cost effectiveness are not conclusive. A randomized clinical trial involving 10,000 women with the goal of measuring the effect of FPO as an adjunct to EFM on overall cesarean delivery rate is being initiated.

A study by Luttkus et al.[1] calls into question the diagnostic power and technology precision of the FPO. One hundred seventy (170) fetuses with nonreassuring FHR tracings were evaluated. Fetal blood samples (blood gas analysis and lactate analysis) and distribution and duration of desaturation periods to <30% were compared for those fetuses defined as being academic. The authors found an overestimation of FPO in the low range of saturation values and an underestimation of FPO values in the higher ranges of saturation. Thus, the authors conclude, the advantage of FPO is limited by its diagnostic power and technology precision.

In a separate study, the same authors[2] suggest that simultaneous monitoring with a combination of fetal ECG and FPO is feasible and reliable in indicating signs of intermittent hypoxia. They suggest that development of technology combining these two modalities of fetal monitoring may be encouraged as a result of their findings.

Recently, Nellcor Perinatal (manufacturer of the FPO) addressed obstetricians regarding 13 case reports in which parturients with an ominous FHR tracing, but a FPO reading >30%, had poor neonatal outcomes. In this communication, the manufacturer recommends delivery of the fetus in the presence of an ominous tracing, even if FPO values are normal. Thus, the accuracy of fetal pulse oximetry may be inadequate in the diagnosis of fetal acidemia, when the FHR tracing suggests an ominous pattern.

Fetal Electrocardiogram Monitoring

Fetal ECG monitoring may also be used as an adjunct to EFM. Fetal hypoxemia during labor can alter the shape of the fetal ECG. Changes may be seen in the relation of the PR to RR intervals, and ST segment elevation or depression may occur. A recent review of trial data involving 8357 women supports the restricted use of fetal ST segment analysis in those fetuses displaying a nonreassuring electronic FHR tracing to improve fetal outcome. The major disadvantage of fetal ECG monitoring is that it requires an internal scalp electrode.

A new fetal monitoring system, the STAN method, combines electronic FHR monitoring and fetal ST analysis. Recent Swedish multicenter randomized controlled trials involving 6826 women showed improvement in perinatal outcome when using combined intrapartum cardiotocography (CTG) with fetal ST segment wave form analysis compared with CTG alone. This new monitoring methodology may reduce fetal exposure to intrapartum hypoxia and decrease the number of operative deliveries for fetal distress. The most important finding of this randomized controlled trial is a significant reduction in fetal metabolic acidosis at birth (0.7%) in the fetuses monitored with both CTG and ST analysis compared with CTG alone (1.5%). At this time, 10 major European university clinics use the STAN method of fetal monitoring.

Ultrasound

The ultrasound scan is a basic essential obstetric tool throughout pregnancy, labor, and delivery. Intrapartum fetal ultrasonographic assessment often guides clinical management and is a useful adjunct to electronic FHR monitoring.

Ultrasound examination may be useful in the accurate determination of fetal head position when digital examination is difficult or uncertain (i.e., caput, molding, asynclitism, excessive scalp hair). If instrumental vaginal delivery is considered, it is essential that the obstetrician know the accurate fetal head position to avoid trauma. Should fetal position in the laboring patient come into question, ultrasound examination is important if vaginal delivery is contraindicated.

During the intrapartum period, ultrasound scanning may be useful in confirming suspected diagnoses. If fetal heart tones are undetectable using a Doppler device, ultrasound may confirm intrauterine fetal health or demise. Premature (23 to 28 weeks gestation) fetal position may be confirmed in the laboring obese patient. Intrauterine growth restriction can be recognized in the premature fetus. Quantity of amniotic fluid may be determined. Undiagnosed breech presentation may be confirmed. Fetal positions in multifetal gestations can be elucidated. Placental abnormalities may be recognized. The diagnosis of significant acute placental abruption accompanied by fetal distress is crucial to fetal survival. Placenta previa may initially present in the laboring patient with vaginal bleeding. Adherent placental tissue (accreta, increta, percreta) as well as an anterior low-lying placenta may also be recognized by ultrasound. Ultrasound guidance may also be used in the patient with postpartum uterine atony/retained placenta, to locate and aid in the evacuation of retained products of conception.

NEWBORN EVALUATION—THE APGAR SCORE

Immediate evaluation of the neonate is essential to both ensure newborn well-being and/or diagnose any problems, which may result in increased morbidity and mortality. In addition, the newborn's condition should be quickly assessed to determine whether immediate resuscitation is necessary.

Currently, the universally accepted scoring system used to evaluate newborn well-being is the Apgar score (Table 5-5). This scoring system is simple and repro-

Table 5-5   The Apgar Score

	0	1	2
Heart rate	Absent	<100 bpm	>100 bpm
Respirations	Absent	Irregular, shallow	Good, crying
Reflex irritability	No response	Grimace	Cough, sneeze
Muscle tone	Flaccid	Good tone	Spontaneous flexed arms/legs
Color	Blue, pale	Body pink, extremities blue	Entirely pink

From Chantigan RC: Neonatal Evaluation. In Ostheimer GW (ed): Manual of Obstetric Anesthesia. New York: Churchill Livingstone, 1992, p 49.

ducible and addresses five vital parameters: heart rate, respiratory effort, muscle tone, reflex irritability, and color. Each physiologic variable is assigned a numeric score ranging from 0 to 2. This score reliably identifies infants who are depressed and require resuscitation. Scoring of each parameter occurs at 1 and 5 minutes of life (following an infant's progress over time).

Heart rate and respiratory effort are the most important physiologic parameters in identifying a compromised neonate. Neonatal heart rate should be >100 bpm at birth. Usually, heart rate is determined by auscultation, palpation of the umbilical cord stump, or observation of the precordium. A heart rate <100 bpm may reflect hypoxia. Reflex bradycardia may occur with pharyngeal suctioning. Uncommonly, congenital heart block may cause bradycardia.

Quality of respiratory effort is evaluated rather than respiratory rate *per se*. A good strong cry receives a score of 2, whereas an absent cry is assigned a score of 0. Poor respiratory effort may require immediate mask ventilation and intubation with 100% oxygen administration. If poor O_2 saturation persists, anatomic causes (e.g., pulmonary hypoplasia) may be present.

Muscle tone is evaluated by observation. A newborn with vigorous movement and whose extremities are flexed and resistant to extension receives a score of 2. A score of 0 is assigned if the neonate is flaccid. Drugs given to pregnant women, such as magnesium sulfate, may cause decreased muscle tone in the neonate at birth.

Reflex irritability is evaluated by vigorous stimulation of the newborn. Common methods include flicking the soles of the feet, nasal catheter insertion, or vigorous rubbing of the newborn's body. If no response is elicited, a score of 0 is assigned. If the newborn sneezes or cries, a score of 2 is assigned.

Newborns are normally cyanotic at birth. Prompt resolution of this cyanosis occurs with normal ventilation and adequate perfusion. A cold delivery room environment can cause peripheral vasoconstriction, resulting in cyanotic extremities. A pink newborn receives a score of 2 for color, whereas a persistently cyanotic child receives a score of 0. Hypovolemia and hypotension may result in a pale-appearing newborn. If a newborn remains cyanotic despite adequate respirations and administration of 100% oxygen, acidosis and pulmonary vasoconstriction may be present. Other causes may include hypoplastic lungs or congenital heart disease.

The Apgar score quickly, reliably, and easily identifies newborns who require resuscitation and thereby aims to reduce perinatal morbidity and mortality. This score also has prognostic significance in terms of neonatal mortality. If a neonate shows progressive improvement in Apgar score, this evaluation should continue through every 5 minutes until a score of 7 is obtained.

Generally speaking, the 1-minute score relates to the degree of neonatal depression and need for resuscitation. Infants with scores >8 at 1 minute usually do not require ventilatory assistance. Infants scoring 3 to 7 are mild to moderately depressed and usually respond quickly to mask ventilation with 100% oxygen. Severely depressed infants (score 0 to 2) usually require aggressive resuscitation, including endotracheal intubation and cardiac massage. Mortality within the first month of life is, generally speaking, inversely related to both 1- and 5-minute Apgar scores and increases in low-birth-weight infants. In addition, Apgar scores correlate with neurologic morbidity. The incidence of neurologically abnormal infants varies inversely with both 1- and 5-minute Apgar scores. Low birth weight is also an extremely significant factor, increasing the incidence of neurologic abnormalities sixfold in infants weighing <2000 grams.

FETAL RESPIRATORY AND CIRCULATORY CHANGES AT BIRTH

Understanding the respiratory and circulatory changes that occur at birth underlies effective resuscitation of the newborn. Fewer than 10% of newborns require active resuscitation to establish adequate respiration, heart rate, color, and tone. Yearly, over one million neonatal deaths are due to neonatal asphyxia. Implementation of basic resuscitative techniques may be the cornerstone to improving neonatal outcome.

Normally, the fetal lung is filled with an ultrafiltrate of plasma produced by the lungs in utero. Most reabsorption of this fluid takes place with the onset of contractions and throughout the process of labor and delivery. During the second stage of labor, squeezing of the thorax in its transit through the vaginal canal pushes approximately two-thirds of the remaining pulmonary fluid out of the lungs. Newborn capillaries and lymphatics remove the remainder of this fluid after birth. Newborns delivered by cesarean section do not always benefit from the aforementioned process and may have more difficulty establishing normal ventilation. Following delivery of the thorax, normal infants take their first breath within a few seconds. This is partially due to normal elastic recoil of the lungs following birth. Up to 80 mL of air is inspired with the first breath as a negative pressure of 60 to 100 cm H_2O is generated. A normal term neonate has a tidal volume of 5 to 7 mL/kg and a respiratory rate of 30 to 60 breaths/min. Rhythmic ventilation is normally established approximately 90 seconds after birth and depends upon peripheral chemoreceptors, which normally respond to low PO_2 and low pH.

A comprehensive description of normal fetal circulation is beyond the scope of this chapter. At birth, fetal systemic vascular resistance increases, left atrial pressure increases, and foramen ovale flow decreases as the umbilical cord is clamped and the low-resistance placenta is removed from the fetal systemic circulation. Simultaneously, pulmonary vascular resistance decreases as the first breaths are taken. As a result, pulmonary perfusion is instituted as >90% of the right ventricular output perfuses the lungs. Physiologic closure of the foramen ovale occurs with pulmonary venous return into the left atrium. Until the foramen ovale is anatomically closed (several months after birth), any condition increasing right atrial pressure may open the foramen ovale, causing a right-to-left shunt and cyanosis. With normal oxygenation and ventilation, arterial oxygen tension and pH increase, the pulmonary vasculature dilates further, and pulmonary vascular resistance decreases. The right-to-left shunt through the ductus arteriosus ceases.

Both the pulmonary and circulatory changes that normally occur at birth do so spontaneously, as an adaptation for extrauterine survival. Failure of these physiologic adaptations to occur may impede neonatal resuscitative efforts.

Neonatal Resuscitation

The ultimate goal of neonatal resuscitation is to reduce perinatal morbidity and mortality. Both acute and chronic fetal asphyxia may result in cognitive impairment, developmental delay, organ failure, cardiomyopathy, bone marrow depression, and/or ischemic encephalopathy (cerebral palsy). Prompt evaluation and appropriate resuscitation are the cornerstone of newborn well-being.

Newborn resuscitation may be categorized into four basic steps: rapid assessment/evaluation, establishment of ventilation (via mask or endotracheal tube), chest compressions, and fluid/medication administration.

Rapid assessment of the newborn includes the evaluation of breathing, color, heart rate, muscle tone, the presence of meconium staining, and a classification of gestational age. Routine care, including drying, warming, and airway clearing, may be the only necessary intervention if the newborn's assessment is normal. Some newborns may require physical stimulation to improve ventilation (back rubbing, flicking of the feet) and/or oxygen administration. Most newborns only require the preceding interventions.

BASIC NEWBORN CARE

Basic routine newborn care is essential to newborn well-being. Hypothermia increases oxygen consumption and may thereby make effective resuscitation more difficult. Hypothermia is associated with respiratory depression. To maintain normothermia, newborns should be delivered in a warm area and placed under a radiant warmer. Thoroughly drying the skin and wrapping the newborn in warm blankets helps prevent heat loss. Newborns should be placed in a supine or lateral position with the neck slightly extended to facilitate ventilation. Secretions should be suctioned to avoid airway obstruction. An 8 Fr or 10 Fr suction catheter should be used to clear secretions from the mouth and then the nose. Care should be taken to avoid both deep suctioning (this may cause laryngospasm and/or vagal stimulation/ bradycardia) and prolonged suctioning. Negative pressure should not exceed 100 mm Hg. Meconium staining of the amniotic fluid requires intrapartum suctioning of the fetal nose, mouth, and posterior pharynx prior to delivery of the body. This can be accomplished with a bulb syringe or a large suction catheter (12 Fr to 14 Fr) and prevents meconium aspiration (in a passive manner or as the newborn initiates spontaneous respirations). *In utero* meconium aspiration occurs in up to 30% of meconium-stained newborns. Tracheal suctioning should only be performed in those newborns who are depressed (inadequate respirations, depressed muscle tone or bradycardia). Direct laryngoscopy should be immediately performed prior to the initiation of spontaneous respirations. Any residual meconium directly visualized from the hypopharynx should be suctioned and intubation performed. Further suctioning via the endotrachial tube (ETT) should be accomplished as the ETT is withdrawn from the airway. This process should be repeated as necessary until little meconium is suctioned. Should bradycardia persist or respirations remain depressed, positive pressure ventilation may become necessary despite the presence of meconium. It is important that the newborn receive tracheal suctioning prior to positive pressure ventilation, as this may cause meconium to travel down the respiratory tree.

Subsequent evaluation of respiratory effort, heart rate, and color may indicate that further resuscitative efforts are necessary. Establishment of adequate ventilation is the most important resuscitative maneuver. At birth, regular respirations normally improve color, and heart rate remains >100 bpm. Free-flow oxygen may be delivered. Assisted ventilation (via bag or mask) is indicated if gasping or apnea is present. Positive pressure ventilation is also indicated if the heart rate remains <100 bpm or if central cyanosis persists despite 100% oxygen administration. In newborns, inflation pressures of 30 to 40 cm H_2O (or higher) may be necessary to establish visible expansion of the chest. Assisted ventilation should be delivered at a rate of 40 to 60 breaths/min (30 breaths/min if chest compressions are being delivered). Administration of 100% oxygen is indicated to achieve normoxia (pink mucous membranes and a normal oxygen saturation). Adequate ventilation is established when bilateral chest expansion, breath sounds, and improvement in heart rate and oxygen saturation are observed. Causes of inadequate ventilation include poor mask seal, airway obstruction, and abnormal pulmonary anatomy (e.g., pulmonary hypoplasia, diaphragmatic hernia). Gastric distention with prolonged mask ventilation may occur and compromise ventilation, at which point decompression with an 8 Fr orogastric tube may be indicated. Assisted ventilation with 100% oxygen should continue if inadequate respirations or bradycardia persist. If the heart rate is below 60 bpm, chest compression should be initiated and endotracheal intubation performed. Traditionally, 100% oxygen has been utilized to correct hypoxia. Currently, preliminary evidence suggests that lower oxygen concentrations may be utilized. However, the evidence currently available does not justify adopting this measure in a routine manner.

Resuscitative Equipment

The equipment used in newborn resuscitation must be of appropriate size for successful intervention. Ventilation bags for neonatal resuscitation are either self inflating or flow inflating and should be no larger than 750 mL. The tidal volume delivered with each breath is small (5 to 8 mL/kg). Face masks should seal around the mouth and nose and not cover the eyes or overlap the chin. The mask should have a low dead space and preferably have a cushioned rim to avoid excess pressure on the face, while maintaining a good seal. At this time, the laryngeal mask airway may be used in the full-term neonate when bag-mask ventilation is ineffective and endotracheal intubation has failed. There are no studies supporting its use in the presence of meconium, and its use in small preterm neonates has not been adequately studied.

For intubation, a laryngoscope with a straight blade (size 0 for premature newborns, size 1 for infants) is used. The tip of the laryngoscope is inserted into the vallecula or under the epiglottis, and gentle elevation (with or without cricoid) should bring the vocal cords into view. The ETT should be of appropriate size and depth to result in adequate ventilation. ETT position should be confirmed by checking for breath sounds bilaterally over the chest and over the stomach. A CO_2 detector may be used if clinical assessment is not definitive. If a stylet is used, it should not extend beyond the tip of the ETT.

Improvement in the color, heart rate, and activity of the newborn is reassuring. Neonatal weight and gestational age determine the ETT size and depth of ETT insertion. Alternatively, depth of ETT insertion can be calculated by the following formula: weight (kg) + 6 cm = insertion depth at lip in centimeters (Table 5-6).

Chest Compressions

Chest compressions may be needed during resuscitation of the newborn. In general, vital signs will be restored, in most neonates, once adequate oxygenation and ventilation are established. Persistent hypoxia may result in generalized vasoconstriction and poor tissue perfusion and oxygenation. This may lead to acidosis, decreased myocardial contractility, bradycardia, and asystole. Currently, the indication for initiating chest compressions, in most cases, is a heart rate of <60 bpm for 30 seconds, in the presence of adequate ventilation. Oxygenation and ventilation always takes priority in the resuscitation of a neonate. This should always be considered when tempted to start chest compressions, as they may decrease the effectiveness of ventilation.

There are two acceptable techniques for the delivery of chest compressions. The preferred technique is the two thumb-encircling hands technique. Two thumbs are placed on the lower one third of the sternum. They may be superimposed or adjacent to one another. The health care provider's other fingers should circle the chest on their respective sides and support the newborn's back. Most providers prefer this technique, as it appears to promote coronary perfusion and peak systolic pressures. In large newborns, the use of this technique may be limited. Another technique used to deliver chest compressions in neonates is the two-finger technique. Two fingers from one hand are placed at a right angle to the lower one third of the sternum. The provider's other hand supports the child's back. With respect to depth of compression, the current recommendation is to compress the sternum to one third the anterior-posterior diameter of the chest. In so doing, a palpable pulse should be generated. If no pulse is appreciated, further compressions, up to one half the diameter of the chest may be delivered. Producing a palpable pulse is the goal of chest compression delivery. Compressions should be delivered smoothly and at a specific rate. The relaxation phase should be slightly longer than the compression phase so as to permit maximum blood flow throughout the body.

Chest compressions to ventilations should be delivered in a 3:1 ratio. Thus, 90 chest compressions and 30 breaths are delivered per minute. Each three compression cycle should be followed by one breath. Heart rate should be assessed every 30 seconds (i.e., carotid artery pulse, umbilical cord pulse, brachial artery pulse). Discontinuation of chest compressions should occur once the spontaneous heart rate is >60 bpm.

Medications

Medications are infrequently indicated during neonatal resuscitation. Generally speaking, the establishment and provision of adequate oxygenation and ventilation correct bradycardia in the newborn. Pharmacologic therapy is indicated for a spontaneous heart rate <60 bpm despite adequate oxygenation/ventilation and chest compressions.

Epinephrine is indicated when the spontaneous heart rate is <60 bpm for 30 seconds, despite adequate ventilation and chest compressions and in the presence of a systole. α-adrenergic effects include vasoconstriction, which increases perfusion pressure during chest compression. Thus, oxygen delivery to the heart and brain is improved. β-adrenergic stimulation results in enhanced

Table 5-6	Neonatal Weight, Gestational Age, ETT Size, and Depth of ETT Insertion		
Weight (g)	Gestational age, (weeks)	ETT size, mm (ID)	Depth of insertion from upper lip (cm)
<1000	<25	2.5	6.5 to 7
1000 to 2000	26 to 34	3.0	7 to 8
2000 to 3000	34 to 38	3.5	8 to 9
>3000	>38	3.5 to 4.0	10

ID, Internal diameter.

cardiac contractility and an increase in heart rate. Spontaneous contractions of the heart may be induced. Delivery of epinephrine may take place intravenously or via the endotracheal tube. Currently, a dose of 0.01 to 0.03 mg/kg (0.01 to 0.03 mL/kg of a 1:10,000 solution) every 3 to 5 minutes is recommended. Higher doses may result in hypertension, decreased cardiac output and intracranial hemorrhage.

Volume expanders may be indicated in the neonate who is hypovolemic or is not responding to resuscitation. Hypovolemia may be due to blood loss or shock (i.e., pale, weak pulse). Isotonic crystalloid solutions, such as normal saline or Ringer's lactate, are the fluids of choice for volume expansion. If large volume blood loss has occurred, O-negative red blood cells may be the volume expander of choice (remember total blood volume is approximately 90 mL/kg in neonates). Initial volume expansion is rarely accomplished with albumin-containing solutions, due to their potential for transmitting infectious disease and their association with increased mortality in this patient population. The initial volume expander dose is 10 mL/kg given intravenously, and slowly, over 5 to 10 minutes. Before repeating this dose, the clinical response to the first dose should be noted. Inappropriate volume expansion in the hypoxic or preterm neonate may cause volume overload or intracranial hemorrhage.

Naloxone hydrochloride is a narcotic antagonist indicated to reverse neonatal respiratory depression within 4 hours of delivery, secondary to maternal narcotic administration. Prior to naloxone administration, adequate ventilation should be established, as narcotic duration may exceed that of naloxone. Repeated doses may be needed to prevent recurrent episodes of respiratory depression. Care should be taken not to administer naloxone to a neonate whose mother may have recently abused narcotics, as neonatal withdrawal symptoms may occur. Currently, the recommended dose is 0.1 mg/kg of a 0.4 mg/mL or 1.0 mg/mL solution. It may be administered intravenously or endotracheally. Intramuscular or subcutaneous administration is acceptable if perfusion is adequate.

Routine use of bicarbonate in neonatal resuscitation is not currently recommended. Its use during brief CPR is discouraged. Bicarbonate's hyperosmolarity and its potential to generate CO_2 may be detrimental to cardiac and cerebral function. Bicarbonate may be used after initial CPR to correct documented persistent metabolic acidosis and hyperkalemia. After adequate ventilation is established, a dose of 1 to 2 mEq/kg (of a 0.5 mEq/L solution) may be given slowly (over a 2-minute period) via the intravenous route.

Medication Administration Routes

During resuscitation, the tracheal route is usually most accessible. Epinephrine and naloxone may be given via ETT. Sodium bicarbonate is caustic and should not be given intratracheally. Administration of medication via the ETT results in a more variable systemic response than drugs given intravenously.

Intravenous access in the newborn may be established through the umbilical vein or a scalp or peripheral vein. The most accessible vein is the umbilical vein. A 3.5 Fr or 5 Fr radiopaque catheter is inserted so that its tip is at the level of the skin. Catheter aspiration should result in blood return. Epinephrine, naloxone, volume expanders, and bicarbonate may be given by this route. Care should be taken not to permit the introduction of air into the catheter, as a venous air embolism may result. Peripheral or scalp veins may be difficult to cannulate in the newborn, thus delaying emergency drug administration. Intraosseous lines are rarely used for resuscitative purposes. They can, however, be used for medications and volume expanders if other routes of access are not available.

Withholding Resuscitation

The question of whether to resuscitate an extremely premature neonate or a neonate with severe congenital anomalies may be a difficult one. Withholding resuscitation for neonates of <23 weeks gestational age or who weigh <400 g is generally regarded as being appropriate. In addition, it is appropriate to withhold resuscitation in neonates in which anencephaly and trisomy 13 or 18 are confirmed. Resuscitation of newborns with these conditions is unlikely to increase chance of survival or may result in survival of a neonate with severe disabilities. If antenatal information or confirmation of the preceding is incomplete or questionable, a trial of resuscitation should be undertaken. It can be discontinued once further neonatal evaluation has taken place. Once resuscitation has been initiated, its continuation is not mandatory. The neonate should be continuously evaluated, and a discussion with the parents should take place with regard to these decisions. If time allows, neonatal evaluation and parental participation in decision making may occur prior to birth.

Termination of Resuscitation

Appropriate termination of resuscitation occurs if there is no spontaneous return of circulation within 15 minutes after cardiopulmonary arrest and resuscitation. After 10 minutes of asystole, survival without severe disability is very unlikely.

INDEX 5-1: Recommendations of the National Institute of Child Health and Human Development Research Planning Workshop for Standardizing FHR Tracing Definitions (1997)

Baseline FHR: Mean FHR rounded to increments of 5 bpm during a 10-minute segment (excluding periodic changes, episodes of marked FHR variability)

    bradycardia: FHR < 110 bpm
    tachycardia: FHR > 160 bpm

Baseline FHR Variability: No distinction between short- and long-term variability.

- FHR baseline fluctuations of ≥ 2 cycles/minute, irregular in amplitude and frequency
- Absent FHR variability: Undetectable amplitude range
- Minimal FHR variability: > Undetectable amplitude range: amplitude range ≤ 5 bpm
- Moderate FHR variability: amplitude range 6 to 25 bpm
- Marked FHR variability: amplitude range > 25 bpm

Acceleration: Sudden increase (onset to peak in <30 seconds) in FHR above baseline. FHR baseline change occurs if an acceleration lasting ≥10 minutes is present.

Early Deceleration: Visually observed gradual decrease (onset of deceleration to nadir ≥ 30 sec) in FHR with a return to baseline occurring with a uterine contraction. The nadir of the deceleration coincides with the peak of the contraction.

Variable Deceleration: Visually noted sudden decrease (onset of deceleration to beginning of nadir < 30 seconds) in FHR below baseline. FHR decrease ≥ 15 beats/minute below baseline and < 2 minutes from its onset to return to baseline.

Late Deceleration: Visually noted gradual decrease and return to FHR baseline occurring with a uterine contraction. Respectively, the onset, nadir, and recovery of the deceleration occur after the beginning, peak, and ending of a contraction, in most cases.

Prolonged Deceleration: Visually noted FHR decrease below the baseline of ≥15 bpm lasting ≥2 minutes but is <10 minutes from onset to baseline return.

Quantification: All decelerations should be quantified based on the depth of the nadir (bpm) below baseline and duration (min, sec) from the beginning to the end of the deceleration. Likewise, accelerations should also be quantified.

From the National Institute of Child Health and Human Development Research Planning Workshop: Electronic fetal heart rate monitoring: Research guidelines for interpretation. Am J Obstet Gynecol 177:1385-1390, 1997.

REFERENCES

1. Luttkus AK, Callisen TA, Stupin JH, Dudenhausen JW: Pulse oximetry during labour—does it give rise to hope? Value of saturation monitoring in comparison to fetal blood gas status. Eur J Obstet Gynecol Reprod Biol 22:110-111, 2003.

2. Luttkus AK, Stupin JH, Callsen TA, Dudenhausen JW: Feasibility of simultaneous application of fetal electrocardiography and fetal pulse oximetry. Acta Obstet Gynecol Scand 82:443-448, 2003.

SUGGESTED READING

Dildy GA: A guest editorial: Fetal pulse oximetry. Obstet Gynecol Survey 58(4):225-226, 2003.

East CE, Colditz PB, Begg LM, Brennecke SP: Update on intrapartum fetal pulse oximetry. Aust NZ J Obstet Gynaecol 42(2):119-124, 2002.

Garite T, Nageotte M, Porreco R, Boehm F: Fetal pulse oximetry. Obstet Gynecol 99(3):514-515, 2002.

Ibrahimy MI, Mohd Ali MA, Zahedi E, Tsuruoka S: A comparison of abdominal ECG and Doppler ultrasound for fetal heart rate deceleration. Front Med Biol Eng 11(4):307-322, 2002.

Kattwinkel J, Van Reempts P, Nadkarni V, et al: International guidelines for neonatal resuscitation: An excerpt from the guidelines 2000 for cardiopulmonary resuscitation and emergency cardiovascular care: International consensus on science. Pediatrics 106(3):e29, 2000.

Kilpatrick S, Laros Jr. RK: Fetal Evaluation: Routine and Indicated Tests. In Hughes SC, Levinson G, Rosen MA (eds): Shnider and Levinson's Anesthesia for Obstetrics, Fourth edition. Philadelphia, Lippincott, Williams and Wilkins, 2002, pp 613-622.

Kryc JJ: Evaluation of the Pregnant Patient: Preoperative Concerns. In Dewan DM, Hood DD (eds): Practical Obstetric Anesthesia. Philadelphia, W.B. Saunders, 1997, pp 19-47.

Leszcynska-Gorzelak B, Poniedzialek-Czajkowska E, Oleszczuk J: Fetal blood saturation during the 1st and 2nd stage of labor and its relation to the neonatal outcome. Gynecol Obstet Invest 54(3):159-163, 2002.

Levinson G, Hughes SC, Rosen MA: Evaluation of the neonate. In Hughes SC, Levinson G, Rosen MA (eds): Shnider and Levinson's Anesthesia for Obstetrics, Fourth edition. Philadelphia, Lippincott, Williams and Wilkins, 2002, pp 657-670.

Lockwood CJ: Fetal pulse oximetry. Obstet Gynecol 99(3): 515-516, 2002.

Luttkus AK, Lubke M, Buscher V, et al: Accuracy of fetal pulse oximetry. Acta Obstet Gynecol Scand 81(5):417-423, 2002.

Neilson JP: Fetal electrocardiogram (ECG) for fetal monitoring during labor. Cochrane Database Syst Rev 2:CD000116, 2003.

Olofsson P: Current status of intrapartum fetal monitoring: Cardiotocography versus cardiotocography and ST analysis of the fetal ECG. Eur J Obstet Gynecol Reprod Biol 110(1): 5113-5118, 2003.

Parer JT, King TL: Electronic Fetal Monitoring and Diagnosis of Fetal Asphyxia. In Hughes SC, Levinson G, Rosen MA (eds): Shnider and Levinson's Anesthesia for Obstetrics, Fourth edition. Philadelphia, Lippincott, Williams and Wilkins, 2002, pp 623-638.

Sniderman SH, Levinson G, Gregory GA: Resuscitation of the Newborn. In Hughes SC, Levinson G, Rosen MA, (eds): Shnider and Levinson's Anesthesia for Obstetrics, Fourth edition. Philadelphia, Lippincott, Williams and Wilkins, 2002, pp 657-670.

Ugwumadu A: The role of ultrasound scanning on the labor ward. Ultrasound Obstet Gynecol 19:222-224, 2002.

Vitoratos N, Salamalekis E, Saloum J, et al: Abnormal fetal heart rate patterns during the active phase of labor: The value of fetal oxygen saturation. J Matern Fetal Neonatal Med 11(1):46-49, 2002.

Williams KP, Galerneau F: Intrapartum fetal heart rate patterns in the prediction of neonatal academia. Am J Obstet Gynecol 188(3):820-823, 2003.

Anesthesia for Cesarean Delivery

JASON SCOTT

PAMELA FLOOD

The developments of asepsis and anesthesia in the nineteenth century paved the way for the introduction of cesarean delivery. The name "cesarean" is probably derived, not from Julius Caesar, but from the Latin *caedere*, to cut. The Roman law Lex Caesare stated that a woman who died in late pregnancy should be delivered soon after her death, and if the baby died they should be buried separately.

The first cesarean delivery of modern times is attributed to a Swiss sow gelder, Jacob Nufer, who in the year 1500 gained permission from the authorities to operate on his wife after she had been in labor for several days. She subsequently had five successful vaginal deliveries, leading some to doubt the authenticity of the story.

After Nufer, the first cesarean deliveries with survival of the mother were performed in Ireland by Mary Donally in 1738; in England by Dr. James Barlow in 1793; and in America by Dr. John Richmond in 1827. The "first" in the British Empire outside the British Isles was performed in South Africa before 1821 by James Miranda Barry (an Edinburgh graduate who masqueraded successfully as a man from 1809 until her death in 1865), though in fact cesarean deliveries had been performed in Africa by indigenous healers for many years.

All these operations, however, were performed without anesthesia. In the mid-nineteenth century, death rates remained high, and cesarean delivery was often combined with hysterectomy. In the 1880s, with the advent of the concept of asepsis, a more conservative operation was developed, and the "classical" operation—a vertical incision in the upper part of the uterus—became more frequently used. This incision does not heal well, however, and in 1906 the modern "lower segment" operation was introduced, which carries less risk of subsequent uterine rupture.

The evolution of anesthesia for this procedure was initially slow—ether and chloroform were the only two agents available until the addition of cyclopropane during the 1950s. Regional anesthesia was first available around 1900 but did not gain popularity until much later. Since 1960, physicians have gained a greater understanding of the physiology of pregnancy, the pharmacology of anesthetic drugs, and the attendant risks of anesthesia to the mother and fetus. Obstetricians have begun performing cesarean delivery more frequently to treat both maternal and fetal problems, and anesthesiologists have striven to produce improved anesthetic techniques that protect the mother and have the least possible effect on the child.

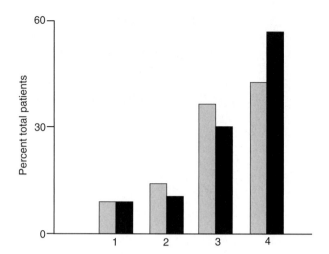

Figure 6-1   Distribution of Mallampati grades to show changes between 12 (shaded lines) and 38 (solid black) weeks gestation. The percentage of grade 4 cases is seen to increase at 38 weeks with corresponding reductions in the other three grades. (From Pilkington S, Carli F, Dakin M, et al: Increase in Mallampati score during pregnancy. Br J Anaesth 74(6):638–642, 1995.)

PREOPERATIVE ASSESSMENT

As for any patient undergoing anesthesia for surgery, a full medical and surgical history and examination of relevant systems is performed. Some assessment points unique to the parturient include the following:
- Guided obstetric and gynecologic history. The indication for cesarean delivery is important. Common indications are scarring from prior cesarean delivery, impression of cephalo-pelvic disproportion, dystocia, maternal medical problems that may be worsened by labor, abnormal presentation of the fetus, fetal intolerance of labor, and maternal hemorrhage (placenta previa, placental abruption). The urgency of the cesarean delivery might also influence the choice of anesthetic and other elements of patient care. Also important are the gravidity and parity of the mother, and, if the surgery is secondary, the type of previous caesarean delivery (lower segment/classic). The gestational age and anticipated medical problems of the fetus need to be considered to plan successful delivery and care of the neonate.
- Airway examination AT THE TIME of cesarean delivery (to include usual assessment—Mallampati score, thyromental distance, neck flexion, Wilson score). Exams done even days prior to the date of anesthesia can change (usually for the worse) during pregnancy—particularly in the presence of conditions associated with edema such as pre-eclampsia. The presence of large breasts should also be noted, as they make use of an ordinary laryngoscope difficult for intubation in the supine position (Fig. 6-1).

- Fasting state should be recorded as time of last food/clear fluids before the onset of labor, as the pain of contractions arrests gastric emptying, as do parenteral or neuraxial opioids. All pregnant women are treated as if they present an increased risk of aspiration (mechanical effect of uterus on stomach, decreased LES tone, increased acidity of stomach contents, and delayed gastric emptying); however, when possible it is best to minimize gastric volume. It was previously thought that pregnancy itself reduced gastric emptying. However, recent evidence from studies using the absorption of nonmetabolized substances suggests that stomach emptying in pregnancy may not be delayed and that residual gastric volume and acidity also remain unchanged. However, labor can decrease gastric transit time.

CHOICE OF ANESTHETIC TECHNIQUE

The increased risks during pregnancy of aspiration, and of encountering a "difficult airway" with potential inability to intubate and/or ventilate, have made regional anesthesia a more attractive option for most cesarean deliveries. Regional anesthesia for cesarean delivery has also become increasingly popular over the past decades, as more experience has been gained and initial fears that epidural and spinal anesthesia would negatively affect fetal well-being were allayed. Early studies in sheep suggested that sympathetic inhibition from regional anesthesia would impair uteroplacental perfusion independent of maternal hypotension. Studies conducted in the 1980s, however, demonstrated that if maternal blood pressure is maintained, regional anesthesia has no negative effects on fetal perfusion. Currently, the indication for cesarean delivery, the urgency, the medical conditions of both mother and fetus, and the mother's wishes, will all influence the choice of anesthetic technique.

For most elective or urgent cesarean deliveries in patients without an epidural in place, a spinal technique offers the best risk/benefit ratio. Blood loss at cesarean delivery may be less with a regional technique, though studies in support of this finding have been criticized for selection bias because patients in whom excessive blood loss is predicted are more likely to be selected for general anesthesia. However, the avoidance of volatile anesthetic agents will eliminate these agents as a cause of uterine atony postdelivery. Postoperative opioid requirements are lower in those who have received axial opioids than in patients who receive a general anesthetic. As a result, postoperative recovery is better with the mother more mobile the next day, and better able to breast-feed and care for her baby. Fewer postoperative complications are likely to develop, such as pyrexia and chest infections. There is also less depression in mothers both immediately postpartum and at 1 week. If there are indications that the surgery may be prolonged, a combined spinal-epidural (CSE) technique can be used for anesthesia. In patients with an epidural, the block can usually be used for cesarean delivery. Epidurals may also provide an advantage in minimizing maternal hypotension, or when trying to avoid motor blockade of the thoracic segments and intercostal muscles in patients with respiratory compromise, as the dose can be titrated to the desired sensory/motor level.

In cases of nonreassuring fetal assessment, the anesthesiologist and obstetrician must together weigh the severity of the fetal compromise against the maternal risks of general anesthesia. General anesthesia may be indicated for an emergency cesarean delivery. However, clinical studies have shown that fetal outcome is not affected by the decision to administer regional anesthesia in cases of moderate fetal distress. As such, in an emergency, the anesthesiologist must decide to proceed with general or regional anesthesia based on his or her assessment of the likely speed of administration of the anesthetic for each individual parturient.

In parturients with medical illness, the nature and severity of the comorbid condition will influence the choice of anesthesia. Patients with a coagulopathy are at increased risk for epidural hematoma after a regional technique.

Low platelets are associated with pre-eclampsia, HELLP syndrome, and other complications of pregnancy such as thrombotic thrombocytopenic purpura (TTP). Though controversial, most anesthesiologists consider a platelet count between 80 and 100×10^9/L as a cutoff below which a regional technique is contraindicated.

The American Society of Regional Anesthesia (ASRA) has produced guidelines regarding the administration of regional anesthesia in patients receiving anticoagulant prophylaxis or therapy (Fig. 6-2).

Anatomic abnormalities such as severe kyphoscoliosis (with or without Harrington rod fixation) and spina bifida may make regional anesthesia impossible or impractical. General anesthesia is usually considered best in cases of severe maternal hemorrhage when fluid repletion is not possible prior to induction. However, it is acceptable to use regional anesthesia in cases of placenta previa with no evidence of hypovolemia—recent studies do not support the idea that blood loss is increased in these cases when regional anesthesia is employed.

Local anesthesia in the form of abdominal field block, though not a first-line technique, may be useful in urgent cases when an anesthesiologist is unavailable. Local anesthesia may also be a useful adjunct in cases of incomplete or "patchy" spinal or epidural anesthesia.

PREOPERATIVE PREPARATION

Premedication

Surgical delivery, whether planned or unplanned, can be anxiety provoking for the parturient and her family. Sedative drugs are not usually required in the parturient about to undergo cesarean delivery, although this is a good setting for psychoprophylaxis. Verbal reassurance and education are usually sufficient to facilitate the anesthetic procedures. Benzodiazepines can cause amnesia, and most mothers wish to be able to remember the birth of their child. Small doses of a benzodiazepine, such as midazolam 0.5 to 2 mg intravenous, can be used to reduce maternal anxiety if nonpharmacologic methods are not sufficient. An opioid such as fentanyl 25 to 50 μg intravenous may also be used to expedite painful procedures if required. If an oral route is preferred, 5 mg of diazepam 1 to 2 hours prior to surgery is an effective anxiolytic. Small doses of these drugs are safe and will produce minimal fetal depression.

Occasionally, it may be appropriate to administer an anticholinergic drug to reduce secretions and/or prevent bradycardia induced by regional or general anesthesia. Glycopyrrolate does not cross the placenta to the same extent as atropine and is the anticholinergic agent of choice, although it should be noted that it retains the potential to reduce lower esophageal tone in the mother and thus theoretically increases the risk of aspiration. If regional anesthesia is used and the mother's airway reflexes are maintained, this should not be problematic.

Aspiration of gastric contents during general anesthesia has been a major cause of maternal morbidity and

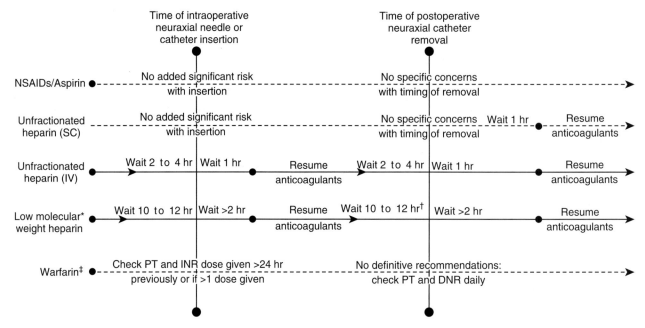

Figure 6-2 Timing of neuraxial manipulation and anticoagulation (based on the American Society of Regional Anesthesia's [ASRA] Neuraxial Anesthesia and Anticoagulation Consensus Statements. See complete guidelines [www.asra.com] for full details). *Based on prophylactic and not treatment doses. Delays of 24 hours rather than 10 to 12 hours are considered appropriate on bid dosing regimens. Consider delaying catheter removal for at least 24 hours after the last low-molecular weight heparin (LMWH) dose. †ASRA recommends that indwelling catheters be removed before initiation of LMWH prophylaxis. ‡Refers to patients receiving low-dose warfarin for perioperative thromboprophylaxis, not chronic oral anticoagulation. Hold warfarin for an international normalized ratio (INR) <3. Continue neurologic monitoring for 24 hours if INR < 1.5. (From Wu CL: Regional anesthesia and anticoagulation. J Clin Anesth 13:49-58, 2001.)

mortality. In 1986, a large Swedish study reported an aspiration incidence of one in 661 cases of general anesthesia for cesarean delivery, four times higher than the incidence for nonobstetric surgery. However, in the last triennial report on maternal death from the UK, there was only one case of aspiration, and this complication occurred in a woman with multiorgan failure in an intensive-care setting. Other western countries have seen a similar decline in morbidity and mortality from gastric aspiration. This success has been a result of the implementation of several measures including recognition of and preparation for difficult endotracheal intubation, NPO, nonparticulate-antacid preparation, and a reduction in the use of general anesthesia for cesarean delivery.

A good preanesthetic assessment identifies patients at greatest risk of difficult intubation and therefore aspiration. The most effective way to minimize the risk of aspiration is to use regional anesthesia and maintain a patent airway with intact reflexes. If regional anesthesia is contraindicated, awake fiber optic intubation should be considered in the patient with an anticipated difficult airway. Application of cricoid pressure and a rapid sequence induction and intubation with a cuffed endotracheal tube

should be performed when a difficult airway is not predicted. Gastric emptying with a nasogastric tube has been utilized before general anesthesia in the parturient who has had a recent meal and requires urgent surgery. It is, however, unpleasant for the patient and does not guarantee either an empty stomach or reduced gastric acidity.

Pharmacologic prophylaxis includes measures to increase gastric pH and decrease gastric volume. A total of 30 mL of 0.3 M sodium citrate will raise the gastric fluid pH above 2.5 for 1 to 2 hours when given 15 to 30 minutes prior to the induction of general anesthesia; however, there is no reduction in gastric volume. Nonparticulate antacids such as sodium citrate are preferred, as particulate antacid aspiration results in pulmonary damage similar to that caused by acid aspiration.

Histamine H_2-receptor antagonists, such as ranitidine, will significantly reduce gastric acid secretion, reducing pH and, to a lesser degree, gastric volume. They have no effect on the volume or acidity of the gastric contents already present. Ranitidine 150 mg administered orally will take 60 to 90 minutes to exert an effect and has duration of action of 6 to 8 hours. The recommended regimen is an oral dose at bedtime and in the morning for patients undergoing elective cesarean delivery. The intravenous administration of ranitidine 50 mg with oral administration of sodium citrate 30 mL resulted in a greater increase in gastric pH than when sodium citrate was used alone, providing 30 minutes had elapsed from the dose of ranitidine to intubation.

Oral omeprazole has been reported to be less effective in raising gastric pH than oral ranitidine or famotidine in patients for scheduled cesarean delivery. Ranitidine and omeprazole administered intravenously were found to be equally effective adjuncts to sodium citrate in reducing gastric acidity for emergency cesarean delivery.

Metoclopramide, a dopamine antagonist, promotes gastric emptying in the pregnant woman, even during labor; raises the lower esophageal tone; and has antiemetic properties. However, it may not affect the delayed gastric emptying associated with opioid administration or the use of anticholinergics. In cases in which urgent general anesthesia is planned, the administration of sodium citrate with intravenous metoclopramide and an H_2-receptor antagonist is highly recommended (Box 6-1).

Fluid Preload

Most patients are given a bolus of fluid before either regional or general anesthesia to ensure that the vasodilation induced by either technique does not result in undue maternal hypotension. Patients who have not been taking oral fluids due to fasting should receive an intravenous preload—those whose last fluid intake was the night before a scheduled cesarean delivery will be relatively dehydrated and should have their fluid deficit replaced. Glucose-containing crystalloid solutions should be avoided for use as bolus or resuscitative therapy. Apart from being less effective as volume expanders, a large glucose bolus can cause both maternal and fetal hyperglycemia and hyperinsulinemia. After delivery, the increased activity level in the infant utilizes the glucose; no additional glucose is being administered; and as the insulin has a longer half-life, the neonate is at risk of hypoglycemia in the second hour of life.

Box 6-1 Acid Aspiration Prophylaxis

30 mL 0.3 M sodium citrate 15 to 20 minutes prior to anesthetic
Ranitidine 150 mg PO 60 to 90 minutes prior to anesthetic or 50 mg IV 30 minutes prior to anesthetic or qhs and qam the night before/morning of scheduled surgery
Metoclopramide 10 mg IV 15 to 20 minutes prior to anesthetic

CURRENT CONTROVERSIES: FLUID PRELOADING

- 75% incidence of spinal hypotension after 1.5-L crystalloid
- Question larger volumes →↓ oncotic pressure →↑ pulmonary edema in susceptible patients
- Colloids: anaphylaxis risk, alter coagulation, expensive
- No effect on fetal outcome if hypotension treated promptly

Controversy exists regarding the necessity of administering a fluid "preload" prior to the administration of regional anesthesia. The widespread prophylactic use of crystalloid solution resulted from work in gravid ewes, demonstrating restoration of uterine blood flow after rapid intravenous fluid administration following spinal hypotension. Since then, there have been many clinical studies assessing the incidence of spinal hypotension after crystalloid preload, some indicating a benefit from preloading and others none. Recently Ueyama et al.[1] used the indocyanine green dilution method to measure blood volume and cardiac output as well as the incidence of spinal-induced hypotension following three different fluid preload regimens: 1.5-L lactated Ringers (LR), 0.5-L Hydroxyethylstarch solution (HES) 6%, and 1-L HES 6%. The incidence of spinal hypotension was 75%, 58%, and 17% respectively. The incidence of hypotension correlated inversely with the degree of volume expansion and increased cardiac output achieved using the different regimens. The authors concluded that "the augmentation of blood volume with preloading, regardless of the fluid used, must be large enough to result in a significant increase in cardiac output for effective prevention of hypotension." While colloid-based fluids are used extensively and efficiently for volume expansion, particularly outside of the United States, expense and alteration of blood rheology and platelet function are concerns. Dextran is associated with a small risk of anaphylaxis. However, the volume of crystalloid required to produce the same increase in intravascular volume is larger, is only transiently effective, and may exacerbate the normal decrease in colloid osmotic pressure that occurs during the first 6 to 12 hours postpartum. Such a change may predispose patients with concomitant pre-eclampsia or cardiovascular disease to development of pulmonary edema. Furthermore, many point out that anesthetic-induced hypotension is not always severe, is readily treated, and if short-lived does not significantly affect neonatal outcome.

As there is no guaranteed method to prevent spinal hypotension and improve neonatal outcome, we advocate vigilant monitoring of maternal blood pressure every 2 minutes after spinal injection with immediate pharmacologic treatment of hypotension.

Maternal Position

Aortocaval compression, also known as maternal supine hypotensive syndrome, occurs when the pregnant woman lies supine. The etiology is multifactorial. The gravid uterus compresses the inferior vena cava and the aorta against the bodies of the lumbar vertebrae. The decreased venous return may result in decreased maternal cardiac output and blood pressure. Compression of uterine venous drainage results in an increased uterine venous pressure and therefore a reduced uterine perfusion pressure. Compression of the aorta or common iliac arteries also results in a reduced uterine artery perfusion pressure. For these reasons, left uterine displacement must be maintained during cesarean delivery. This can be effected by placing a wedge underneath the right buttock or tilting the operating table to the left by 15 degrees. This practice results in a similar incidence of maternal hypotension and fetal bradycardia as that seen if anesthesia is performed in the lateral decubitus position. Adequacy of tilt can also be assessed by palpation of the left femoral artery while displacing the uterus to the left; if the position is adequate, there should be no significant increase in pulse quality.

Monitoring

The American Society of Anesthesiologists (ASA) "Standards for Basic Anesthetic Monitoring" must be observed for all anesthetics, including those for cesarean delivery. First and foremost is Standard I: "Qualified anesthesia personnel shall be present in the room throughout the conduct of all general anesthetics, regional anesthetics, or monitored anesthesia care." Standard II states that "During all anesthetics the patient's oxygenation, ventilation, circulation, and temperature shall be continually evaluated."

During administration of general anesthesia, the concentration of oxygen in the patient's breathing system should be measured with an oxygen analyzer with a low oxygen concentration alarm operating. A method for continual and quantitative measurement of end tidal CO_2 should also be employed during general anesthesia. Failure to detect CO_2 after endotracheal tube placement signals esophageal intubation. In pregnant patients, it is desirable to avoid hyperventilation, as acute respiratory alkalosis can cause a reduction in uterine blood flow.

Capnography is also used by many anesthesiologists to measure respiratory rate during regional anesthesia. Because a high thoracic sensory level is required in cesarean delivery with regional anesthesia, some patients have the sensation that they are not breathing because they cannot feel their chest rise and fall nor-

mally. Showing the patient the capnographic tracing of her breaths or simply placing her hand on her upper chest can be reassuring.

During the administration of both general and regional anesthesia, pulse oximetry should be used as a quantitative method of assessing oxygenation; this is of particular importance during the induction of general anesthesia. The electrocardiogram (ECG) should be continuously displayed during the administration of anesthesia for surgery. Many have noted, however, the surprisingly frequent occurrence of ST-depression after delivery of the infant during cesarean delivery, one study noting an incidence of 25% in young, healthy parturients. The same study noted that these changes did not occur during vaginal delivery, and transthoracic echocardiography did not show any associated wall motion abnormalities or other indication of myocardial ischemia. Authors have speculated on a number of etiologies, including tachycardia, acute hypervolemia, coronary vasospasm, vasopressor administration, and venous air/amniotic fluid embolism; the exact cause remains unclear.

The detection of venous air emboli by Doppler ultrasonography has been advocated by some. The method is extremely sensitive and detects venous air emboli of 0.1 mL or more in 30% of patients, so it is probably best reserved for use in patients with intracardiac shunts. Chest pain, oxyhemoglobin desaturation, and arrhythmias will diagnose significant venous air embolism during cesarean delivery. Venous air embolism can be minimized by maintaining good intravascular volume and maintaining 5 to 10 degrees of reverse Trendelenburg position during surgery.

In cases of severe cardiac disease or pre-eclampsia, it may be useful to place a pulmonary artery catheter to provide information on cardiac output and filling pressures. In the asleep intubated patient, noninvasive methods of measuring cardiac output, such as transesophageal Doppler, may also be helpful.

REGIONAL ANESTHESIA FOR CESAREAN DELIVERY

General Considerations

If there is suspicion of fetal compromise, oxygen should be administered either by mask or nasal cannulae during the administration of regional anesthesia to improve maternal and thus fetal oxygenation. A support person of the patient's choice can also be present during the surgery to provide comfort and emotional support. Many anesthesiologists prefer to administer the regional anesthesia first and test the block, before inviting the support person into the room. It should be stressed that the guest must leave the room immediately on request of the medical personnel, should administration of general anesthesia become necessary.

A bilateral sensory block to T4 including sacral roots accompanied by motor block is generally accepted as necessary for cesarean delivery. Zones of differential blockade exist at the upper and lower edges of a regional block. Loss of sensation to cold is two dermatomes higher than loss of sensation to pinprick, which is in turn two dermatomes higher than loss of sensation to light touch. Loss of sensation to light touch from S1 to at least T5, and a dense motor block of hips and ankles are good signs that anesthesia is adequate for surgery. The sensation of cold can be measured with ice or ethyl chloride spray, pin prick with a neurologic pin, and light touch with a nylon filament (Von Frey hair) or tissue. Measuring with these techniques is highly anesthesiologist-dependent, and consistency of technique is important.

Rates of onset and regression are different for spinal and epidural blockade. Alahuhta[2] compared these rates using pinprick. Spinal blockade rose to T5 by 10 minutes and peaked at T3 at 20 minutes and by 90 minutes had regressed to T9; it completely anesthetized the sacral roots. Epidural blockade reached a maximal height at 30 minutes and remained at T6 after 2 hours. In some cases, epidurals loaded with bupivacaine failed to completely anesthetize the sacral roots.

After delivery of the baby and umbilical cord clamping, intravenous oxytocin should be administered to the mother to aid uterine involution and to reduce blood loss. Bolus oxytocin can cause maternal hypotension and tachycardia; 20 to 40 U of oxytocin should be diluted in 1000 mL of crystalloid and run at 40 to 80 mU/min (approximately 120 to 180 mL/hr).

In cases of refractory uterine atony, methylergonovine 0.2 mg intramuscularly, or 15-methyl prostaglandin F_2-alpha 0.25 mg intramuscularly may be required to enhance uterine contraction. Ergot derivatives may produce severe hypertension and occasionally coronary vasospasm, myocardial infarction, or cerebrovascular accidents. In cases of life-threatening hemorrhage, methylergonovine may be given by slow intravenous bolus of 60 seconds or longer. The prostaglandins may cause nausea, vomiting, diarrhea, fever, tachycardia, tachypnea, hypertension, and bronchoconstriction, and should be avoided in patients with asthma.

Spinal Anesthesia

Spinal anesthesia is popular because of its relative simplicity, fast onset time, reliability, and "density" of block.

Technique

Patient position for administration of spinal blockade can influence the rate of onset and spread of the drug, but has little effect on the ultimate height of the block. The sitting position is commonly used, as many anesthesiologists can perform a dural tap more easily in this posi-

tion, but spread of anesthesia may be slower. One study found that the time from start of injection to completion of anesthesia was similar in the sitting and lateral groups because the more rapid identification of cerebrospinal fluid (CSF) in the sitting group offset the longer time taken for the block to spread. If the lateral decubitus position is used, the right lateral decubitus position is preferred to ensure a similar level of anesthesia bilaterally, given that the patient will be positioned after anesthetic induction with left lateral tilt.

Lumbar puncture is performed at the L2-L3 or L3-L4 interspace. Smaller 25 to 27 G atraumatic pencil point needles such as Sprotte or Whittacre result in headache rates of >1% (Fig. 6-3). The selection of local anesthetic depends on duration of surgery and the plan for postoperative analgesia (Table 1). Doses of bupivacaine required for spinal anesthesia during pregnancy are about 25% less than those required in nonpregnant women; venocaval obstruction resulting in engorged epidural veins and therefore decreased epidural and CSF volume probably contribute to this effect, and it is even more pronounced in pregnancies with multiple fetuses. The dose of bupivacaine used for cesarean delivery range from 7.5 to 15 mg. The patient's height and weight may affect the dose required though evidence for consistent variation is sparse. If the dose of bupivacaine is reduced to >10 mg with no opioid the incidence of intraoperative pain is 70%.

Isobaric solutions tend to spread farther and wear off faster than hyperbaric solutions in the nonpregnant population. However, in pregnant patients subarachnoid injections of 12.5 mg of both solutions have both been shown to reliably reach the upper thoracic dermatomes. The number of milligrams of drug affects the block height rather than the volume of injectant; no difference between final block height or rate of onset was detected between 12 mL of 0.125% bupivacaine and 3 mL of 0.5% bupivacaine. The

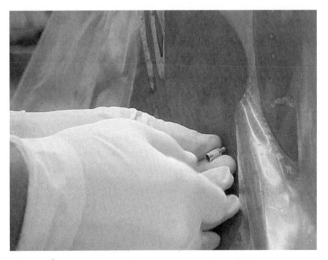

Figure 6-3   Insertion of a 25-gauge spinal needle for an anesthetic for cesarian delivery.

Table 6-1	Drugs Used for Spinal Anesthesia for Cesarean Section	
Drug	**Dosage range (mg)**	**Duration (min)**
Lidocaine	60 to 75	45 to 75
Bupivacaine	7.5 to 15.0	60 to 120
Tetracaine	7 to 10	120 to 180
Procaine	100 to 150	30 to 60
Adjuvant Drugs		
Epinephrine	0.1 to 0.2	—
Morphine	0.1 to 0.25	360 to 1080
Fentanyl	0.010 to 0.025	180 to 240

quality and duration of the block may be improved by the addition of epinephrine 0.1 to 0.2 mg, though some controversy exists as to whether there is a prolongation of the effects of lidocaine or bupivacaine.

Epidural Anesthesia

Most cesarean deliveries performed under epidural blockade are urgent or emergent cases where the epidural catheter is *in situ* having been used for labor analgesia. There remain some indications for the establishment *de novo* of an epidural (see Choice of Anesthetic Technique section).

Technique

Epidural catheters are usually placed at L2-L3 or L3-L4 to avoid potential injury to the spinal cord from unintentional dural puncture. In obese women, the sitting position often allows easier identification of the midline. Infiltration of the skin and subcutaneous tissues with 1% lidocaine helps allow easy and pain-free insertion of the Tuohy needle, and helps the mother to remain still and comfortable during epidural insertion.

The midline approach is used by most anesthesiologists, with the paramedian approach being used by some practitioners in difficult patients, as there is less risk of dural puncture. With the midline approach, the epidural needle passes through skin, subcutaneous fat, supraspinous ligament, interspinous ligament, and finally ligamentum flavum before entering the epidural space. The epidural space is most often located using a loss-of-resistance technique. Either saline or air can be used. Saline has been advocated as having a lower incidence of accidental dural puncture; however, this may make identification of a small dural puncture less reliable. Glucose testing may give false positives as CSF drains into the epidural space. Both techniques are acceptable, and anesthesiologists should use whichever technique is more reliable in their hands. Multiorifice

catheters seem to provide more reliable anesthesia than single orifice catheters—though their safety has been questioned, as they have the potential to allow multicompartment spread of local anesthetic.

CURRENT CONTROVERSIES: EPIDURAL TEST DOSE

- Bupivacaine 7.5 to 12.5 mg or lidocaine 45 to 60 mg: +/−15 µg epinephrine or isoprenaline 5 µg
- Fentanyl 100 µg
- 10 mL of low dose epidural mixture (e.g., 0.0625% to 0.125% bupivacaine + 2 µg/mL fentanyl
- 1 to 2 mL air

Having inserted the epidural catheter, the catheter should be aspirated observing for blood or fluid, and then an epidural test dose may be administered. The local anesthetic dose should be equivalent to the intrathecal dose used for cesarean delivery (e.g., bupivacaine 7.5 to 12 mg or lidocaine 45 to 60 mg) to detect inadvertent intrathecal administration. The addition of epinephrine 15 µg may help identify intravascular placement as baseline heart rate increases by about 10 bpm, though this test is not particularly sensitive or specific in pregnancy. Some recommend the addition of 100 µg of fentanyl to the test dose, and patients may then report the central effects of lightheadedness if the dose is intravascular, though this may interfere with the assessment of the level of block. Air 1 mL combined with cardiac Doppler has also been put forward as a substrate for a test dose. A subdural block is harder to detect. It comes on relatively slowly (like an epidural block), usually extends higher than expected (may extend intracranially producing cranial nerve palsies), and is patchy. No technique is completely reliable, and it should be remembered that catheters can migrate to a different space at any time, so vigilance should be maintained whenever a drug is bolused through the epidural catheter.

Dosing

Between 3 and 5 minutes after the test dose there should be no evidence of motor blockade or dense sensory blockade (a band of anesthesia may be present in the upper lumbar and lower thoracic dermatomes), or hemodynamic disturbances. If this is the case, the therapeutic dose can be administered. The pregnant woman requires approximately 1 mL of local anesthetic solution for each level of anesthetic blockade. Therefore, a block to T4 will require 18 segments and usually 20 to 25 mL of local anesthetic. We titrate the total dose in 5-mL increments of local anesthetic with at least 2 minutes between boluses.

The choice of anesthetic agent depends on the desired speed of onset and the duration of action. Both lidocaine

2% and bupivacaine 0.5% have durations of action that should be sufficient for cesarean delivery (75 to 100 min and 120 to 180 min, respectively). Lidocaine has a faster onset of action, requiring about half of the onset time as bupivacaine. Bupivacaine 0.5% 10 mL + 10 mL given as a two-stage top-up took an average of 42 minutes until block completion. Lidocaine, however, has been associated with a higher incidence of inadequate block. The addition of epinephrine to the local anesthetic to achieve a concentration of 1 in 200,000 or 1 in 400,000 (0.1 mL or 0.05 mL of 1 in 1000 epinephrine) may decrease vascular absorption of the local anesthetic and improve the quality and duration of the block, and it is particularly efficacious when used with lidocaine. It is better to add the epinephrine just before giving the lidocaine epidurally, as this allows the solution to maintain a higher pH and contains less sodium metabisulfate than the commercially prepared lidocaine and epinephrine solutions. The addition of 1 mEq of sodium bicarbonate to each 10 mL of lidocaine 2% speeds the onset of action of the solution, making it comparable to 2-chloroprocaine 3%.

Dosing a labor epidural for emergency cesarean delivery means that a large dose of local anesthetic may have to be given quickly, as there may not be time to dose incrementally. Lucas[3] used 20 mL of whatever drug the patient had been receiving with rapid and complete results in the majority of mothers. There were no problems with high blocks—although there were some reports of loss of sensation to cold in the cervical dermatomes in some cases. The block is assessed, and if there is any inequality then the mother is placed in the full lateral position on that side and given additional drug. Unless there has been a recent top-up of the epidural, 15 to 20 mL of local anesthetic is required. Topping up in the delivery room is controversial but saves time. Once the top-up has been given, it is imperative to stay with the mother and have a means of measuring her blood pressure and administering appropriate vasopressors. Transfer to the operating room should be expedited.

Three percent 2-chloroprocaine has the fastest onset of action but only a 40-minute duration of anesthesia. It also decreases the subsequent efficacy of epidural opioid analgesia. For these reasons, it is only really considered for dosing of an existing labor epidural when time is of the essence. Alkalinized lidocaine 2% with epinephrine is also a good choice for emergent cesarean delivery. In Europe, an alkalinized mixture of 50:50 lidocaine: bupivacaine with epinephrine is popular, combining rapid onset with an improved quality of block and decreased need for intraoperative supplementation.

Combined Spinal-Epidural Anesthesia

The combined spinal-epidural (CSE) technique is useful, as it both increases the reliability of the epidural and allows for prolongation of the block in cases of prolonged cesarean delivery such as a tertiary delivery or

delivery and tubal ligation. Brownridge[4] first described combined spinal epidural anesthesia in 1981. He inserted an epidural catheter at the L1–L2 interspace, gave a test dose, and then performed spinal anesthesia at the L3–L4 interspace. The technique has since been adapted by locating the epidural space with the Tuohy needle, inserting a long spinal needle through the Tuohy needle into the subarachnoid space to deliver the intrathecal dose of drug, and then passing the epidural catheter. Success is improved when using a conic needle and feeling the dural puncture as a slight click.

The Sequential Block

Ten minutes after a spinal injection, 10 mL of epidural saline can produce a more cephalad spread of the block. This has been confirmed by myelography to be a volume effect, a squeezing of the dural sac resulting in a decrease in CSF volume. This allows a smaller initial spinal dose to be used and then supplemented by injection into the epidural space. One advantage of this is that the length of time the mother is blocked after her cesarean delivery is reduced. Another advantage is a decrease in the incidence of hypotension, though not all authors have found this benefit. A drawback of the technique is the fear of producing a high or total spinal block. Volumes should be limited to 5 mL every 5 minutes, with 10 minutes before the first injection. Care should be taken to assess the level of the block between each top-up.

Spinal Injection After Epidural Injection

Placing a spinal block after an epidural block raises concerns about the production of a high or total spinal block. However, in an audit of 72 spinal blocks after failed epidural anesthesia, in which half the women received 12.5 mg of bupivacaine, there were no reports of high blocks. If spinal is being considered because an epidural has not been topped up, then a standard dose should be considered. If it is to supplement an epidural block that has failed to spread to the sacral or thoracic dermatomes, then 75% of the usual dose should be used and the mother positioned to control the height of the block with pillows under the shoulders and head (Fig. 6-4).

Neuraxial Opioids

Epidural fentanyl improves intraoperative comfort for the mother. Doses of 0 to 100 µg of fentanyl have been studied with 50, 75, and 100 µg found to be equally efficacious, providing 4 hours of postoperative pain relief. Intrathecal fentanyl has been studied in doses of 6.25 to 25 µg. Doses over 20 µg may increase the incidence of pruritus. Epidural morphine 3 mg is efficacious for postoperative pain but takes about

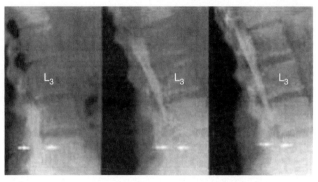

Figure 6-4   Lateral view of myelogram. The white arrows point to the diameter of the subarachnoid space. The diameter diminished to one quarter of the original diameter after a 10 ml epidural injection of saline. (From Takiguchi T, Okano T, Egawa H, et al: The effect of epidural saline injection on analgesic level during combined spinal and epidural anesthesia assessed clinically and myelographically. Anesth Analgesia, 85:1097–1000, 1997.)

60 minutes to have maximal effect, the comparable intrathecal dose is 0.2 mg.

Complications of Regional Anesthesia

Hypotension

The reduction in systemic vascular resistance (SVR) and increase in venous capacitance after regional anesthesia may cause hypotension. Hypotension is defined as a decrease in systolic of 25% or any absolute value below 100 mm HG systolic. Uteroplacental perfusion is dependent on maternal perfusion pressure, and the maintenance of a good mean arterial pressure results in better cord gases at delivery. Hypotension is more likely to occur in women who are not in labor. Treatment includes oxygen, IV fluids, left uterine displacement, and vasopressors.

Many anesthesiologists use a prophylactic dose of intramuscular ephedrine 25 to 50 mg or 5 to 10 mg intravenously, prior to spinal anesthesia, to maintain hemodynamic stability. It has been demonstrated to decrease the hypotension associated with spinal, but not epidural, anesthesia. It has not been demonstrated to affect fetal outcome, and many anesthesiologists

---

CURRENT CONTROVERSIES: VASOPRESSOR THERAPY FOR HYPOTENSION

- Ephedrine: α- and β-agonist, currently first-line vasopressor.
- Theoretical fear of uterine artery vasoconstriction with phenylephrine: α-agonist.
- Clinical evidence shows less fetal acidosis and less maternal nausea and vomiting with phenylephrine than with ephedrine.

---

prefer the rapid treatment of hypotension should it occur, rather than prophylaxis.

For vasopressor treatment of hypotension, ephedrine has long been preferred. Animal studies have demonstrated maintenance of uterine blood flow. Concerns about using the α-agonist phenylephrine have been that it may cause vasoconstriction of the uterine vessels—and therefore it has been used more sparingly—usually to avoid extreme tachycardia, in patients where this may be a concern, for example, mitral stenosis. However, in a recent study comparing infusions of ephedrine, phenylephrine, or a combination of both, given as an infusion to treat hypotension, Cooper[5] found that, "Giving phenylephrine alone by infusion at cesarean delivery was associated with a lower incidence of fetal acidosis and maternal nausea and vomiting than giving ephedrine alone. There was no advantage to combining phenylephrine and ephedrine because it increased nausea and vomiting, and it did not further improve fetal blood gas values, compared with giving phenylephrine alone."

High Spinal Anesthesia

An unexpectedly high block can result if an epidural dose is inadvertently given to the subarachnoid space, or there is unexpectedly large rostral spread of an intrathecal dose. In 1985, an incidence of 1 in 4500 was reported. Early warning signs of a total spinal may be agitation, dyspnea, and a husky voice, progressing to complete sensory and motor blockade, hypotension, bradycardia, unconsciousness, and cardiorespiratory arrest. Treatment includes endotracheal intubation and positive pressure ventilation with 100% oxygen, the maintenance of maternal circulation with left uterine displacement, fluids, and ephedrine. Epinephrine should be used without hesitation if there is a poor response to ephedrine or if cardiac arrest.

Local Anesthetic Toxicity

This may occur if an epidural dose of local anesthetic is inadvertently injected into an epidural vein. Early signs are numbness, circumoral tingling, slurred speech, confusion, and dizziness. This may progress to loss of consciousness, convulsions, and cardiovascular collapse. The treatment is similar to that for total spinal anesthesia. Seizures should be controlled with diazepam 2 to 10 mg and cardiopulmonary resuscitation (CPR), and Advanced Cardiac Life Support (ACLS) should be commenced if necessary.

Failed Regional Anesthesia

There are a number of causes of failed spinal. These include placement of drug somewhere other than the subarachnoid space, an inadequate dose of local anesthetic, caudal pooling of a hyperbaric drug, omitting the local anesthetic from the drug mixture, a low potency drug lot, or anatomic enlargement of the lumbar dural sac. If delivery is urgent or the patient does not wish to repeat the subarachnoid block, epidural or general anesthesia may be administered. If there is little or no evidence of anesthesia, the spinal can be repeated with the same dose. If there is insufficient caudal spread, a sequential block may be suitable.

Failed epidural occurs in 2% to 6% of cases and is caused by malposition or displacement of the epidural catheter, inadequate amount of local anesthetic, or anatomic barriers to local anesthetic spread. Options here include general anesthesia, repeat epidural, or spinal injection. If the epidural is repeated, care must be taken not to administer a toxic dose of local anesthetic, as often a large dose has already been given. Assessment for signs of local anesthetic toxicity is important. If a spinal is chosen, the risk of high spinal anesthesia exists due to reduced CSF volume, and either a reduced dose should be given or the procedure delayed before spinal injection. Parenteral analgesic drugs may be used for the treatment of breakthrough pain during regional anesthesia. 50% nitrous oxide (N_2O), intravenous fentanyl 1µg/kg, and intravenous ketamine 0.25 mg/kg are all useful adjuncts because they do not greatly depress central airway reflexes. Clinical judgment must be used to decide when supplementation has failed and general anesthesia is required.

GENERAL ANESTHESIA

Neither general anesthesia nor regional anesthesia (which is always accompanied by the potential need to institute general anesthesia) should be considered in the absence of a minimum equipment requirement. All equipment must be checked regularly by a designated trained person and must include the following: oxygen analyzer, end tidal carbon dioxide (CO_2) analyzer, ventilation disconnect alarm, pulse oximeter, noninvasive blood pressure monitor with a 1 minute cycle, ECG, suction, and a tilting table. An assistant trained in applying cricoid pressure is essential for airway management, and it is recommended that there should also be the following (Fig. 6-5):
• One standard and one long-bladed laryngoscope
• A short-handled/polio blade laryngoscope (useful if blade insertion is difficult)
• McCoy levering laryngoscope, which may improve a poor view at laryngoscopy or other noninvasive device
• A gum elastic bougie and stylet
• Tracheal tubes cut to the required length size 6 to 8 mm
• Oral airways
• Size 3 laryngeal mask
• A minitracheostomy set or the equivalent

The McCoy laryngoscope has a levering tip, which may lift the epiglottis forward and aid in the visualization of the vocal cords. The laryngeal mask may be useful when there has been a failure to secure the airway using a tracheal tube. However, it does not prevent regurgitation of gastric contents into the oropharynx, and cricoid pressure must be maintained unless this interferes with oxygenation.

Cricothyrotomy is the last resort when the patient cannot be oxygenated any other way, and there are a variety of packs available to perform this. Minitracheostomy sets are good because they are relatively easy to insert, the 15 mm connector will attach to the breathing circuit, and the 4-mm internal diameter is sufficient to provide oxygenation. In cases of a completely obstructed upper airway, resistance through the small diameter airway will result in hypoventilation, and the CO_2 will rise. A more definitive airway must be provided within 30 to 45 minutes.

Induction of General Anesthesia

Left uterine displacement should be instituted as previously discussed. In nonpregnant patients, preoxygenation, otherwise known as denitrogenation, will allow approximately 3 minutes before oxygen saturation begins to fall. At term, there is an increase in oxygen consumption of 20%, a further increase of 20% during labor, and an increase of up to 100% over nonpregnant controls during the second stage of labor. Therefore, desaturation occurs much more rapidly in pregnant women. If the mask is not tightly fitted, room air can enter, decreasing the efficacy of denitrogenation. Normal tidal volume breaths for 3 minutes will decrease alveolar nitrogen to 1%; four vital capacity breaths decrease alveolar nitrogen to 5%. The tidal volume method buys about 15 seconds more time.

Rapid Sequence Induction

Cricoid pressure was first described by Sellick in 1961 and is often referred to as Sellick's maneuver. He described a two-handed technique. The thumb and middle finger of one hand are placed either side of the cricoid, and backward pressure compresses the esophagus on the vertebral column at C6, thus occluding it. The other hand is placed behind the neck, and forward pressure is applied, placing the head in the sniffing position and making the esophagus easier to occlude. In practice, when only one assistant is present, the second hand of the assistant is more usefully employed in reaching for additional equipment, and one-handed cricoid pressure is most commonly used. If cricoid pressure is badly applied, it may make intubation more difficult.

It has been found that a constant backward pressure of 44 Newtons (N) will prevent passive regurgitation of

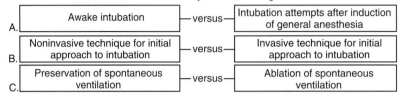

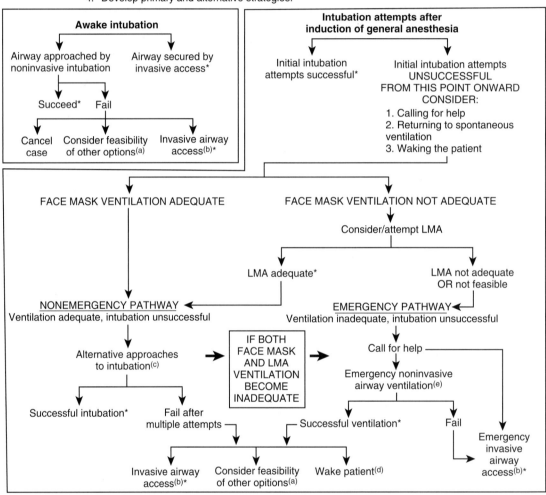

*Confirm tracheal intubation or LMA placement with exhaled CO_2.

Figure 6-5   Difficult airway algorithm. (a) Other options include (but not limited to): surgery utilizing face mask or LMA anesthesia, local anesthesia infiltration or regional nerve blockade. Pursuit of these options usually implies that mask ventilation will not be problematic. Therefore, these options may be of limited value if this step in the algorithm has been reached via the emergency pathway. (b) Invasive airway access include surgical or percutaneous tracheostomy or cricothyrotomy. (c) Alternative noninvasive approaches to difficult intubation include (but are not limited to): use of different laryngoscope blades, LMA as an intubation conduit (with or without fiberoptic guidance), fiberoptic intubation, intubating stylet or tube changer, light wand, retrograde intubation, and blind oral or nasal intubation. (d) Consider repreparation of the patient for awake intubation or canceling surgery. (e) Options for emergency noninvasive airway ventilation include (but are not limited to): rigid bronchoscope, esopageal-tracheal combitube ventilation, or transtracheal jet ventilation.

stomach contents. If vomiting occurs, cricoid pressure should be released, as intraesophageal pressures could otherwise lead to rupture. Cricoid pressure should be established before induction of anesthesia. Most patients will tolerate a pressure of 20 N, which should be increased after consciousness is lost.

The Failed Intubation

Careful positioning of the mother is important to optimize the chances of a successful intubation. This includes adjusting the table height to one most comfortable for the anesthesiologist, placing pillows under the mother's head to provide support, good head extension on the neck, and ensuring that the mother's arms are not resting on her chest, as this may exacerbate difficulty in inserting the laryngoscope blade.

If a failed intubation is encountered, it is important to have a plan of action; failed intubation algorithms can be useful for this. Failure to intubate the mother will cause no harm as long as oxygenation can be maintained and passive regurgitation prevented. If intubation has failed, a second dose of succinylcholine should not be given. Repeated attempts at intubation will increase the chance of aspiration, and in the presence of hypoxemia the second dose may produce profound bradycardia.

If it remains possible to maintain oxygenation and ventilation via a laryngeal mask or face mask, then a decision needs to be made regarding whether to awaken the mother. This will be based on an evaluation of the mother and fetus, and the reliability of the airway. If the mother's life depends on completion of the surgery, as in massive hemorrhage or cardiac arrest, then surgery should continue. In the case of sudden and severe fetal distress with no recovery between contractions—for example, with placental abruption or prolapsed cord—and where the airway is manageable, then to save the life of the fetus it is reasonable to continue with anesthesia, though such an anesthetic may be extremely difficult. The inhalation agent should be increased to 2 to 3 times minimum alveolar concentration (MAC) in the spontaneously breathing patient, as light anesthesia may precipitate coughing, vomiting, and breath-holding. If the mother's life is deemed to be at risk, she should be awakened. In all other cases, the safest course of action is to wake the mother and form an alternative plan. This will be spinal, epidural, or awake fiber-optic intubation.

Prevention of Awareness

There is a reduction in MAC of 28% in pregnant women at 8 to 12 weeks gestation when compared to nonpregnant controls, and this reduction in MAC is seen with all volatile anesthetic drugs. This effect may be mediated by increased endorphin levels in pregnancy and is reversed by naloxone. Progesterone and its metabolites have anesthetic effects and may also contribute to the reduction in MAC during pregnancy. Concerns about failure of uterine involution and subsequent bleeding due to the presence of volatile anesthetics led to the practice of using only 70% nitrous in oxygen in the 1970s and 1980s. There followed a spate of awareness cases. Now at least 0.5 MAC of inhalational agent is used in conjunction with 70% N_2O to prevent awareness.

Because of the lower blood/gas partition coefficients of the newer agents—isoflurane, desflurane, and sevoflurane—it is easier to achieve 0.5 MAC rapidly following an intravenous induction. Using a high initial concentration (overpressure) and measuring the end tidal concentration facilitate rapid achievement of 0.5 MAC anesthetic at the effect site.

Considerations for Maternal Ventilation

A higher oxygen concentration should be used during cesarean delivery, as mothers have an increased metabolic demand. An inspired oxygen concentration of 50% should be used with the woman in the left lateral tilt position. Mechanical hyperventilation may increase intrathoracic pressure, exacerbating the effects of aortocaval compression, decreased venous return, and decreased cardiac output, and should be avoided. Furthermore, it has been shown that a maternal $PaCO_2$ less than 27 mm Hg (3.6 kPa) results in vasoconstriction of the umbilical vessels and fetal acidosis. Conversely, if the maternal $PaCO_2$ is allowed to rise above its term value of 31 mm Hg (4.1 kPa), the concentration gradient from fetus to mother is abolished, and the fetus may develop a "respiratory" acidosis.

Induction–Delivery Interval

It is possible for the baby to become acidotic during the time from induction of anesthesia until delivery if placental perfusion is impaired or high concentrations of N_2O are used, resulting in diffusion hypoxia. Some evidence shows that higher concentrations of oxygen 60% to 70% may improve the condition of the baby at delivery. If precautions against aortocaval compression and maternal hypotension are taken and a high FiO_2 is used, Crawford[6] showed that an interval of up to 30 minutes should not adversely affect fetal outcome.

All lipid-soluble anesthetic agents will cross the placenta, and the longer the baby is exposed to a concentration gradient the greater the uptake will be. Intravenous induction agents do not accumulate in the baby because of rapid redistribution into the larger maternal volume of distribution. Maternal levels of inhalation agents are relatively constant, and a maternal–fetal gradient will be maintained until delivery. Prolonged induction–delivery times may therefore be detrimental to the baby in this respect.

Common practice is to allow the surgeons to scrub and drape the patient prior to induction to minimize fetal exposure to the inhalation agent. Unlike induction-delivery times, long uterine incision to delivery time is particularly hazardous to the baby, with times in excess of 3 minutes being associated with lower Apgar scores and fetal acidosis.

ANESTHETIC AGENTS

Induction Agents

When choosing an induction agent, one should consider the preservation of maternal blood pressure and cardiac output, and thus umbilical blood flow, the avoidance of fetal depression, and also the reliability of maternal hypnosis and amnesia.

Thiopental

At a dose of 4 mg/kg, thiopental provides prompt reliable induction of anesthesia, has few adverse effects, and allows a smooth emergence from anesthesia. Although it is detected in the umbilical vein, the circution through the fetal liver protects the fetus from sedation. At higher doses of 8 mg/kg, fetal depression does occur. The main advantage of thiopental is that while it doesn't produce neonatal compromise, it has a relatively long duration of action when given at 4 mg/kg, and may therefore help protect against early awareness at the time when the induction agent is wearing off and the end tidal concentration of volatile agent is rising toward equilibrium.

Propofol

Propofol allows a rapid smooth induction of anesthesia. Propofol attenuates the hypertensive response to laryngoscopy and intubation more effectively than other induction agents, making it a good choice for the induction of general anesthesia in hypertensive patients. Some studies have noted a greater decrease in blood pressure with propofol than with thiopental, though other studies have not found this. After an induction dose of 2.5 mg/kg, propofol was not found to cause more neonatal depression than thiopental. A major advantage is that the mother may be less sedated during the emergence from anesthesia. However, there is some concern that its more rapid offset produces a risk of maternal waking before adequate inhalational anesthesia has been achieved. Propofol can be administered as an infusion to maintain anesthesia, allowing the administration of 100% oxygen. At a low-maintenance dose of 6 mg/kg/hr, the condition of the neonate was found to be good.

Ketamine

Ketamine's powerful sympathomimetic action makes it useful in hypovolemic patients and those with severe asthma. It reliably produces hypnosis, amnesia, and analgesia at doses of 1 mg/kg, and the condition of the neonate compares favorably with thiopental at this dose. At a dose of 2 mg/kg, neonatal depression does occur. Ketamine can cause delirium and hallucinations on emergence, especially in the unpremedicated patient.

Etomidate

Etomidate causes less myocardial depression than thiopental or propofol and less histamine release, making it a good choice in patients with asthma or who are hemodynamically unstable. It is partially hydrolyzed by cholinesterases, found in high concentrations in the placenta, and its concentration in the fetal circulation after induction of anesthesia is less than with other agents. In a dose of 0.3 mg/kg, it produces rapid wakening in the mother and good neonatal Apgar scores. Its major disadvantages are pain on injection, myoclonic rigidity with involuntary movements, postoperative nausea and vomiting, and a reduction in plasma cortisol concentration in the baby at 1 hour of life, a potential disadvantage in an already stressed baby.

Midazolam

Midazolam has limited use due to a slow onset of action and side effects, which include neonatal hypothermia, hypotonia, jaundice, lethargy, respiratory depression, and poor feeding. It should be used for induction only when there are contraindications to the use of other agents. The induction dose is 0.2 mg/kg.

Maintenance of Anesthesia

Nitrous Oxide

Nitrous oxide (N_2O) does not interfere with oxytocin-induced uterine involution, and its low blood solubility allows for a rapid effect. It is therefore a useful component of an inhalational anesthetic, but due to its high MAC must be used in conjunction with other volatile anesthetic agents. If more than 50% is used, diffusion hypoxia and deteriorating acid base status of the neonate becomes a potential risk.

Volatile Anesthetic Agents

Halothane, enflurane, isoflurane, desflurane, and sevoflurane have all been used successfully for cesarean delivery. Isoflurane is probably the best established and popular current choice, although the newer more soluble volatile anesthetics are gaining popularity. If used at a one MAC equivalent with N_2O and if the induction delivery interval is >11 minutes, neonatal depression is unusual. Although all produce uterine relaxation and decreased sensitivity to oxytocin, if used at 0.5 MAC following delivery, bleeding should not be a problem. Sevoflurane and desflurane have lower blood solubility, allowing for very rapid induction and recovery from anesthesia, but no specific benefits over isoflurane have been shown. Elevated serum levels of fluoride ions, a byproduct of sevoflurane metabolism, have been detected in babies 24 hours after anesthesia, without clinical sequelae.

Neuromuscular Blockers

Succinylcholine

Succinylcholine, a depolarizing neuromuscular blocker, in a dose of 1 to 1.5 mg/kg, is the muscle relaxant of choice for most patients. It is the only agent that combines rapid onset, allowing intubation within 90 seconds, with rapid offset, allowing spontaneous respiration to return 1 to 5 minutes after administration. It is metabolized by pseudocholinesterase, and although concentrations of pseudocholinesterase are decreased by 30% due to a dilutional effect in pregnancy, this appears to be of little clinical significance. However, there are a number of contraindications. The prevalence of pseudocholinesterase deficiency in the population is 0.3%; the use of succinylcholine in these patients results in prolonged paralysis requiring postoperative ventilation. If succinylcholine is used in patients with burns, demyelinating neurologic conditions, or recent cord transections, it can result in hyperkalemia. In patients with myotonia, succinylcholine may produce rigidity. Finally, in susceptible patients, succinylcholine may trigger malignant hyperthermia. A personal or family history of these condition should be elicited prior to induction of general anesthesia for cesarean delivery as for any surgery.

Rocuronium

Rocuronium, a nondepolarizing neuromuscular blocker, at a dose of 0.6 mg/kg, can achieve intubating conditions at about 80 seconds. McCourt[7] found that intubating conditions were significantly better after a dose of 1 mg/kg, comparing more favorably with succiny choline. The disadvantage of rocuronium is that at these doses neuromuscular blockade lasts 50 to 60 minutes.

Vecuronium and Atracurium

These nondepolarizing muscle relaxants are not well suited to a rapid sequence induction, as even at relatively high doses they have an onset of action of about 3 minutes. Atracurium, though not its isomer cisatracurium, also causes histamine release. Vecuronium 0.05 mg/kg or atracurium 0.25 mg/kg can be used to provide 20 to 30 minutes of muscle relaxation after succinylcholine has worn off. Residual neuromuscular blockade should be reversed at the end of the procedure with neostigmine and an anticholinergic agent, such as glycopyrrolate, to blunt the muscarinic side effects.

Interactions with Magnesium Sulphate

Patients receiving magnesium sulphate may not fasciculate after the intubating dose of succinylcholine, even though the action of succinylcholine is unaffected. Magnesium sulphate also prolongs the neuromuscular blockade produced by nondepolarizing neuromuscular blockers. The phenomenon of "recurarization" may occur in mothers who have received magnesium sulphate, particularly those who remain on infusions in the postoperative period. It is therefore important to monitor patients for signs of muscle weakness for several hours postoperatively.

Opiates

Opiates rapidly cross the placenta to the baby and can potentially result in neonatal depression. For this reason, they are not routinely used as part of a rapid sequence induction. They may, however, be used to help obtund the hypertension and tachycardia associated with laryngoscopy and intubation if this is considered appropriate; a dose of 1 μg/kg of fentanyl is considered safe for the neonate, but higher doses may cause respiratory depression. If opiates have been given to the mother prior to delivery of the baby, it is important to inform the pediatrician. This will prepare him for the possibility of respiratory depression. After delivery of the baby and cord clamping, opiates (100 to 200 μg of fentanyl or 10 to 20 mg morphine) can be administered to the mother as part of the anesthetic, and to allow a smooth, pain-free emergence from anesthesia.

Opiates should be continued for postoperative pain control after general anesthesia. Patients receiving general anesthesia for cesarean delivery seem to suffer more postoperative pain than those who received regional anesthesia for the procedure, despite using short-acting local anesthetics. Long-acting opioids such as meperidine or morphine can be given by intramuscular injection or intravenously via a patient-controlled pump. Nonsteroidal anti-inflammatory drugs, such as tenoxicam 20 mg intravenously, ketordac 15 mg intravenously, or diclofenac 100 mg pr, are good adjuncts to opiate analgesia and reduce opioid requirements without adverse effect to mother or baby.

CONCLUSION

The modern anesthetic for cesarean delivery is regional rather than general in the large majority of cases. As discussed, there are sound medical reasons for this trend. These reasons are not limited to concerns about the maternal airway and transfer of anesthetic drugs to the newborn. In addition to these issues are the psychological well-being of the parturient and her partner. Cesarean delivery is not the birth route of choice normally, but a regional anesthetic can help to make the birth experience "family friendly." Often, the parents can experience the birth of their child together, and see and hold the baby nearly immediately after birth. With the knowledge of the physiologic and pharmacologic changes in pregnancy, and importantly a supportive bedside manner, the obstetric anesthesiologist can provide a safe and pleasant environment for what are the most memorable days in many people's lives.

REFERENCES

1. Ueyama H, He YL, Tanigami H, et al: Effects of crystalloid and colloid preload on blood volume in the parturient undergoing spinal anesthesia for elective cesarean section. Anesthesiology 91(6):1571-1576, 1999.

2. Alahuhta S, Kangas-Saarela T, Hollmen AI, Edstrom HH: Visceral pain during caesarean section under spinal and epidural anaesthesia with bupivacaine. Acta Anaesthesiol Scand 34(2):95-98, 1990.

3. Lucas DN, Ciccone GK, Yentis SM: Extending low-dose epidural analgesia for emergency Cesarean section. A comparison of three solutions. Anaesthesia 54(12):1173-1177, 1999.

4. Brownridge P: Epidural and subarachnoid analgesia for elective caesarean section. Anaesthesia 36(1):70, 1981.

5. Cooper DW, Carpenter M, Mowbray P, et al: Fetal and maternal effects of phenylephrine and ephedrine during spinal anesthesia for cesarian delivery. Anesthesiology 97(6):1582-1590, 2002.

6. Crawford JS, James FM 3rd, Davies P, Crawley M: A further study of general anaesthesia for Cesarean section. Br J Anaesth 48(7):661-667, 1976.

7. McCourt KC, Salmela L, Mirakhur RK, et al: Comparison of rocuronium and suxamethonium for use during rapid sequence induction of anaesthesia. Anaesthesia 53(9):867-871, 1998.

SUGGESTED READING

Fernando R, Jones HM: Comparison of plain and alkalinized local anaesthetic mixtures of lignocaine and bupivacaine for elective extradural caesarean section. Br J Anaesth 67(6):699-703, 1991.

Pilkington S, Carli F, Dakin M, et al: Increase in Mallampati score during pregnancy. Br J Anaesth 74(6):638-642, 1995.

Sellick BA: Cricoid pressure to control regurgitation of stomach contents during induction of anaesthesia. Lancet 2:404-406, 1961.

Stuart JC, Kan AF, Rowbottom SJ, et al: Acid aspiration prophylaxis for emergency caesarean section. Anaesthesia 51(5):415-421, 1996.

Thomas TA, Cooper GM: Maternal deaths from anaesthesia. An extract from Why Mothers Die 1997-1999, the Confidential Enquiries into Maternal Deaths in the United Kingdom. Br J Anaesth 89(3):499-508, 2002.

Wu CL: Regional anesthesia and anticoagulation. J Clin Anesth 13(1):49-58, 2001.

CHAPTER 7

Postcesarean Analgesia

FERNE R. BRAVEMAN

INTRODUCTION

Effective pain management has become a benchmark for the adequacy of health care in the United States, with pain now termed the "fifth vital sign." As with other vital signs, recording a pain score and "reporting" a pain score higher than a predetermined number are not the endpoint of care. The goal, in the postoperative period, is to assess and treat pain in a manner which allows the patient to be satisfied with her pain control. The cesarean delivery patient presents a unique challenge for those managing her pain. Unlike other postoperative patients, new mothers are motivated to be out of bed and caring for their newborns. Postcesarean patients not only want to be comfortable; they expect to be clearheaded and experience few side effects. They look to become quickly unencumbered by intravenous and epidural catheters and infusion pumps, with the goal to interact with the newborn. Further, breast-feeding necessitates the use of analgesics that are minimally excreted in breast milk and that have little effect on the newborn.

In the United States, the cesarean delivery rate is now approaching 30% of all deliveries. In some other countries, it is more than twice this rate. The goals of postoperative care thus become multifactorial: patient satisfaction and an uncomplicated postoperative course are important, as are rapid mobilization and patient discharge.

Hospital stays after cesarean delivery are longer than after vaginal delivery. A reduced length of stay following cesarean section would be helpful to create beds for newly delivered patients, as the size of postpartum units have not increased with the increase in the cesarean delivery rate! Nikolajsen[1] has suggested that patients with recall of severe postoperative pain are more likely to experience chronic pain following cesarean delivery. This pain can interfere with the patient's daily activities. Better pain control would minimize the occurrence of chronic pain complaints.

POSTCESAREAN ANALGESIA

The current trend in providing postoperative analgesia is to use a multimodal approach. The goal is to use drugs with different mechanisms/sites of action to create additive or supra-additive effects, while at the same time a lower incidence of side effects is seen as the dosage of individual drugs may be reduced. The choice of therapies in the patient undergoing cesarean delivery is often predicated by the choice of anesthetic for the procedure.

In the United States, most cesarean sections are performed with regional anesthesia. The coadministration of neuraxial opioids to augment intraoperative anesthesia and to treat postoperative pain control is very common. More than 90% of obstetric anesthesiologists administer neuraxial opioids in this setting.[2] Patients who have general anesthesia for cesarean delivery will not be administered neuraxial opioids. For these patients, parenteral or oral opioid administration will still be the mainstay of postoperative analgesia.

Multimodal therapy for postcesarean analgesia includes opioid therapy—neuraxial, parenteral, or oral. Transdermal administration is not routinely used in this population. Nonsteroidal Anti-inflammatory Drugs (NSAIDs), with a different side effect profile than opioids, are often coadministered with opioids. Metoclopramide, clonidine, and ondansetron have all been used as analgesic adjuvants for postcesarean analgesia, with varying degrees of efficacy.

Neuraxial Opioids

The large majority of patients undergoing cesarean delivery, as previously mentioned, have regional anesthesia and thus will be administered neuraxial opioids. Short-acting opioids such as fentanyl and sufentanil provide improved intraoperative anesthesia but have little effect on postoperative analgesia, unless administered epidurally as a continuous infusion or via patient-controlled epidural analgesia (PCEA). Hydromorphone, morphine, diamorphine, and meperidine have all been administered for postoperative analgesia, all with good analgesic results (Table 7-1).

Intrathecal morphine administered in doses of 0.1 to 0.4 mg provides a duration of analgesia between 18 to 24 hours. Yang[3] recommends the optimal analgesic dose of 0.1mg of morphine, administered with hyperbaric bupivacaine. This dose is associated with a lower incidence of side effects and no greater pain relief than 0.25 mg. The most frequent side effects are pruritus (up to 60% incidence) and nausea and vomiting. Studies have not shown problems with hypoxemia or respiratory depression in this population. Side effects respond to therapy (Table 7-2). Therapy should be included as part of the postoperative orders to facilitate rapid treatment of side effects and greater patient satisfaction.

Optimal epidural morphine administration is with 2 to 5 mg for a duration of action of 18 to 24 hours. Again, lower doses were associated with a better side-effect profile. Longer durations of analgesia can be obtained with PCEA. Some studies suggest PCEA is associated with better analgesia and fewer side effects.[4] Longer duration of action can also be achieved with a sustained release preparation of morphine (DepoDur), administered as a single dose of 10 to 15 mg, which has a duration of analgesia of 24 to 48 hours.[5]

Meperidine, an opioid of intermediate lipid solubility with local anesthetic properties, has been added to spinal bupivacaine for intraoperative and early postoperative analgesia. Ten milligrams intrathecally provides approximately 4 hours of postoperative analgesia and facilitates the transition to other forms of postoperative analgesia. A 50-mg dose administered epidurally provides similar duration of analgesia and may be used to transition to other analgesics or as a bolus prior to beginning an epidural opioid/local anesthetic infusion or PCEA.

Short-acting opioids (e.g., fentanyl and sufentanil) are useful for postoperative analgesia as an epidural infusion or PCEA. Bolus doses are short acting, thus not efficacious for postoperative analgesia. Table 7-1 provides guidelines for administration.

Other opioids administered epidurally, although less frequently, include butorphanol, methadone, and hydromorphone. The agonists/antagonist butorphanol is associated with significant sedation, which makes its use in the obstetric population less popular than other

Table 7-1   Neuraxial Opioid Administration

Opioid	Spinal Bolus (with Intraoperative LA)	Epidural Bolus	PCEA/CI
Morphine	0.1 to 0.4 mg (Duration: 18 to 24 hr)	2 to 5 mg (Duration: 8 to 24 hr)	Loading: 1 to 3 mg CI (50 µg/mL) @ 6 to 12 mL/hr PCEA 2 to 4 mL q10 to 15 min 50 to 60 mL 4 hr lockout
Sustained Release Morphine (DepoDur)	Not recommended	10 to 15 mg (Duration: 24 to 48 hr)	Not recommended
Meperidine	10 mg (Duration: 4 hr)	50 mg (Duration: 4 hr)	Loading: 200 to 300 µg
Hydromorphone	Not recommended	200 to 300 µg (Duration: 8 to 12 hr)	CI (3 to 5 µg/mL) @ 6 to 12 mL/hr PCEA 2 to 4 ml q4 to 6 min 50 to 60 mL 4 hr lockout
Diamorphine	0.25 to 1 mg (Duration: 6 to 8 hr)	2 to 5 mg (Duration: 8 to 12 hr)	Not recommended
Sufentanil	15 µg (Duration: 2 hr)	25 µg (Duration: 2 to 3 hr)	Loading: 25 µg CI (2 µg/mL) @ 5 to 10 mL/hr PCEA 2 to 4 mL q4 to 6 min 40 to 50 mL 4 hr lockout
Fentanyl	10 µg (Duration: 2 hr)	50 µg (Duration: 2 to 3 hr)	Loading: 50 to 100 µg CI (5 µg/mL) @ 10 to 15 mL/hr PCEA 2 to 4 mL q4 to 6 min 40 to 50 mL 4 hr lockout
Butorphanol	Not recommended	2 to 4 mg (Duration: 4 to 6 hr)	Not recommended

CI, Continuous infusion; PCEA, patient-controlled analgesia.

Table 7-2 Treatment of Side Effects of Neuraxial Opioids

Pruritus (Incidence 40% to 60%)	
Naloxone	0.04 to 0.08 mg intravenous or 400 µg/L maintenance IVF
Nalbuphine	5 mg intravenous
Propofol	10 mg intravenous
Diphenhydramine	12.5 to 25 mg intravenous
Nausea and Vomiting (Incidence 25% to 30%)	
Cyclizine[10]	50 mg intravenous
*Metoclopramide	10 mg intravenous
*Ondansetron	4 mg intravenous
Acupressure	@ P6 point[11]
Dexamethasone	5 to 10 mg intravenous

IVF, Intravenous fluid.
*Author's preference

medications. Preservative-free methadone is difficult to obtain, thus limiting its use neuraxially. In our institution, hydromorphone is routinely used as a single epidural dose or as an epidural infusion/PCEA for postoperative analgesia. Advantages include a lower incidence of side effects than with morphine and analgesia with very low opioid/local anesthetic concentrations. Hydromorphone is more lipophilic than morphine, but less so than fentanyl; thus, it has less systemic effects than fentanyl.

Spinal administration, single-dose, and continuous epidural administration are all accepted therapies for neuraxial opioid administration. What, however, is the preferred route? Much of the decision is predicated on the anesthetic choice for cesarean delivery. Rapid onset and ease of administration are advantages for the use of spinal anesthesia for cesarean delivery, and thus, spinal opioids are used, with morphine as the "gold standard."[6] Others preferentially use CSE for cesarean delivery and epidural postoperative analgesia. Certainly, patients with epidural labor analgesia who then proceed to cesarean delivery will receive epidural postoperative analgesia. A single dose after which the catheter is removed is less labor intensive, although postoperative PCEA or continuous

epidural infusion may be used if a pain management service is available to manage the patient. Some patients do not wish to be encumbered by the infusion pump and thus request that a catheter technique not be used. Advantages of PCEA or continuous infusion epidural analgesia over bolus epidural or spinal opioid are reported by some as increased patient satisfaction and possibly improved analgesia.[7] In all cases, neuraxial analgesia will be followed by intravenous, intramuscular, or oral opioid therapy. In most cases, other analgesics will be coadministered as part of a multimodal analgesic plan.

Patient-Controlled Intravenous Analgesia (PCA)

PCA provides for patient autonomy in administration of pain medication. A programmable infusion pump allowing the patient to self-administer incremental intravenous doses of medication allows her to maintain analgesia independent of the hospital staff. The key to successful PCA therapy is achieving analgesia prior to beginning PCA therapy. This can be with an IV loading dose or with previously administered spinal opioid, as already discussed. Also important to successful therapy are prevention of and treatment of side effects. Therapies suggested for neuraxial opioid side effects are appropriate for PCA side effects as well. Table 7-3 provides dosing guidelines for IV-PCA opioids.

Maternal use of PCA carries the concern of neonatal effects secondary to excretion in the breast milk. Studies comparing meperidine and morphine[8] suggest greater neurobehavioral effects with meperidine. Thus, PCA with morphine or hydromorphone may be better choices in nursing mothers.

Intramuscular and Subcutaneous Opioid Administration

Intramuscular and subcutaneous administration typically do not provide the consistent level of analgesia obtained with intravenous or neuraxial administration of opioids. Unpredictable blood levels are seen when these routes of administration are used. If pro re nata (PRN) administration is used, this unpredictability can be still

Table 7-3 IV-PCA Opioids

Drug	Bolus Dose (mg)	Interval (min)	CI (mg/hr)	4 hr Lockout (mg)
Fentanyl	0.01 to 0.05	3 to 5	0.02	≤1
Meperidine	5 to 10	6	5 to 10	300
Morphine	1 to 1.5	6	1 to 2	30
Hydromorphone	0.1 to 0.2	6	0.1 to 0.5	5 to 10

CI, Continuous infusion.

greater. Advantages of this approach include ease of administration and low cost. In 2004, this would not be the preferred route of administration.

Oral Opioid Administration

Typically, following cesarean delivery oral intake is begun within 12 hours of surgery. Sips of fluids are often tolerated and requested by the patient in the Post Anesthesia Care Unit. Thus, the use of oral analgesics can be an effective, inexpensive, and labor-saving method of achieving postoperative analgesia. Oral therapy with opioid, nonopioid, or opioid/nonopioid combinations has been shown effective for analgesia when administered around the clock (RTC) with additional PRN dosing for breakthrough pain. Therapy is especially efficacious when combined with a single-dose neuraxial opioid. Table 7-4 lists commonly used medications.

Nonopioid Therapies

Nonopioid therapies are best used as part of multimodal therapy, although Jacobi[9] reports successful use of oral NSAIDs as the sole analgesic following cesarean delivery. Local anesthetic wound infiltration has been used to decrease opioid requirements. NSAIDs, administered parenterally or orally, have an additive or supra-

additive effect when administered with opioids. Clonidine, administered neuraxially or orally, has been used successfully as an adjunct to opioid therapy.

Nonopioids provide opioid sparing effects and result in lower incidences of opioid-related side effects; the site of action of these medications is not at the opioid receptor. The NSAIDs act to decrease inflammation and prostaglandin release, both centrally and at the periphery. Local anesthetics block pain transmission. Clonidine provides analgesia by its effect on the α-receptors. Table 7-5 provides dosage and site of administration for commonly used nonopioid therapies.

Table 7-4   Oral Opioid Therapy

Opioid	Dose	Interval (hr)
Morphine	10 to 30 mg	3 to 4
Oxycodone	5 to 10 mg	3 to 4
Percocet (Oxycodone/		
Acetaminophen)	*5/325 to 15/1000*	3 to 4
Hydromorphone	2 to 6 mg	3 to 4
Hydrocodone	5 to 15 mg	4 to 6
(Lortab) (Hydrocodone/		
Acetaminophen)	*5/500 to 15/1000*	4 to 6
Vicoprofen (Hydrocodone/		
Ibuprofen)	*7.5/200 to 15/400*	4 to 6

Table 7-5   Nonopioid Therapy

Drug	Doses	Route	Interval (hrs)	Comments
Ketorolac	15 mg	IV/IM	4 to 6	
Diclofenac	75 mg	IM	12	
	100 mg	PR	8	
Ibuprofen	400 mg	PO	3 to 4	• First dose 3 hr postoperative.
Clonidine	60 to 150 µg	Spinal	Single dose	• Multimodal therapy with spinal opioid provides 6 hr of analgesia.
				• Higher doses (alone or with opioid) have unacceptable incidences of side effects.
	150 to 300 µg	Epidural	Single dose	• In combination with opioids, clonidine will prolong the duration of analgesia.
	4 µg/kg	PO	Single dose	• Give 1 hr preoperatively.
Bupivacaine	Varies	Skin infiltration	—	• Can also be administered via a SQ infusion pump (On-Q).

Multimodal Therapy

Multimodal therapy allows for lower doses of all agents administered. Analgesia is comparable or better than that with single-drug therapy but with less dose-related side effects.

Following general anesthesia, a combination of local anesthetic wound infiltration with IV-PCA opioids and ketorolac administered intravenously every 6 hours will provide good analgesia for the first 24–36 hours postoperatively. By 36 hours, the patient can take oral therapy and thus can be administered oral opioids in combination with acetaminophen or ibuprofen, or either class of drugs can be administered alone (Fig. 7-1).

If a patient receives regional anesthesia for cesarean delivery, intrathecal morphine or the meperidine with or without clonidine should be administered (Fig. 7-2). If epidural anesthesia is used, morphine, sustained release morphine (DepoDur) (Fig. 7-3) or any agent listed in Table 7-1 can be administered (Figs. 7-4 and 7-5). Ketorolac may be used as an adjuvant. At 24 to 36 hours oral therapy can be administered as previously described.

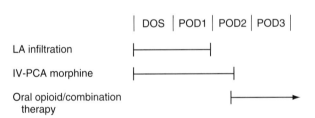

Figure 7-1 Pain management following general anesthesia. DOS, Day of surgery; POD, postoperative day.

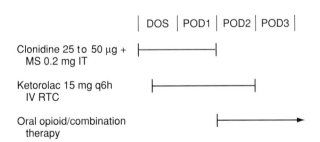

Figure 7-2 Multimodal therapy. DOS, Day of surgery; IT, intrathecal; POD, postoperative day; RTC, around the clock.

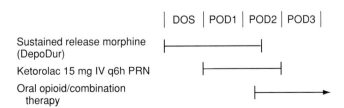

Figure 7-3 DepoDur multimodal therapy. DOS, Day of surgery; POD, postoperative day.

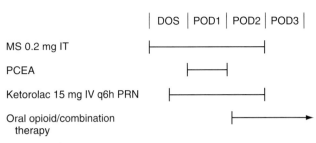

Figure 7-4 CSE–PCEA multimodal therapy. DOS, Day of surgery; IT, intrathecal; POD, postoperative day.

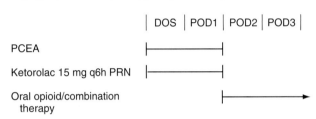

Figure 7-5 PCEA multimodal therapy. DOS, Day of surgery; POD, postoperative day.

PAIN THERAPIES AND OUTCOME

To date, we have been unable to demonstrate that any therapy, individual or multimodal, improves outcome following cesarean delivery. This may be due to the nature of the population—young patients who are relatively healthy in whom significant morbidity is rare. The choice for analgesia thus should be influenced by those factors previously discussed, which are unique to obstetric patients; that is, the need for excellent analgesia which does not impact maternal–neonatal interactions. Minimal encumbrance and minimal neonatal effects are important.

Regarding the cost of analgesic therapies in the United States, postoperative PCEA costs average $180 more than IV-PCA. This in turn is two to three times greater than the cost of oral therapy. Single-dose neuraxial therapy is less costly than either PCA therapy but more expensive than oral therapy. Extrapolating this expense to the millions of cesarean deliveries performed each year, it may be difficult to justify the higher expenses of more "complex" therapies without improved outcomes.

CLINICAL CAVEAT

PCEA should be reserved for patients with comorbid disease.

To conclude, in 2004, single-dose neuraxial opioid therapy with the coadministration of clonidine or a NSAID followed by oral NSAIDs and/or opioids provided state-of-the-art analgesia without encumbering the patient with anything more than an IV and without effect on the infant. Maternal side effects should be minor and readily treated. The cost of this care is not excessive. In circumstances in which the patient has significant comorbid disease, PCEA may be warranted.

CASE REPORT

A 26-year-old G_2P_1 patient is to undergo elective repeat cesarean delivery. Discuss management as relates to postoperative analgesia.

Spinal anesthesia is logical choice for intraoperative care.

For postoperative management, morphine 0.1 to 0.2 mg with or without 25 to 50 µg of clonidine can be administered with:

- Ketorolac 15 mg IV q6hr × 24 hrs
- Then oral Percocet or Vicoprofen beginning at approximately 24 hr
  If CSE or epidural is used for surgical anesthesia, postoperative management could be with 5 mg DepoDur administered epidurally followed by intravenous and oral therapy as above.

REFERENCES

1. Nikolajsen L, Sorensen HC, Jensent TS, et al: Chronic pain following caesarean section. Acta Anaesthesiol Scand 48:111-116, 2004.

2. Chen B, Kwan W, Lee C, et al: A national survey of obstetric post-anesthesia care in teaching hospitals (abstract). Anesth Analg 76:543, 1993.

3. Yang T, Breen TW, Archer D, et al: Comparison of 0.25 mg and 0.1 mg intrathecal morphine for analgesia after cesarean section. Can J Anesth 46(9):856-860, 1999.

4. Cooper DW, Ryall DM, McHardy F, et al: Patient controlled extradural analgesia with bupivacaine, fentanyl, or a mixture of both after caesarean section. Br J Anaesth 176:611-615, 1996.

5. Hartrick CT, Manvelian G: Sustained-release epidural morphine (Depodur): A review. Today's Therapeutic Trends 22(3):167-180, 2004.

6. Ayoub CM, Sinatra RS: Postoperative analgesia: Epidural and spinal techniques. In Chestnut DH (ed): Obstetric Anesthesia, Third edition. Philadelphia, Elsevier Mosby, 2004, pp 480-482.

7. Sinatra RS: Post cesarean analgesia. In Birnbach DJ, Gatt SP, Datta S (eds): Textbook of Obstetric Anesthesia. Philadelphia, Churchill Livingstone, 2000, p 325.

8. Wittels B, Glosten B, Faure EA, et al: Postcesarean analgesic with both epidural morphine and intravenous patient-controlled analgesia. Neurobehavioral outcomes among nursing neonates. Anesth Anal 85(3):600-606, 1997.

9. Jakobi P, Solt I, Tamir A, Zimmer EZ: Over the counter analgesic for post-cesarean pain. Am J OB Gyn 187(4):1066-1069, 2002.

SUGGESTED READING

Parker RK: Postoperative Analgesia: Systemic Techniques. In Chestnut DH (ed): Obstetric Anesthesia, Third edition. Philadelphia, Elsevier Mosby, 2004, pp 461.

CHAPTER 8

The High-Risk Obstetric Patient

REGINA Y. FRAGNETO

Anesthetic care of the high-risk obstetric patient is challenging and requires knowledge of both the pathophysiology of the condition causing the parturient to be classified as high risk as well as an understanding of how this condition is affected by pregnancy. High risk obstetric patients include women with pre-existing medical problems as well as pregnant women experiencing complications of the pregnancy itself. A myriad of conditions and complications will cause a pregnancy to be considered high risk. This chapter will address the problems most commonly encountered among high-risk parturients, including pre-eclampsia, obstetric hemorrhage, multiple gestation, diabetes, morbid obesity, and cardiac disease. Although some of these patients, such as those with cardiac disease, will nearly always be cared for at high-risk perinatal centers, anesthesiologists practicing at any facility that provides obstetric services will certainly encounter some of these high-risk parturients.

PRE-ECLAMPSIA

Definition and Risk Factors

Pre-eclampsia is defined as the development of hypertension and proteinuria after the twentieth week of gestation. Specifically, systolic blood pressure of at least 140 mm Hg or diastolic blood pressure of 90 mm Hg must be present as well as proteinuria of at least 300 mg in a 24-hour period. The presence of nondependent edema is no longer included in the definition of pre-eclampsia. Approximately 6% to 8% of all pregnancies are complicated by pre-eclampsia. The disease affects multiple organ systems and is the second leading cause of maternal mortality in the United States for pregnancies that result in a live birth. Its adverse effects on uteroplacental perfusion may also prove deleterious to the fetus. The majority of women with pre-eclampsia are nulliparous. Several other common risk factors for the disease are listed in Box 8-1.

Pre-eclampsia is defined as mild or severe. The presence of any of the conditions listed in Box 8-2 establishes the diagnosis of severe pre-eclampsia.

HELLP syndrome is a variant of pre-eclampsia in which *h*emolysis, *e*levated *l*iver enzymes, and *l*ow *p*latelets are present. Women with pre-eclampsia who develop grand mal seizures have eclampsia.

Obstetric Management

The definitive treatment for pre-eclampsia is delivery of the fetus. When a parturient is diagnosed with the disorder at term, delivery is indicated. When the disorder develops remote from term, the risks to the neonate of premature delivery must be weighed against the risks to mother and fetus of continuing the pregnancy. In women with mild disease remote from term, conservative therapy with bedrest and close monitoring is recommended until signs of maternal or fetal deterioration appear or gestational age of 37 weeks is reached. Traditionally, expeditious delivery of women with severe pre-eclampsia has been recommended, regardless of gestational age. However, expectant management beyond the 48 hours required to administer corticosteroids for fetal lung maturation is increasingly gaining acceptance in patients with severe pre-eclampsia remote from term. The use of high-dose dexamethasone

---

Box 8-1   Common Risk Factors for Preeclampsia

Nulliparity
African-American race
Age >40 years
Pre-eclampsia with previous pregnancy
Chronic hypertension
Diabetes
Multiple gestation
Lupus
Chronic renal disease
Obesity

Box 8-2   Criteria for Severe Pre-eclampsia

Systolic blood pressure of at least 160 mm Hg or diastolic blood pressure at least 110 mm Hg on two occasions at least 6 hours apart
Proteinuria of at least 5 g in a 24-hr period
Oliguria
Pulmonary edema
Impaired liver function
Visual or cerebral disturbances
Epigastric or right upper quadrant pain
Thrombocytopenia
Intrauterine growth restriction

---

may also stabilize and improve laboratory abnormalities in patients with HELLP syndrome. However, if the maternal or fetal status deteriorates at any time during the course of expectant management, delivery must be expedited.

CLINICAL CAVEAT: EXPECTANT MANAGEMENT OF SEVERE PRE-ECLAMPSIA REMOTE FROM TERM

- Has been shown to prolong pregnancy by 2 weeks
- Should only be utilized in patients with stable disease
- Decreases neonatal complications
- No apparent increased maternal morbidity or mortality
- Requires intensive monitoring of mother and fetus in hospital with adequate blood pressure control
- High-dose dexamethasone (10 mg IV q12hr) may improve laboratory abnormalities and accelerate postpartum recovery in patients with HELLP syndrome.

Magnesium sulfate is administered to pre-eclamptic parturients for seizure prophylaxis. It exerts its anticonvulsant effect centrally via N-methyl-D-aspartate (NMDA) receptors. Recent studies have demonstrated that it is more effective in preventing seizures than other drugs, including phenytoin and diazepam. Usually, an intravenous bolus of 4-g magnesium sulfate is administered, followed by a continuous infusion of 1 to 2 g/hr. The goal of therapy is to achieve a magnesium concentration of 4 to 6 mEq/L. While magnesium sulfate is administered to prevent seizures, it does produce other beneficial effects. A sustained decrease in systemic vascular resistance and an increase in cardiac index occur in pre-eclamptic patients receiving magnesium sulfate. This can lead to improved uteroplacental perfusion.

The administration of magnesium sulfate is not without risk. A major concern is the development of magnesium toxicity, especially in patients with oliguria. The clinical signs of toxicity with corresponding serum magnesium concentrations are listed in Table 8-1. Careful monitoring of patients for the continued presence of

Table 8-1	Signs of Magnesium Toxicity
Clinical Sign	**Magnesium Level**
Loss of deep tendon reflexes	10 mEq/L
Respiratory depression	12 to 15 mEq/L
Respiratory arrest	15 mEq/L
Cardiac arrest	20 to 25 mEq/L

deep tendon reflexes will help prevent this complication. If toxicity is suspected, the magnesium sulfate infusion should be discontinued, and the patient should receive calcium gluconate 1 g or calcium chloride 300 mg intravenously.

Peripherally, magnesium effects changes at the neuromuscular junction, resulting in abnormal neuromuscular function. It causes a decrease in motor endplate sensitivity to acetylcholine and a decrease in the release of acetylcholine at the neuromuscular junction. Sensitivity to nondepolarizing and depolarizing muscle relaxants is enhanced. Magnesium sulfate is also used for tocolysis of labor and does affect uterine activity. Although studies have found that it does not prolong labor in pre-eclamptic parturients, increased doses of oxytocin may be required for induction of labor, and these patients may be at increased risk for uterine atony in the postpartum period.

Parturients with severe hypertension will require antihypertensive therapy. Most obstetricians recommend treatment for systolic blood pressure >160 to 170 mm Hg or diastolic blood pressure >105 to 110 mm Hg. The aim of therapy is to maintain systolic blood pressure between 140 and 155 mm Hg and diastolic blood pressure between 90 and 105 mm Hg. Greater reductions in blood pressure could compromise uteroplacental perfusion, leading to a nonreassuring fetal status. Intravenous hydralazine and labetalol are the most common antihypertensive agents used in pre-eclamptic patients. The recommended dose of hydralazine is 5 to 10 mg every 20 minutes as needed, up to a cumulative dose of 30 mg. The recommended initial dose of labetalol is 10 mg. It has a faster onset of action than hydralazine and can be repeated every 10 minutes. If the initial dose does not achieve the desired blood pressure, each subsequent dose can be increased up to a dose of 40 mg. The maximum cumulative dose of labetalol is 300 mg. Nifedipine, a calcium-channel blocker, is also an effective antihypertensive drug in pre-eclampsia. Its recommended dose is 10 to 20 mg orally every 30 minutes, with a cumulative dose of 50 mg. Although hydralazine has been the most popular antihypertensive drug of obstetricians in the past, a recent meta-analysis suggested that labetalol and nifedipine are as effective as hydralazine with fewer side effects.

In patients with severe refractory hypertension, continuous infusion of an antihypertensive drug may be required. Blood pressure monitoring with an intra-arterial catheter is indicated in such situations. Labetalol can be administered as a continuous infusion, beginning with a dose of 40 mg/hr. Nitroglycerin and sodium nitroprusside are also useful for the management of severe hypertension, especially when only short-term treatment is required. Both drugs can be administered at an initial dose of 0.5 μg/kg/min and then titrated until a satisfactory response is achieved. Placental transfer of sodium nitroprusside does occur, but fetal cyanide toxicity is unlikely if the drug is used at low doses for a short time. The drug is not a good choice in situations in which a high-dose infusion for several hours is needed to manage hypertension.

Anesthetic Management

A thorough preanesthetic evaluation of the pre-eclamptic parturient is necessary before the anesthesiologist can develop an appropriate anesthetic plan. On physical examination, particular attention should be paid to evaluation of the patient's airway. Signs of possible severe upper airway edema, such as the presence of facial edema or stridor, may indicate increased difficulty with tracheal intubation. Attention should also be paid to the fluid balance of the patient. Many pre-eclamptic patients are hypovolemic and prone to hypotension during the administration of neuraxial anesthesia. However, these patients are also at increased risk for developing pulmonary edema if excessive fluids are administered, so maintaining appropriate fluid balance can be challenging. The anesthesiologist must look for signs that will help assess the patient's fluid status and determine whether invasive monitoring with a central venous pressure (CVP) or pulmonary artery catheter is needed. Although most pre-eclamptic patients do not require invasive monitoring, pulmonary edema or oliguria unresponsive to an adequate fluid challenge are conditions that may warrant the use of central hemodynamic monitoring.

Some controversy exists about whether a CVP or pulmonary artery catheter should be utilized once the decision has been made that central monitoring is required. Significantly more information about the patient's hemodynamic status, including systemic vacular resistance and cardiac output, can be obtained from a pulmonary artery catheter compared to a CVP catheter. This additional information can assist the anesthesiologist in achieving more optimal volume resuscitation and pharmacologic therapy with vasoactive agents. As a result, many anesthesiologists choose to use a pulmonary artery catheter. However, the risks of pulmonary artery catheter placement are greater than the risks of CVP catheter insertion, so the risks and benefits for each patient must be considered when choosing which type of central monitoring to utilize.

Assessment of laboratory values is another important aspect of the preanesthetic evaluation. An elevated hematocrit suggests hemoconcentration and hypovolemia in a patient with pre-eclampsia. The most important component of the complete blood count, however, is the platelet count. Thrombocytopenia occurs in at least 15% of women with pre-eclampsia, so it is essential that a platelet count be obtained before proceeding with regional anesthesia. In patients with a platelet count <100,000/mm^3, the risks of epidural hematoma must be considered along with the benefits of epidural anesthesia when deciding whether to proceed with a neuraxial technique. Tests that evaluate platelet function might assist the anesthesiologist in making this decision. Thromboelastography measures all phases of coagulation, and the maximum amplitude of the trace is affected by platelet function. Investigators have used this laboratory test to assess coagulation in pre-eclamptic patients and suggest it may be useful for evaluating platelet function in patients with thrombocytopenia. The PFA-100 platelet function analyzer test measures global platelet function. This test gives reproducible results within minutes and is easy to perform. Initial studies in pre-eclamptic patients found that platelet function remains normal in many patients with platelet counts between 70,000 and 100,000/mm^3. This appears to support the practice of many obstetric anesthesiologists who do utilize neuraxial anesthesia in pre-eclamptic patients with platelet counts within this range. The bleeding time is no longer considered a reliable test to measure platelet function or risk of bleeding.

Routine measurement of prothrombin time (PT) and activated partial thromboplastin time (PTT) is not necessary in most patients because disseminated intravascular coagulation is rare in pre-eclampsia. In fact, it is highly unlikely that PT or PTT will be prolonged in parturients with platelet counts >100,000/mm^3. In patients with thrombocytopenia or abnormal liver function tests, it is recommended to document normal PT and PTT before proceeding with regional anesthesia.

Blood urea nitrogen (BUN) and creatinine concentrations should be measured to determine whether renal dysfunction is present. Liver function tests are also essential in the evaluation of pre-eclampsia. Finally, if the patient is complaining of shortness of breath or has findings on physical examination suggestive of pulmonary edema, an arterial blood gas and chest x-ray should be obtained.

Labor Analgesia
Adequate labor analgesia is an important component in the care of pre-eclamptic women. Epidural analgesia is considered the preferred technique by many anesthesiologists if contraindications don't exist. Compared to parenteral medications, epidural analgesia provides superior pain relief. Many other advantages also exist. Uncontrolled labor pain will increase endogenous maternal catecholamine levels. Because pre-eclamptic patients exhibit an exaggerated response to vasopressors, these increased levels of catecholamines can exacerbate hypertension. Epidural analgesia reduces maternal catecholamine levels and can help facilitate blood pressure control during labor. Pre-eclampsia compromises uteroplacental perfusion because of the disease's vasospastic effects, but Doppler studies have documented improved intervillous blood flow when epidural analgesia is administered for labor pain management in severe pre-eclamptic patients. This improved uteroplacental perfusion may benefit the fetus during the stress of labor. Pre-eclamptic patients are also at increased risk for emergency cesarean delivery compared to healthy parturients. Confirmation of a functioning epidural catheter placed early in labor to provide analgesia will facilitate the use of epidural anesthesia in such an emergency situation and avoid the risks associated with general anesthesia in pre-eclamptic patients, including severe hypertension during laryngoscopy and difficult intubation that may be exacerbated by increased airway edema.

It is important to avoid hypotension associated with epidural analgesia because this could worsen the status of a fetus that may already be affected by the compromised uteroplacental perfusion that characterizes pre-eclampsia. Adequate intravenous hydration with crystalloid is necessary although it may be a challenge to determine how much volume to administer. The majority of pre-eclamptic parturients are hypovolemic and should receive at least 500 to 1000 mL of crystalloid before administration of epidural local anesthetics. However, the volume of intravenous prehydration should be decreased in patients with signs of overhydration or pulmonary edema, and central hemodynamic monitoring may be needed to guide appropriate fluid management in these patients. The same local anesthetic drugs and doses used to initiate and maintain epidural analgesia in healthy parturients can be used in pre-eclamptic parturients, but the block should be established slowly and blood pressure monitored at intervals of 1 to 3 minutes during drug administration to avoid hypotension.

If hypotension does occur, prompt treatment is needed. A drop in blood pressure that is 20% or greater below the patient's baseline requires treatment. An additional bolus of crystalloid should be infused, and administration of a vasopressor should be considered. Although ephedrine has traditionally been the vasopressor of choice to treat hypotension in obstetric anesthesia, a recent meta-analysis that compared ephedrine and phenylephrine for the treatment of hypotension found that umbilical artery pH was higher in neonates whose mothers received phenylephrine, suggesting the preferred use of ephedrine is not supported by the available data. However, all of the studies that have compared ephedrine and phenylephrine included only healthy parturients. No data are available about the use of phenylephrine in pre-eclamptic women. Therefore, it remains logical to avoid a pure α-agonist such as phenylephrine in patients with pre-eclampsia, and ephedrine remains the vasopressor of choice. Because patients with pre-eclampsia do exhibit increased sensitivity to vasopressors, the initial dose of ephedrine should not exceed 5 mg to avoid a rebound hypertensive response. Further doses should be titrated to effect.

Combined spinal-epidural (CSE) analgesia is another popular labor analgesia technique that provides rapid and superior pain relief. The initial analgesia is produced by an intrathecal opioid that does not produce a sympathectomy, thus decreasing the risk of hypotension compared to epidural analgesia. However, until the initial intrathecal analgesia has dissipated, the epidural catheter remains unproven. If emergency cesarean delivery were required during this interval, the anesthesiologist could be faced with a nonfunctioning catheter, thus necessitating the induction of general anesthesia. Therefore, while CSE analgesia may be a reasonable technique to use in a patient with mild pre-eclampsia and a reassuring fetal heart rate tracing, some prefer epidural analgesia in patients with severe pre-eclampsia.

Anesthesia for Cesarean Delivery

Many factors must be considered when deciding on the type of anesthesia to use for cesarean delivery. Assessment of the mother's airway, coagulation, and hemodynamic status must occur. Any evidence of fetal compromise and the reason for and urgency of surgery must also be evaluated as the anesthesiologist develops a plan for the anesthetic management of a pre-eclamptic patient undergoing cesarean delivery. Epidural anesthesia is the preferred anesthetic for nonurgent delivery unless a severe coagulopathy is present. If an epidural catheter is already in place for labor, an attempt to utilize it for surgery should be made even in an emergent situation, unless the patient exhibits signs of hemodynamic instability. Various advantages are associated with the use of epidural anesthesia for cesarean delivery. The anesthetic level required for surgery (T4–T6) can be obtained slowly. This will decrease the likelihood of hypotension, which might not be tolerated well by a fetus already affected by the compromised uteroplacental perfusion of pre-eclampsia. Compared to general anesthesia, it blunts the hemodynamic and neuroendocrine stress responses to surgery in patients with severe pre-eclampsia. Finally, it avoids the risks of general anesthesia that include not only the risks of aspiration and difficult intubation present in all parturients but also the risk of severe hypertension and associated cerebral hemorrhage.

In patients with severe pre-eclampsia, it is advisable to avoid an epidural test dose containing epinephrine because a significant rise in blood pressure could occur if the epidural catheter were intravascular. Instead, a dose of plain local anesthetic can be administered and symptoms of intravascular injection elicited from the patient. Once intravascular placement of the catheter has been ruled out, it is preferable to slowly administer 2% lidocaine with epinephrine 1:200,000 to achieve anesthesia adequate for surgery. This provides a dense block for surgery, and the amount of epinephrine that is absorbed systemically from the epidural space results in a β-adrenergic effect (e.g., vasodilation). Because one advantage of epidural anesthesia is the ability to slowly raise the anesthetic level, adding sodium bicarbonate to the local anesthetic solution should be avoided in the setting of nonurgent cesarean delivery. If epidural anesthesia is being utilized for an urgent cesarean delivery with a nonreassuring fetal heart rate pattern, 3% 2-chloroprocaine should be used to establish surgical anesthesia. The more rapid onset of this drug will expedite delivery, and its rapid maternal metabolism avoids the possible "ion trapping" of local anesthesia in an acidotic fetus that may occur with other agents, such as lidocaine and bupivacaine.

The use of spinal anesthesia for cesarean delivery in pre-eclamptic patients has previously been discouraged because of concerns that marked hypotension may occur with the rapid onset of sympathectomy. However, some investigators have recently questioned the validity of this clinical teaching. Many anesthesiologists now consider spinal anesthesia a reasonable choice in patients with mild pre-eclampsia although its use in patients with severe disease remains quite controversial.

While general anesthesia for cesarean delivery should be avoided in pre-eclamptic parturients whenever possible, some clinical circumstances will require its use. Sustained fetal bradycardia, clinical signs of coagulopathy, obstetric hemorrhage secondary to placental abruption, and patient refusal of regional anesthesia are situations that may require general anesthesia. Careful evaluation of the patient's airway is mandatory before proceeding with induction of general anesthesia. If examination suggests a high probability that intubation will be difficult, awake fiber-optic intubation should be accomplished before inducing general anesthesia. Otherwise, the increased risk of aspiration in pregnancy requires that aspiration prophylaxis be administered preoperatively and a rapid sequence induction with application of cricoid pressure be utilized. All patients should receive sodium citrate, and if time allows, intravenous metoclopramide and an H_2-receptor antagonist should

CURRENT CONTROVERSIES: SPINAL ANESTHESIA FOR CESAREAN DELIVERY IN PATIENTS WITH SEVERE PRE-ECLAMPSIA

- Conventional teaching has been to avoid spinal anesthesia because it may precipitate profound hypotension secondary to the rapid onset of sympathetic blockade. This is more likely to occur in patients with severe pre-eclampsia because they often have a constricted intravascular volume.
- A prospective study that compared epidural, spinal, and general anesthesia and a retrospective study that compared epidural and spinal anesthesia in severely pre-eclamptic women did not find a difference in hypotension or neonatal outcome among the anesthetic techniques.
- A recent prospective study that compared spinal and general anesthesia in pre-eclamptic patients with a nonreassuring fetal heart rate tracing found a greater umbilical artery base deficit among women who received spinal anesthesia. However, the mean base deficit in the spinal group was within the range reported after uncomplicated vaginal delivery.
- Based on the data currently available, the use of spinal anesthesia in urgent situations is preferred because it avoids the maternal risks of general anesthesia without obvious compromise to the fetus.
- Until more data become available, epidural anesthesia should probably remain the preferred anesthetic technique for nonurgent cesarean delivery.

DRUG INTERACTION: MAGNESIUM SULFATE AND NEUROMUSCULAR BLOCKING AGENTS

- Magnesium sulfate alters the neuromuscular junction:
  - Decreases motor endplate sensitivity to acetylcholine.
  - Decreases release of acetylcholine at the neuromuscular junction.
  - Enhances sensitivity to all neuromuscular blocking agents, especially nondepolarizing drugs.
- Do not decrease dose of succinylcholine used during rapid sequence induction to ensure optimal intubating conditions.
- Administer small, incremental doses of nondepolarizing agent during surgery only if necessary.
- Closely monitor response with peripheral nerve stimulator.

be administered. Sodium thiopental and succinylcholine are the preferred induction drugs.

Pre-eclamptic patients are at risk for severe hypertension during laryngoscopy and emergence from general anesthesia, which could lead to intracerebral hemorrhage, a leading cause of death due to pre-eclampsia. Therefore, prevention and prompt control of hypertension are important components in the management of patients undergoing general anesthesia for cesarean delivery. If delivery is nonemergent, placement of an intra-arterial catheter before anesthesia induction is advisable in patients with severe pre-eclampsia. Preinduction administration of intravenous labetalol has been shown to attenuate the hypertensive response to laryngoscopy. In patients with severe disease, an antihypertensive drug with rapid onset that is easily titrated to effect and can be administered as a continuous infusion should be immediately available to treat severe hypertension that might occur despite preventive measures. Nitroglycerin and sodium nitroprusside are both effective for the management of refractory hypertension during general anesthesia.

Maintenance of an adequate depth of general anesthesia is essential to not only prevent patient awareness but to also prevent hypertension caused by "light" anesthesia. Careful attention should be paid to the interaction between magnesium sulfate and neuromuscular blocking agents.

OBSTETRIC HEMORRHAGE

Obstetric hemorrhage is a serious complication of pregnancy that contributes significantly to maternal and perinatal morbidity and mortality. Placenta previa, abruptio placenta, and uterine rupture are the most important causes of antepartum bleeding. Uterine atony is the most common cause of postpartum hemorrhage. The Centers for Disease Control's most recent surveillance data from 1991 to 1999 reported that hemorrhage was the second leading cause of all pregnancy-related maternal deaths in the United States. Among pregnancies in which the fetus also died, hemorrhage was the leading cause of maternal death. In developing countries, obstetric hemorrhage is an even greater problem. A systematic review determined that 50% of maternal postpartum deaths in developing countries resulted from hemorrhage. Obstetric hemorrhage also contributes significantly to maternal morbidity and is a common reason for transfer of obstetric patients to critical care units.

Antepartum hemorrhage also poses risks to the fetus and neonate, accounting for a significant portion of perinatal morbidity and mortality. Poor outcomes and death occur both from the effects of compromised uteroplacental perfusion associated with hemorrhage and the complications of prematurity when maternal hemorrhage necessitates early delivery. Antepartum hemorrhage was reported as the third leading cause of delivery of very low-birth-weight infants (<1500 g). In these infants, the risks of death and disability are increased when hemorrhage is the obstetric factor precipitating premature delivery. The cause of hemorrhage is also an important factor affecting perinatal mortality rates. Death rates are significantly higher for infants whose mothers had abruptio placenta compared to placenta previa.

Because of the physiologic changes of pregnancy, including increased blood volume, pregnant patients tolerate mild to moderate hemorrhage with little change in vital signs. This contributes to an underestimation of blood loss by anesthesiologists and likely contributes to the maternal morbidity and mortality caused by obstetric hemorrhage. Classification of hemorrhage in parturients can help anesthesiologists more accurately estimate blood loss and provide adequate resuscitation.

CLINICAL CAVEAT: CLASSIFICATION OF OBSTETRIC HEMORRHAGE

Class 1:
- Blood loss approximately 15% of blood volume (900 mL)
- No clinical signs or symptoms of significant volume deficit

Class 2:
- Blood loss 20% to 25% of blood volume (1200 to 1500 mL)
- Clinical signs: Increased heart rate, orthostatic hypotension, narrowed pulse pressure, prolonged capillary refill times

Class 3:
- Blood loss 30% to 35% of blood volume (1800 to 2000 mL)
- Clinical signs: Hypotension, marked tachycardia, cold and clammy skin

Class 4:
- Blood loss 40% or greater of blood volume
- Clinical signs: Profound shock that requires immediate and aggressive resuscitation

---

Abruptio Placenta

Abruptio placenta is one of the two leading causes of serious antepartum hemorrhage. Placental abruption is the premature separation of a normally implanted placenta from the decidua basalis. Bleeding occurs from the torn decidual vessels, causing formation of a retroplacental hematoma. The expanding hematoma often causes further separation of the placenta. Because the uterus is distended by the fetus, the normal hemostatic mechanism within the uterus (e.g., contraction of the uterus compressing the torn decidual vessels) is ineffective, and hemorrhage results.

Abruptio placenta occurs in approximately 0.6% to 1% of all pregnancies. Several risk factors exist for placental abruption and are listed in Box 8-3.

The signs and symptoms of abruption are listed in Box 8-4. Not all symptoms will be present in every

---

Box 8-3   Risk Factors for Abruptio Placenta

Hypertension (chronic or pre-eclampsia)
Premature rupture of membranes
Abdominal trauma
Cigarette smoking
Cocaine use
Advanced maternal age
Advanced parity
Previous abruption

Box 8-4   Signs and Symptoms of Placental Abruption

Vaginal bleeding
Abdominal pain
Uterine tenderness
Uterine hypertonus
Fetal distress
Fetal demise

---

patient. In addition, inspection of the amount of vaginal bleeding may lead to underestimation of the actual degree of hemorrhage because substantial blood loss can be concealed within the uterus, especially when a large retroplacental hematoma is present. Presence of such a hematoma can sometimes be identified by ultrasound examination.

Placental abruption places the fetus at significant risk. Separation of the placenta decreases the surface area available for oxygen delivery to the fetus, and fetal hypoxia may result. The incidence of both fetal distress and fetal demise are greater with abruptio placenta than with placenta previa, the other leading cause of antepartum hemorrhage. Recent data reported a perinatal mortality rate of 119 per 1000 births when abruption was present compared with 8 per 1000 among all other births. Although a significant portion of the perinatal deaths occurring with abruptio placenta are related to preterm delivery, babies born at term are also at high risk. The mortality rate was 25-fold higher for babies born at term with normal birth weights if the pregnancy was complicated by abruption.

Abruptio placenta also places the mother at significant risk. Maternal complications associated with placental abruption include disseminated intravascular coagulation (DIC), acute renal failure, and uterine atony that may lead to postpartum hemorrhage. Abruptio placenta is the most common cause of DIC in parturients. It occurs in approximately 10% of patients and occurs with greater frequency when fetal distress or fetal demise is present.

Anesthetic Management

Initial management of the parturient with abruptio placenta includes the establishment of large-bore venous access and fluid resuscitation with a non-dextrose-containing crystalloid solution to achieve maternal hemodynamic stability. Fetal heart rate monitoring must be initiated to determine fetal status. The anesthesiologist should promptly evaluate any patient who presents to the labor and delivery unit with vaginal bleeding. Emphasis should be placed on the airway examination. A brief medical history, including coexisting diseases, problems with previous anesthetics, drug allergies, current medications, and recent illicit drug use, should be quickly obtained. The availability of blood products also needs to be confirmed.

Further anesthetic management will depend on the obstetric plan. In situations in which a mild abruption is suspected and there is no evidence of severe hemorrhage or nonreassuring fetal status, the obstetrician may decide to attempt labor induction and vaginal delivery. If the patient has normal coagulation studies and no evidence of hypovolemia, epidural analgesia can be offered. In fact, it may be advisable to encourage the initiation of epidural analgesia in such a situation because this patient is at risk for further separation of the placenta, which could then require emergency cesarean delivery due to fetal hypoxia. Once epidural analgesia is established in a patient with abruptio placenta, however, one must be vigilant for signs of additional blood loss. Should acute hemorrhage occur, the anesthesiologist must quickly begin aggressive fluid resuscitation and consider the use of vasopressors, such as ephedrine or phenylephrine, because the sympathectomy produced by epidural analgesia could prevent the normal physiologic compensations for hypovolemia.

In cases of severe placental abruption, maternal hemorrhage or deteriorating fetal status will preclude an attempt at vaginal delivery, and emergency cesarean delivery will be required. In most cases, general anesthesia will be the technique of choice. Reasons to avoid regional anesthesia in such a situation include a time factor (general anesthesia can usually be achieved more quickly than epidural or spinal anesthesia), concern about sympathectomy-induced hemodynamic instability in a hypovolemic patient, and risk of spinal hematoma formation in a patient with possible DIC. If the patient is already receiving epidural analgesia for labor when emergency cesarean delivery becomes necessary, it is acceptable to utilize epidural anesthesia for cesarean delivery if maternal hemorrhage is not severe and the patient has remained hemodynamically stable. Otherwise, general anesthesia is recommended.

After the patient has received a nonparticulate antacid, rapid sequence induction of general anesthesia should proceed. Because significant hemorrhage is probable in a parturient requiring emergency delivery secondary to abruptio placenta, etomidate or ketamine are preferred as induction agents compared to thiopental or propofol because they are less likely to produce hypotension. However, if uterine hypertonus is present, ketamine should be avoided because large doses can increase uterine tone further and possibly jeopardize uteroplacental perfusion.

Maintenance of general anesthesia will depend largely on the hemodynamic status of the patient. Until delivery of the infant, FiO_2 of at least 50% should be administered. Nitrous oxide (N_2O) and a volatile anesthetic such as isoflurane or desflurane can be used in the relatively stable patient. In the parturient experiencing uterine hypertonus, initial use of a volatile agent may be beneficial by producing some decrease in uterine tone. Once delivery has been accomplished, the concentration of N_2O can be increased, and opioids can be administered. The concentration of the volatile agent should be decreased after delivery to ensure adequate uterine tone. This is especially important in parturients with abruptio placenta because they are at increased risk for developing uterine atony.

Aggressive fluid resuscitation is another important component of the anesthetic management of emergency cesarean delivery for abruptio placenta. The availability of blood products must be confirmed. If cross-matched blood cannot be quickly obtained, the use of type-specific or O-negative blood may be necessary. In addition to packed red blood cells, the patient with DIC will require other blood components, including fresh frozen plasma, cryoprecipitate, and platelets.

Placenta Previa

Placenta previa is the other leading cause of serious antepartum hemorrhage. Placenta previa occurs when the placenta implants over the cervical os. Placenta previa is classified as total, partial, or marginal (Fig. 8-1). A total, or complete, placenta previa completely covers the cervical os whereas a partial previa covers only part of the cervical os. When the placenta lies close to but does not cover the cervical os, it is considered a marginal previa.

The incidence of placenta previa is approximately 1 in 200 births. The incidence is higher in twin gestations than in singleton pregnancies. The greatest risk factor for placenta previa is previous cesarean delivery. The risk increases as the number of previous cesarean deliveries increases. Other risk factors that have been identified are advanced maternal age, multiparity, previous placenta previa, and other uterine surgeries, including abortions. Unlike abruptio placenta, maternal mortality resulting from placenta previa is rare. The perinatal mortality rate is also markedly lower with placenta previa compared to placental abruption. A recent study reported 12 perinatal deaths per 1000 births, which is 10-fold lower than the rate reported for abruptio placenta.

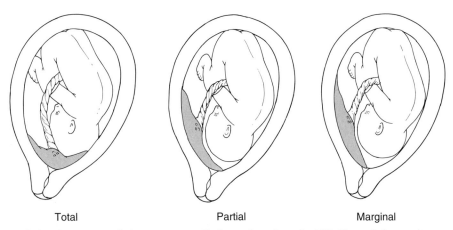

Total   Partial   Marginal

Figure 8-1 Three types of placenta previa. (Redrawn from Benedetti TJ: Obstetric hemorrhage. In Gabbe SG, Niebyl J, Simpson JL [eds]: Obstetrics: Normal and Problem Pregnancies, Fourth edition. Philadelphia, Churchill Livingstone, 2002, p 515.)

The typical presentation for placenta previa is painless vaginal bleeding during the second or third trimester. The first bleeding episode usually stops spontaneously without causing hemodynamic or fetal compromise. The diagnosis is determined by ultrasound examination. Whereas a double set-up vaginal examination was sometimes required to confirm the diagnosis in the past, improved ultrasonographic technology has nearly eliminated the need to perform this high-risk procedure.

Anesthetic Management

Once the diagnosis of placenta previa has been established, the anesthesiologist must determine the obstetric management plan so care of the parturient can be coordinated appropriately. Gestational age, maternal and fetal condition, amount of bleeding, and type of placenta previa are all factors that will be considered when the obstetrician decides on the timing and mode of delivery. If the fetus is premature and bleeding has stopped, expectant management is usually chosen to allow time for fetal maturation. Throughout the patient's hospitalization, intravenous access and a valid type and screen should be maintained. Continuous availability of cross-matched blood is not necessary for most patients, however. When either fetal lung maturation has been achieved or the pregnancy has reached 37 weeks gestation, delivery of the fetus will proceed. When a patient experiences ongoing hemorrhage, or there is evidence of maternal instability or nonreassuring fetal status, urgent cesarean delivery will be required regardless of gestational age. All parturients with a total or partial placenta previa undergo cesarean delivery because massive hemorrhage would occur with vaginal delivery. In some cases, the obstetrician will attempt a vaginal delivery when a marginal placenta previa is present. The use of epidural analgesia is recommended in this situation, and the anesthesiologist must be prepared for the possibility of hemorrhage and the need for an emergent cesarean delivery.

Anesthetic management of the patient undergoing cesarean delivery will depend on maternal and fetal status and the urgency with which surgery must proceed. In parturients who have not experienced recent bleeding and are undergoing elective delivery, regional anesthesia is preferred for the same reasons it is preferred in all pregnant women. Either epidural or spinal anesthesia is acceptable for elective cesarean delivery in the patient with placenta previa. The type and dose of local anesthesia should be chosen in the same manner as they are chosen for any nonurgent cesarean delivery. These patients are at higher risk for intraoperative bleeding and cesarean hysterectomy than other parturients undergoing elective cesarean delivery. Therefore, it is essential to establish reliable large-bore intravenous access. The anesthesiologist should also consider having cross-matched blood immediately available before proceeding with surgery.

If maternal hemorrhage or nonreassuring fetal status necessitates emergency cesarean delivery in a parturient with placenta previa, general anesthesia is usually the anesthetic technique of choice. Induction and maintenance of anesthesia are similar to those described for emergency delivery with abruptio placenta. After administration of a nonparticulate antacid (Bicitra), rapid sequence induction is performed. Ketamine and etomidate are the preferred induction agents in the setting of maternal hemorrhage because they are less likely than other induction drugs to produce adverse hemodynamic effects in a hypovolemic patient. Unlike patients with abruptio placenta, there are no concerns about the use of ketamine in these patients because there is no association between placenta previa and uterine hypertonus. Succinylcholine is the muscle relaxant of choice during induction. Maintenance of general anesthesia will be determined by the hemodynamic status of the mother, and generally consists of N_2O and a volatile anesthetic before delivery with the addition of opioids after delivery of the fetus.

The current sophistication of obstetric ultrasonography available in the United States has nearly eliminated the need for a double set-up cervical examination to confirm the diagnosis of placenta previa. There may still be the rare situation where this examination is required, however. The anesthesiologist must be prepared to handle massive hemorrhage as well as the need to proceed immediately with cesarean delivery if the vaginal examination determines the presence of a placenta previa. Before the obstetrician is allowed to perform the cervical examination, all preparations necessary to proceed with emergency cesarean delivery must be completed. Aspiration prophylaxis should be administered. Two large-bore intravenous catheters should be inserted and maternal monitors must be applied. Blood needs to be available in the operating room. All equipment and drugs for rapid-sequence induction of general anesthesia must be ready and preoxygenation of the patient accomplished.

Placenta Accreta

Placenta accreta is defined as a placenta that is abnormally adherent to the myometrium. When the obstetrician attempts to remove the placenta after delivery, massive hemorrhage ensues. Three types of abnormal placentation exist, with placenta accreta occurring most frequently (Fig. 8-2). Placenta accreta describes a placenta that is adherent to the myometrium without invading it. In placenta increta, the placenta actually invades the myometrium. The most serious abnormal placentation, placenta percreta, invades all the way through to the uterine serosa and can also extend into other pelvic structures, such as the bladder.

Over the past 50 years, the incidence of placenta accreta has increased 10-fold. It is still a relatively rare obstetric complication, occurring in approximately one in every 2500 deliveries. Certain women, however, are at significantly increased risk for developing placenta accreta. Among parturients with placenta previa, an incidence of 5% to 9% has been reported. The risk increases even further if a patient with placenta previa has a history of previous cesarean delivery with the risk of accreta increasing as the number of previous cesarean deliveries increases. The location of the placenta previa also affects risk. Among women with anterior or central placenta previa who have had at least two cesarean deliveries, the risk of developing placenta accreta is almost 40%.

Physicians should have a high index of suspicion for placenta accreta when a parturient presents with placenta previa and a history of previous cesarean delivery. Both magnetic resonance imaging and ultrasound with color flow mapping have successfully identified placenta accreta antenatally. However, the predictive value for both tests is poor. As a result, antenatal diagnosis is difficult, and often the diagnosis is made at the time of surgery, especially in patients without placenta previa.

Placenta accreta requires obstetric hysterectomy in the majority of cases. In fact, it is the most common indication for obstetric hysterectomy in many hospitals. The blood loss with this surgical procedure is substantial. In cases where separation of the placenta has been attempted before the diagnosis of accreta was made, massive hemorrhage may have occurred even before hysterectomy is begun.

Anesthetic Management

When caring for the patient at risk for placenta accreta, preoperative preparation and anticipation of potential problems by both the anesthesiologist and obstetrician can significantly improve outcome for the patient. At least two large-bore intravenous catheters should be inserted, and the placement of arterial and central venous catheters should be strongly considered. Packed red blood cells should be immediately available in the operating room before surgery begins, and discussion with the blood bank should confirm that other blood products, including platelets and fresh frozen plasma, will be readily available if needed. The use of cell saver technology should also be considered after delivery has been accomplished. Because arterial embolization has been reported to reduce the intraoperative blood loss, preoperative consultation with an interventional radiologist may be advisable. Finally, the obstetric operating room's resources should be assessed and a decision made as to whether the resources of the general operating room suite could better serve the needs of a potentially complicated surgery.

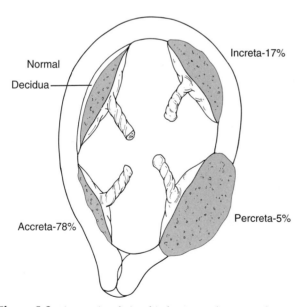

Normal
Decidua

Increta-17%

Accreta-78%

Percreta-5%

Figure 8-2 Anatomic relationship between placenta and myometrium in abnormal placentations. (Redrawn from Benedetti TJ: Obstetric hemorrhage. In Gabbe SG, Niebyl J, Simpson JL [eds]: Obstetrics: Normal and Problem Pregnancies, Fourth edition. Philadelphia, Churchill Livingstone, 2002, p 519.)

When placenta accreta is suspected, anesthesiologists don't agree about the anesthetic of choice. Many anesthesiologists believe all these patients should receive general anesthesia. The presence of a sympathectomy from regional anesthesia could predispose the patient to hypotension and inadequate perfusion of vital organs if massive hemorrhage occurs. If cesarean hysterectomy is necessary, patient discomfort caused by the additional surgical manipulation might require conversion to general anesthesia. Intubation could also become necessary if blood loss results in patient instability. Because of these potential situations, many anesthesiologists prefer to induce general anesthesia in a controlled situation at the beginning of surgery rather than during a time of crisis.

Other anesthesiologists argue, however, that regional anesthesia will provide adequate anesthesia for obstetric hysterectomy in many patients. If all patients at risk for placenta accreta were required to undergo general anesthesia, many women would unnecessarily face the increased risks of general anesthesia associated with pregnancy. In addition, they would not have the opportunity to be awake for the birth of their infants. In patients in whom there is concern that intubation could be difficult, it is prudent to utilize general anesthesia so that intubation can be performed in a controlled, nonurgent setting. In some patients at risk for placenta accreta, however, it is probably reasonable to offer regional anesthesia. If regional anesthesia is chosen, epidural anesthesia is recommended over spinal anesthesia because the duration of surgery could be prolonged.

Uterine Rupture

Uterine rupture is a less common cause of obstetric hemorrhage. However, when it does occur, significant morbidity and mortality can occur for both the mother and fetus. Presence of a uterine scar is the most common risk factor for uterine rupture. The type of scar also affects the incidence of rupture. Women with a previous classic uterine incision (vertical incision that extends into the upper portion of the uterus) have a 10% to 12% risk of experiencing uterine rupture during labor and are, therefore, not allowed to labor. The risk is also significantly greater for a myomectomy scar compared with a low transverse scar. Most studies that have assessed the risk of uterine rupture during labor in patients with a low transverse scar have reported an incidence of at least 1%, with one study reporting an incidence of 1.6%. Although it is rare, rupture of an unscarred uterus can occur. Risk factors in these patients include oxytocin or prostaglandin use, abdominal trauma, grand multiparity, fetopelvic disproportion, fetal malpresentation or macrosomia, and instrument-assisted vaginal delivery.

Fetal bradycardia is the most common sign of uterine rupture and is present in nearly 70% of cases. Other signs and symptoms of rupture include sudden onset of abdominal or suprapubic pain, vaginal bleeding, hemodynamic instability, maternal tachycardia, uterine tenderness, recession of the presenting fetal part, and abrupt change in uterine activity or pressure. Many of these signs and symptoms do not occur as frequently as many clinicians assume (Fig. 8-3). It is important to differentiate between uterine scar dehiscence and uterine rupture. Dehiscence, which is more common than frank rupture, is a separation of a previous uterine incision that is often asymptomatic and does not result in maternal hemorrhage or fetal distress. Frequently, a dehiscence is found incidentally and does not require additional treatment. Patients with a low transverse scar are more likely to experience dehiscence than rupture. In contrast, uterine rupture is a uterine wall defect that results in maternal hemorrhage or fetal distress. Sometimes the uterine contents (fetus and placenta) have extruded into the abdominal cavity. This can be a life-threatening situation for the mother or fetus and requires emergency cesarean delivery or postpartum laparotomy as well as uterine repair or hysterectomy.

Anesthetic management of a uterine rupture requires the anesthesiologist to simultaneously provide aggressive fluid resuscitation and anesthesia for emergency cesarean delivery or postpartum laparotomy. If the parturient already has an epidural catheter in place for labor analgesia, it is acceptable to use epidural anesthesia for delivery and uterine repair, provided the patient is hemodynamically stable. The emergent

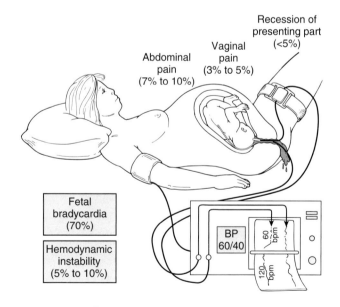

Signs and symptoms of uterine rupture

Figure 8-3 Signs and symptoms of uterine rupture. (Redrawn from Bucklin BA: Vaginal birth after cesarean delivery. Anesthesiology 99:1444–1448, 2003. Copyrighted 2003, American Society of Anesthesiologists.)

nature of the surgery usually requires the use of 2-chloroprocaine to establish surgical anesthesia. If fetal distress is present and an adequate level of epidural anesthesia is not achieved promptly (e.g., by the time the obstetrician is ready to begin surgery), general anesthesia should be induced to expedite delivery of the infant. General anesthesia is also required if an epidural catheter is not in place at the time of rupture or if the mother is hemodynamically unstable. Substantial blood loss should be expected during surgery, and it is likely that significant blood replacement and crystalloid infusion will be required. Once delivery is accomplished, either uterine repair or hysterectomy will be performed, depending on the extent of rupture and degree of hemorrhage. Both procedures require more surgical manipulation than cesarean delivery. As a result, some patients receiving epidural anesthesia will experience significant discomfort, thus necessitating intraoperative conversion to general anesthesia. Development of hemodynamic instability due to severe hemorrhage also may require conversion to general anesthesia. The anesthesiologist should be aware that significant intravascular volume shifts during surgery could alter airway anatomy and increase the risk of difficult intubation.

Vaginal Birth After Cesarean (VBAC)

In the 1970s and 1980s, there was a steady rise in the cesarean delivery rate in the United States. One of the contributing factors was the common practice of performing a repeat cesarean delivery in all women who had previously undergone a cesarean delivery. In response to the continuing rise in cesarean delivery rates, a campaign by the federal government and the American College of Obstetricians and Gynecologists (ACOG) to educate physicians and the public about the option of VBAC was undertaken. ACOG recommended that obstetricians encourage women with one prior cesarean delivery to attempt a trial of labor. ACOG also stated that a woman who had undergone two or more previous cesarean deliveries should not be discouraged from attempting a VBAC if that was what she desired. VBAC was considered to be safe, with some of the earliest studies reporting the incidence of uterine rupture as 0.2% to 0.8%. In addition, the incidence of maternal and perinatal mortality was believed to be similar to that for the general obstetric population while maternal morbidity associated with successful VBAC was decreased compared to patients undergoing elective repeat cesarean delivery. However, as an increasing number of patients attempted a trial of labor in the 1990s, additional data suggested that the safety of VBAC might be more controversial than was initially thought by the medical community.

In the current ACOG practice bulletin for VBAC, women who have undergone one low-transverse cesa-

---

CURRENT CONTROVERSIES: SAFETY OF VBAC

- Although the practice of VBAC was strongly encouraged in the 1990s, no randomized study has proven that VBAC is safer than elective repeat cesarean section for mother or neonate.
- Much of the early evidence suggested that the benefits of VBAC did usually outweigh the risks. However, most of these studies were performed in tertiary care facilities.
- A community hospital-based study reported a uterine rupture rate (1.6%) higher than has been reported in other trials.
- Results of several large studies now indicate the uterine rupture rate is at least 1%.
- Some cases of uterine rupture have resulted in poor outcomes for mother or infant.
- Unsuccessful VBAC requiring cesarean delivery is associated with higher morbidity than elective repeat cesarean delivery.
- Results of population-based retrospective studies and meta-analyses published since 2000 have also raised some concerns. One study found that the risk of delivery-related perinatal death was 11 times greater in women undergoing trial of labor compared to women having a planned repeat cesarean delivery. The rate of perinatal death due to uterine rupture was significantly higher in patients undergoing VBAC compared to other laboring parturients. A meta-analysis that compared patients undergoing trial of labor versus elective repeat cesarean delivery also found a higher incidence of perinatal death in women undergoing trial of labor. However, maternal morbidity, including fever and need for transfusion, was reduced among the women who underwent trial of labor.
- A combination of factors prompted ACOG to revise its practice bulletin for VBAC in 1999.

---

rean delivery and have no other contraindications to a vaginal delivery are considered candidates for VBAC. Women with two previous cesarean deliveries may also be offered a trial of labor, but these patients should be counseled that the risk of uterine rupture increases with the number of previous uterine incisions. It is no longer recommended that women with more than two cesarean deliveries be offered VBAC. The practice bulletin also states that the potential complications of VBAC must be thoroughly discussed with the patient and documented. Finally, both the ACOG practice bulletin and a joint statement issued by ACOG and the American Society of Anesthesiologists entitled *Optimal Goals for Anesthesia Care in Obstetrics* (see Appendix 3) addressed the availability of personnel and facilities when a parturient is attempting VBAC. Of interest, the number of VBAC attempts has declined nationally since the publication of the revised ACOG practice bulletin.

CLINICAL CAVEAT: AVAILABILITY OF PERSONNEL AND FACILITIES DURING VBAC

Both the ACOG practice bulletin on VBAC and an ACOG/ASA joint statement indicate that facilities and personnel, including an obstetrician, anesthetist, and operating room personnel, must be *immediately* available to perform an emergency cesarean delivery when VBAC is being attempted. Although neither document defined the term *immediately available*, many physicians and hospitals have interpreted this to mean that the in-house presence of an obstetrician and anesthesia care provider are necessary whenever a patient attempting VBAC is in active labor.

When VBAC was initially introduced, some obstetricians withheld epidural analgesia from these patients because of a concern that abdominal pain associated with uterine rupture would be masked by the analgesia, and diagnosis would be delayed. However, experience in the management of women attempting a trial of labor has not borne out this concern. First, abdominal pain is not a reliable sign of uterine rupture. Second, when the dilute local anesthetic + opioid solutions that are commonly utilized in current obstetric anesthesia practice are administered, it has been found that pain associated with uterine rupture is not obscured. In fact, when a woman who has been receiving adequate epidural labor analgesia experiences a sudden loss of analgesia, this should be a warning that uterine rupture may be occurring, and the obstetrician should be alerted.

Obstetricians and anesthesiologists now believe that epidural analgesia is an ideal technique of pain relief for parturients attempting a VBAC. Many studies have reported the successful use of epidural analgesia in these patients. Some women are more likely to choose a trial of labor rather than elective repeat cesarean delivery if they know the superior pain relief provided by epidural analgesia is available to them. Because 60% to 80% of patients undergoing a trial of labor have a vaginal delivery, a significant number of VBAC patients will ultimately require a cesarean delivery. Epidural analgesia can quickly be converted to surgical anesthesia in these patients. The dosing strategy used to provide labor analgesia to patients attempting VBAC should not differ from that utilized in the general obstetric population. Attention should be paid to using the smallest doses and concentrations of drugs that provide satisfactory analgesia. Large doses and concentrations that could produce surgical anesthesia rather than analgesia should be avoided because a dense block might mask abdominal pain associated with uterine rupture.

CSE analgesia is another popular technique for providing pain relief during labor. Like epidural analgesia, the pain relief provided by intrathecal opioids and small doses of local anesthetic will not obscure abdominal pain associated with uterine rupture. Because patients attempting VBAC may be at increased risk for requiring emergency cesarean delivery, some anesthesiologists believe that CSE analgesia should not be administered to these patients because adequate functioning of the epidural catheter cannot be determined until the initial intrathecal analgesia has resolved. However, the incidences of both epidural catheter failure after CSE and uterine rupture are very low, so CSE analgesia can be considered a viable option in most patients attempting VBAC.

ABNORMAL PRESENTATION

Many types of abnormal presentation exist, including breech, transverse lie, face, brow, and compound presentations. Pregnancies complicated by an abnormal presentation are associated with an increased incidence of obstetric complications. Optimal management of these patients requires coordination and cooperation among the obstetric care team, including obstetrician, anesthesiologist, obstetric nurse, and pediatrician. Breech presentation is the most common malpresentation and occurs in 3% to 4% of term pregnancies. Among preterm fetuses, the incidence of breech presentation may be as high as 40% although the vast majority of these fetuses assume a vertex presentation by 34 weeks gestation. Three types of breech presentation exist (Fig. 8-4): frank breech, in which the hips are flexed and the knees are extended; incomplete (footling) breech, in which one or both of the lower extremities are extended at the hip; and complete breech, in which both the hips and knees are flexed. Frank breech occurs most commonly. Vaginal breech delivery is only considered with a frank breech presentation.

In the United States, there has been an increasing trend to deliver singleton breech fetuses via cesarean delivery. Obstetricians have chosen this route of delivery because several retrospective studies as well as meta-analyses have reported increased perinatal morbidity and mortality with vaginal breech delivery. However, other studies have not found poorer neonatal outcome with vaginal delivery. Mode of delivery with breech presentation remained controversial throughout the 1990s. The first large, international, multicenter randomized clinical trial that evaluated the effect of mode of delivery on both neonatal and maternal outcome was published in 2000. It found that neonatal mortality and serious morbidity were significantly greater with vaginal breech delivery compared to cesarean delivery. In addition, cesarean delivery was not associated with increased maternal morbidity. As a consequence of these study data, ACOG revised its Committee Opinion on mode of term singleton breech delivery in 2001. They now recommend that a singleton breech fetus be delivered via

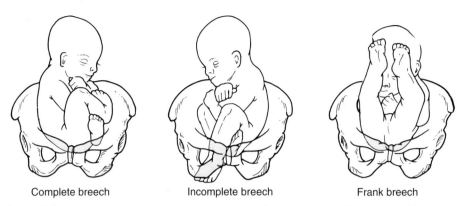

Complete breech   Incomplete breech   Frank breech

Figure 8-4 Three types of breech presentation: complete, incomplete (footling), and frank. (Redrawn from Lanni SM, Seeds JW: Malpresentations. In Gabbe SG, Niebyl J, Simpson JL [eds]: Obstetrics: Normal and Problem Pregnancies, Fourth edition. Philadelphia, Churchill Livingstone, 2002, p 482.)

planned cesarean delivery. They also state that if a vaginal breech delivery is pursued, great caution should be exercised. ACOG does clarify that this recommendation for planned cesarean delivery does not apply to parturients who present in advanced labor in whom delivery is imminent nor in twin gestations where the second twin is in the breech presentation.

Anesthetic Management of Breech Vaginal Delivery

The recent ACOG Committee Opinion has relegated the breech vaginal delivery to a relatively rare procedure. However, because serious complications may occur during a vaginal breech delivery, it is imperative that anesthesia coverage be readily available and the anesthesiologist have a sound understanding of the anesthetic implications associated with this procedure. Umbilical cord prolapse and fetal head entrapment are the two most serious complications associated with breech vaginal delivery. Both are true obstetric emergencies, and the anesthesiologist must be prepared to respond to them emergently.

There are three types of breech vaginal delivery: spontaneous breech delivery in which no traction is applied; assisted breech delivery in which the obstetrician assists delivery of the chest and head with forceps after the neonate spontaneously delivers to the umbilicus; and total breech extraction in which traction is applied on the feet and ankles to deliver the entire body. Total breech extraction is rarely performed in current obstetric practice and is only used to deliver a second twin.

In the past, some obstetricians have not supported the use of epidural analgesia for patients undergoing vaginal breech delivery because they were concerned that it would decrease the woman's expulsive efforts. Currently, most obstetricians and anesthesiologists con-

sider epidural analgesia to be an ideal anesthetic technique for labor and vaginal breech delivery. The advantages of this technique include superior labor analgesia, inhibition of early pushing before the cervix has become fully dilated, provision of a relaxed pelvic wall and perineum at delivery, and the ability to extend the block if an emergency cesarean delivery becomes necessary. Because of the risk of serious obstetric complications, it is advisable to initiate epidural analgesia early in labor.

It can be challenging to effectively meet all the anesthetic goals for providing epidural analgesia to a parturient attempting vaginal breech delivery. During the first stage of labor, the epidural block must be dense enough to prevent early pushing. However, once the second stage of labor is reached, the epidural block must not inhibit the patient's ability to push effectively because it is essential that the infant deliver spontaneously to the umbilicus. The anesthesiologist must also be able to quickly provide dense perineal anesthesia if the obstetrician decides to assist delivery with forceps. Continuous epidural infusion or epidural PCA using a solution of dilute local anesthetic that minimizes motor block (e.g., bupivacaine or ropivacaine) plus a lipid-soluble opioid (e.g., fentanyl or sufentanil) is usually effective for labor and delivery. The administration of 3% 2-chloroprocaine quickly achieves dense perineal anesthesia if forceps need to be applied.

Umbilical cord prolapse is the most common serious obstetric complication associated with vaginal breech delivery. It can occur at any time during labor and requires emergency cesarean delivery. It often results in profound fetal bradycardia. Once the problem is identified, a member of the obstetric team must elevate the fetal head off the umbilical cord until delivery is accomplished to prevent prolonged umbilical cord compression. If an epidural catheter is in place, the anesthesiologist should quickly extend anesthesia with 3%

2-chloroprocaine. However, the anesthesiologist should also be prepared to induce general anesthesia in case adequate surgical anesthesia is not present when the obstetrician is ready to begin surgery. If epidural analgesia is not already established, general anesthesia is nearly always required due to the time factor and the inability to position the patient for regional anesthesia placement while the fetal head is being elevated.

Entrapment of the fetal head, although rare, is probably the most feared complication of vaginal breech delivery. Most of these cases occur in preterm fetuses less than 32 weeks gestation. If the fetal head becomes entrapped after delivery of the body, the obstetrician must choose among three management options to deliver the infant. These include: emergency cesarean delivery after the fetus's body has been returned to the uterus; performance of Dührssen incisions in the cervix, which can result in significant bleeding; or provision of skeletal and cervical/uterine smooth muscle relaxation. Both of the latter maneuvers are used to facilitate vaginal delivery of the entrapped fetus.

The obstetrician may request that the anesthesiologist provide skeletal and cervical/uterine smooth muscle relaxation to assist delivery of the head. If an epidural catheter is in place, skeletal muscle relaxation can quickly be achieved with the administration of 3% 2-chloroprocaine. Although epidural anesthesia will not provide cervical relaxation, the provision of a relaxed pelvic wall and perineum as well as effective pain relief will facilitate delivery of the aftercoming head. For successful delivery of an entrapped head, cervical relaxation is required. Nitroglycerin is a potent smooth muscle relaxant that has successfully provided uterine relaxation for a variety of clinical scenarios. While the uterus is comprised primarily of smooth muscle, only 15% of the cervix is smooth muscle. Therefore, some physicians have suggested that nitroglycerin will not effectively provide the necessary cervical relaxation to deliver an entrapped fetal head. However, two case reports have suggested that administration of intravenous nitroglycerin was primarily responsible for facilitating delivery of the entrapped head of a premature fetus. In these cases, 150 and 600 μg of nitroglycerin were administered. In other obstetric situations, such as retained placenta, doses as low as 50 to 100 μg of intravenous nitroglycerin have provided uterine relaxation. Because rapid sequence induction of general anesthesia and administration of a high concentration (2 to 3 MAC) of a volatile halogenated agent is the only other technique the anesthesiologist can offer to provide cervical/uterine relaxation, it seems reasonable to first administer nitroglycerin when fetal head entrapment occurs, followed by general anesthesia if adequate relaxation is not achieved with nitroglycerin. If epidural analgesia has not already been established in the parturient at the time of fetal head entrapment, general anesthesia will almost certainly be required to provide the skeletal muscle and cervical relaxation as well as the effective analgesia necessary to successfully deliver the entrapped fetal head.

As previously discussed, most women presenting with a fetus in the breech presentation will undergo elective cesarean delivery. Regional anesthesia is the technique of choice unless contraindications exist. Even with an abdominal delivery, uterine relaxation may be required to facilitate delivery of the breech infant. Nitroglycerin should be immediately available. The neonate delivered in the breech presentation is more likely to be depressed at delivery. Therefore, it is essential that personnel trained in neonatal resuscitation be available at all breech deliveries, both vaginal and abdominal.

Anesthetic Considerations in External Cephalic Version

External cephalic version is used to convert a breech or transverse lie presentation to a vertex presentation, thus allowing vaginal delivery. During the procedure, the obstetrician applies manual pressure to the woman's abdomen in an attempt to change the position of the fetus. If version to the vertex presentation is successful, vaginal delivery is accomplished at essentially the same rate as the general obstetric population. External cephalic version is usually performed after 36 weeks gestation before the patient is in active labor. Early labor does not preclude successful version, but the procedure is generally not successful once the presenting part has entered the pelvis. Success rates ranging from 50% to 80% have been reported for the procedure, with an average rate of approximately 60%. Risks of external cephalic version include placental abruption and umbilical cord compression, which could result in acute fetal distress requiring emergency cesarean delivery.

Because vaginal breech delivery is no longer recommended by ACOG, anesthesiologists are likely to see an increase in external cephalic version procedures in an attempt to decrease cesarean delivery rates due to abnormal presentation. Certain maneuvers may increase the success rate for external cephalic version. Uterine tocolysis is frequently administered to facilitate the procedure. Subcutaneous terbutaline 0.25 mg is usually administered 15 to 20 minutes before the procedure is performed. Some obstetricians will also administer nitroglycerin during the version. An anesthesiologist should be available whenever an external cephalic version is being attempted in case emergency delivery is required. The obstetrician and anesthesiologist must also decide whether neuraxial anesthesia should be administered for external cephalic version.

CLINICAL CAVEAT: ANESTHESIA AND EXTERNAL CEPHALIC VERSION

- Preanesthetic evaluation should be performed, even if anesthesia involvement is not planned.
- Epidural or intrathecal analgesia decreases maternal discomfort during the procedure.
- Most studies have found that epidural or intrathecal anesthesia increases the success rate of version.
- When version without anesthesia has failed, a repeat attempt with epidural anesthesia is often successful.
- Some obstetricians discourage the use of neuraxial anesthesia because they believe excessive force that could lead to fetal or uterine injury is more likely to be applied in an anesthetized patient.
- If epidural or CSE anesthesia is used for version, the block can be extended if emergency cesarean delivery becomes necessary, thus avoiding general anesthesia.
- The preferences and practice of the obstetrician and anesthesiologist usually determine whether neuraxial anesthesia is provided.
- When epidural anesthesia is utilized, 2% lidocaine is most commonly administered to achieve a T8-T6 level.
- Intrathecal analgesia with sufentanil 10 μg increased the success rate for version in one study.

Other Abnormal Presentations

Transverse lie, or shoulder presentation, is another malpresentation that sometimes occurs, especially in preterm fetuses. Like a breech presentation, external cephalic version can be attempted in these patients. If the version is unsuccessful, cesarean delivery must be performed. The position of the fetus within the uterus sometimes requires a vertical uterine incision. The risk of umbilical cord prolapse is especially high with the transverse lie presentation.

Other malpresentations that may occur include face, brow, and compound presentations. These are much rarer than breech or transverse lie presentations. Although vaginal delivery may be attempted, these patients are more likely than patients with a vertex presentation to require cesarean delivery.

MULTIPLE GESTATION

With the increasing use of assisted reproductive technologies, there has been a marked rise in the frequency of multiple gestation in the United States. From 1980 to 2001, the incidence of twin pregnancies has risen from <2% of all pregnancies to >3%. The rise in triplet and higher order multiple gestation has been even more dramatic with a more than 500% rise during the same time

period. Both perinatal and maternal morbidity and mortality are increased with multiple gestation. The incidence of cesarean delivery is also increased with multiple gestation. The implications of multiple gestation in the obstetric and anesthetic management of these parturients is significant and presents challenges to obstetricians and anesthesiologists.

Maternal morbidity and mortality are increased with multiple gestation because some complications of pregnancy occur more frequently in these patients (Box 8-5). An increased incidence of obstetric complications (Box 8-6) accounts for the increased perinatal morbidity and mortality also, with preterm delivery the most common etiology. In fact, approximately 10% of all perinatal deaths result from multiple gestation.

In addition to an increased incidence of obstetric complications, some of the maternal physiologic changes of pregnancy are exaggerated by multiple gestation. The larger uterine size of these women results in a greater decrease in functional residual capacity compared to women with singleton gestations. Maternal oxygen consumption is likely increased with multiple gestation. Hypoxemia, therefore, will develop more rapidly if a situation of apnea or hypoventilation occurs. These patients may also be at risk for hypoxemia when they assume the supine position. Exaggerated cardiovascular changes also occur in parturients with multiple gestation. Maternal blood volume is approximately 500 mL greater with twin gestation. The pregnancy-related rise

Box 8-5   Maternal Complications Occurring with Greater Frequency in Multiple Gestation

Pre-eclampsia
Preterm labor
Uterine atony
Postpartum hemorrhage
Anemia
Placental abruption
Placenta previa

Box 8-6   Fetal Complications Occurring with Greater Frequency in Multiple Gestation

Preterm delivery
Intrauterine growth restriction
Malpresentation
Congenital anomalies
Umbilical cord entanglement
Umbilical cord prolapse

in cardiac output is greater in these patients. The most significant cardiovascular change, however, is due to the increased uterine size and weight in multiple gestation. As a result, aortocaval compression and the supine hypotensive syndrome are likely to be more severe. Pregnancy effects on the central nervous system also appear to be exaggerated in multiple gestation, and their significance is of special importance to the anesthesiologist. The spread of spinal anesthesia has been noted to be greater in women with twin gestations compared to singleton gestations. Again, increased uterine size resulting in greater aortocaval compression may contribute to the greater spread. In addition, the higher maternal serum progesterone levels that are present in patients with multiple gestation may contribute to the greater spread of spinal anesthesia because progesterone is known to increase nerve sensitivity to local anesthetics.

Obstetric Management

In planning the obstetric management for a patient with multiple gestation, the route of delivery must first be decided. Cesarean delivery is nearly always chosen for the delivery of triplets and higher order multiple births. For twin gestations, the presentations of Twin A and Twin B are considered when deciding on the mode of delivery. When Twin A is breech, ACOG recommends cesarean delivery because the safety of vaginal birth has not been documented, and the possibility of locked twins exists if Twin B is vertex. Although locked twins rarely occur, fetal mortality is high with this complication. If both twins are vertex, vaginal delivery is generally recommended unless other contraindications to vaginal birth exist. The route of delivery for vertex/nonvertex twins, however, is more controversial. Because ACOG currently recommends planned cesarean delivery for singleton fetuses in the breech presentation, some obstetricians now advocate cesarean delivery when Twin B is breech. However, the ACOG recommendation specifically states that this opinion does not apply to a second twin in the nonvertex presentation. If the estimated fetal weight of Twin B is between 1500 and 4000 g, it is considered reasonable to attempt vaginal delivery of both twins because most studies have not shown improved neonatal outcome of Twin B with cesarean delivery. Regardless of these recommendations, it does appear that the incidence of combined vaginal-cesarean and elective cesarean deliveries for twin gestations is increasing at some hospitals.

When vaginal delivery of a twin gestation is planned, the delivery should occur in an operating room where emergency cesarean delivery can be accomplished. Once Twin A is delivered vaginally, the obstetrician must then decide how to proceed with delivery of Twin B. First, presentation must be confirmed by ultrasound examination because presentation of the second twin can change after delivery of the first twin. Fetal heart tones must be evaluated because fetal bradycardia can also develop after delivery of Twin A. If Twin B is in the vertex presentation and the fetal heart rate pattern is reassuring, the obstetrician will generally proceed with vaginal delivery. If Twin B has a nonvertex presentation, the obstetrician's management options include: external cephalic version followed by vaginal delivery of a vertex infant; internal podalic version with total breech extraction; or cesarean delivery. Delivery of the nonvertex second twin is the one situation in which performance of an internal podalic version and total breech extraction is still considered appropriate obstetric practice. Communication between the obstetrician and anesthesiologist regarding the planned delivery method for Twin B is essential so that appropriate anesthesia and uterine relaxation can be provided, if necessary.

Anesthetic Management

Labor and Vaginal Delivery

Epidural analgesia is usually considered the method of choice for labor and planned vaginal delivery of a twin gestation. It provides effective pain relief, optimal delivery conditions, and the route for a rapid induction of anesthesia should an emergency cesarean delivery be required for Twin B. Epidural drug administration is similar to that used for other laboring parturients. It is essential that the anesthesiologist establish that the epidural catheter is functioning well because these patients are at increased risk for cesarean delivery. Parturients with twin gestation are also more prone to supine hypotensive syndrome. Therefore, particular attention must be paid to maintaining left uterine displacement, and aggressive treatment with intravenous fluids and ephedrine should be instituted if hypotension does develop. Because the incidence of postpartum hemorrhage is increased with multiple gestation, large-bore venous access should be established early in labor, and a current type and screen specimen must be present in the hospital's blood bank. CSE analgesia is less desirable than conventional epidural analgesia in laboring parturients with a twin gestation because the epidural catheter remains unproven during the initial period of intrathecal analgesia.

During vaginal delivery of a twin gestation, some of the anesthetic concerns are similar to those discussed for vaginal breech delivery. After Twin A has been delivered, there is an increased risk of prolapse of the umbilical cord in Twin B that would necessitate emergency cesarean delivery. If a breech delivery of the second twin is attempted, the anesthesiologist must be prepared to respond to an entrapped fetal head.

Because of a significant likelihood that some form of manipulation will be required for delivery of Twin B, augmenting the depth and height of the sensory block during delivery of Twin A should be considered, especially if Twin B is in a nonvertex presentation. Denser anesthesia is required for an internal podalic version with total breech extraction and may also contribute to the success of an external cephalic version. In addition, should emergency cesarean delivery of Twin B become necessary, rapid achievement of adequate epidural anesthesia is more likely to occur if extension of the block was begun before the decision for cesarean delivery was made. A dense anesthetic block can be achieved most quickly if 3% 2-chloroprocaine is administered. However, the anesthesiologist must always be prepared to induce general anesthesia if adequate epidural anesthesia cannot be achieved in a timely manner. The provision of uterine relaxation may also be necessary if the obstetrician is performing external cephalic version or total breech extraction. Usually, intravenous nitroglycerin 50 to 100 μg will provide the necessary relaxation although some physicians have reported administering significantly larger doses.

Anesthesia for Planned Cesarean Delivery

As with any cesarean delivery, maternal and fetal conditions will determine the anesthetic choice for cesarean delivery in multifetal pregnancies. Regional anesthesia is preferred in most cases because of the increased risks of aspiration and airway difficulties during general anesthesia in parturients. The larger uterine size associated with multiple gestation may lead to more severe aortocaval compression and hypotension. As a result, many anesthesiologists prefer epidural anesthesia over spinal anesthesia in these patients because they believe the slower onset of sympathetic blockade that occurs with epidural anesthesia will result in less severe hypotension. In addition, greater cephalad spread of spinal anesthesia has been reported in patients with multiple gestation compared to singleton pregnancies, but no such exaggerated spread of the anesthetic level has been reported with epidural anesthesia. Despite these concerns, spinal and CSE anesthesia have been used safely in many patients undergoing cesarean delivery for multiple gestation. Therefore, epidural, spinal, and CSE anesthesia all seem to be reasonable choices when regional anesthesia is planned. Patient characteristics and anesthesiologist preference should determine the technique chosen.

In some patients with multiple gestation, general anesthesia will be indicated for cesarean delivery. Induction and maintenance of anesthesia should proceed in the same manner as with any parturient. The anesthesiologist should be aware, however, that the greater decrease in functional residual capacity (FRC) and increase in oxygen consumption associated with multiple gestation will place these patients at increased risk for hypoxemia compared to patients with a singleton pregnancy.

DIABETES MELLITUS

Epidemiology and Classification

Diabetes mellitus is one of the most common underlying medical conditions that complicates pregnancy. The incidence of diabetes has been increasing steadily in the United States, largely because of the epidemic of obesity. Currently, diabetes occurs in 2% to 3% of parturients. Approximately 90% of these patients have gestational diabetes, which is present only during pregnancy and results when a woman cannot produce enough insulin to compensate for the enhanced resistance to insulin that occurs during pregnancy. The other 10% of diabetic parturients have pre-existing diabetes, including both Type 1 and Type 2. Type 1 diabetes is an autoimmune disorder. Type 2 diabetes results from an increased resistance to insulin and occurs predominantly in obese patients. In obstetrics, White's classification system is often used to describe a parturient's diabetic status. This system is explained in Table 8-2.

Interaction of Diabetes with Pregnancy

The progressive resistance to insulin that develops during pregnancy results from the pregnancy-related increases in several counter-regulatory hormones, including placental lactogen, cortisol, and progesterone.

Table 8-2	White's Classification System of Diabetes During Pregnancy
Class	**Definition**
A_1	Gestational diabetes that is diet controlled
A_2	Gestational diabetes that requires insulin
B	Pre-existing diabetes with onset >age 20 and duration <10 years without complications
C	Pre-existing diabetes with onset between ages 10 and 19 or duration of ages 10 to 19 without complications
D	Pre-existing diabetes with onset <age 10 or duration >20 years. without complications
F	Pre-existing diabetes complicated by nephropathy
R	Pre-existing diabetes complicated by proliferative retinopathy
T	Pre-existing diabetes and status/post kidney transplant
H	Pre-existing diabetes complicated by ischemic heart disease

Women who are unable to increase insulin production sufficiently to compensate for this resistance develop gestational diabetes. These patients are at increased risk for Type 2 diabetes mellitus later in life. In parturients with pre-existing diabetes, the insulin resistance of pregnancy leads to a progressive increase in insulin requirements. Despite these increased insulin requirements, patients with Type 1 diabetes are at significant risk for developing hypoglycemia, especially during early pregnancy.

Diabetic ketoacidosis (DKA) is another concern in parturients with Type 1 disease. The pregnant state of relative insulin resistance is associated with enhanced lipolysis and ketogenesis. Therefore, DKA can occur at significantly lower glucose levels than is typically associated with DKA in nonpregnant patients. DKA can be diagnosed in parturients with glucose levels as low as 200 to 250 mg/dL. It most commonly occurs in the second and third trimesters. The administration of β-adrenergic drugs for tocolysis and glucocorticoids for fetal lung maturation may precipitate DKA. Infection is another risk factor for DKA, and infection rates in pregnant patients with Type 1 diabetes are higher than rates in nondiabetic parturients. The presence of DKA has also been associated with nonreassuring fetal heart rate patterns. However, these patterns usually resolve once the maternal metabolic abnormalities have been corrected, so every effort is made to avoid fetal intervention and preterm delivery unless the heart rate abnormalities persist after treatment of the DKA.

Several complications, both maternal and fetal, occur more frequently in diabetic pregnancies. The incidence of pre-eclampsia is increased in diabetic patients, both gestational and pregestational. Polyhydramnios is also more common. Diabetic parturients are more likely to require cesarean delivery. Uteroplacental perfusion is decreased 35% to 45% in diabetic patients compared to nondiabetic patients. This decreased blood flow occurs even in women with well-controlled gestational diabetes. An increased incidence of abnormal fetal heart rate patterns is associated with the reduction in uteroplacental perfusion.

The fetal effects of maternal diabetes are numerous. In women with pre-existing diabetes, the risk of congenital anomalies is increased and is now the leading cause of perinatal mortality in diabetic pregnancies. The incidence of major malformations is 8.5% to 10% in large studies, which is a two- to six-fold increase compared to nondiabetic patients. Cardiovascular and central nervous system malformations are the most common. While the etiology of these fetal anomalies is likely multifactorial, the most important factor appears to be poor glucose control during the period of organogenesis. Initiation of strict glycemic control during the preconception period has been found to decrease the incidence of congenital anomalies.

An increased incidence of intrauterine fetal death has been associated with diabetes. Reduced uteroplacental perfusion is felt to be a significant contributing factor. However, aggressive antenatal fetal surveillance in diabetic parturients has been successful in substantially decreasing the number of intrauterine fetal deaths among diabetic women. Fetal macrosomia is another complication of both gestational and pregestational diabetes. This certainly contributes to the increased incidence of cesarean delivery. In addition, during vaginal delivery the risk of shoulder dystocia and birth trauma is increased for the macrosomic fetus.

After delivery, neonates of diabetic mothers face other complications. Neonatal hypoglycemia is the most common problem encountered, occurring in 5% to 12% of these infants. This is a 6- to 16-fold increase compared to infants of nondiabetic mothers. The fetal hyperinsulinemia that develops in response to maternal hyperglycemia is believed to be the cause of neonatal hypoglycemia. Although recent data do not support diabetes as an independent risk factor for infant respiratory distress syndrome (RDS), a variety of factors may increase the incidence of RDS among the neonates of diabetic parturients, especially in those infants whose mothers had poor glycemic control during pregnancy. Obviously, it is important that personnel skilled in the care of neonates be readily available during the delivery of a diabetic woman.

Obstetric Management

Optimal glycemic control is a major focus in the obstetric care of diabetic parturients because it may minimize several complications, including macrosomia, birth injury, fetal lung immaturity, and perinatal death. In patients with pre-existing disease, this management should actually begin in the preconception period because strict glycemic control before conception is associated with a decrease in congenital anomalies. Self-monitoring of fingerstick blood glucose measurements is performed several times each day throughout pregnancy. Tight control with a blood glucose concentration of 60 to 120 mg/dL is desired. Frequent changes in insulin therapy are usually required to maintain adequate glycemic control, with insulin requirements generally increasing progressively throughout pregnancy. The treatment regimen may require three to four daily insulin injections or use of a continuous subcutaneous insulin pump. Strict glycemic control is also necessary during labor and delivery to decrease the risk of neonatal hypoglycemia. The recommended strategy for glucose control during labor is summarized in Box 8-7.

Insulin requirements decrease significantly in the postpartum period, and glycemic control does not need to be as tight as during labor and delivery. If an insulin infusion is utilized during labor, it should be discontinued after delivery to avoid maternal hypoglycemia.

Box 8-7 **Regimen for Glucose Control During Labor and Delivery**
Withhold A.M. dose of insulin. Establish intravenous infusion with normal saline (avoid lactated Ringer's solution because it may contribute to elevated glucose levels). Measure fingerstick blood glucose levels hourly. If glucose < 70 mg/dL, change intravenous infusion to 5% dextrose and consider initiating a second non-dextrose-containing infusion for fluid boluses and drug administration. If glucose > 140 mg/dL, initiate insulin infusion at 0.5 to 2 U/hr and titrate to effect.

When DKA develops in a pregnant patient, the management is similar to that for nonpregnant patients. Laboratory assessment should include arterial blood gases to determine the degree of acidosis and frequent measurement of serum glucose and electrolytes. These patients are volume depleted and require intensive intravenous hydration with normal saline. Intravenous insulin is administered to control glucose levels. If the serum potassium level is normal or reduced, an intravenous potassium infusion of 10 to 20 mEq/hr should be initiated. The administration of bicarbonate is reserved for cases of severe acidosis (i.e., pH < 7.10). Fetal heart rate abnormalities are commonly present, and maneuvers to optimize the fetal status, including left uterine displacement and supplemental oxygen, should be utilized. However, in most cases intervention with delivery of the infant is avoided because the fetal condition usually improves with appropriate medical management of the mother.

In patients with gestational diabetes, the diagnosis must first be made because these women had normal glucose tolerance before pregnancy. In the United States, universal screening with a 1-hour glucose tolerance test is advocated. If the results of this test are abnormal, a 3 hour glucose tolerance test is administered to determine whether the patient has gestational diabetes. Once the diagnosis is made, initial therapy includes a diabetic diet. If glycemic control cannot be achieved with diet, insulin therapy will be initiated.

Diligent antenatal fetal surveillance during the third trimester to decrease the risk of intrauterine fetal death is another important component in the obstetric management of diabetic women. Beginning at 28 to 32 weeks gestation, most obstetricians will begin twice weekly nonstress tests. A nonreactive nonstress test will usually lead to performance of a biophysical profile to further evaluate fetal status. Obstetricians must also make decisions concerning the timing and route of delivery in diabetic parturients. The goal is to deliver an infant with mature lungs while avoiding an intrauterine fetal death late in pregnancy. Results of antenatal fetal monitoring and tests of fetal lung maturation are used to assist obstetricians in making decisions concerning timing of delivery. If amniotic fluid analysis indicates mature fetal lungs and antenatal testing suggests fetal compromise, delivery should proceed promptly. If the fetal lungs are immature and antenatal monitoring suggests fetal compromise, the decision to proceed with delivery is usually made after other tests have also confirmed deterioration in the fetal condition. Even when antenatal fetal surveillance is reassuring, many obstetricians advocate elective induction of labor at 38 to 40 weeks gestation to avoid not only the dreaded complication of late stillbirth but also the risks associated with a macrosomic infant, including shoulder dystocia, birth trauma, and an increased likelihood of cesarean delivery. Fetal condition and estimated fetal weight are two especially important factors considered by the obstetrician when deciding upon a route of delivery in the diabetic patient.

Anesthetic Management

In addition to the usual components of preanesthetic evaluation, the anesthesiologist should focus on the diabetic parturient's glycemic control. In women with pre-existing disease, evidence of diabetes-related complications should be sought. Particular attention should be paid to possible cardiac, vascular, and renal involvement as well as autonomic neuropathy. In patients with long-standing disease, it is advisable to obtain an electrocardiogram (ECG) because it might help identify ischemic heart disease or autonomic dysfunction. In the anesthetic management of diabetic patients, major concerns associated with autonomic neuropathy include a greater propensity to develop hypotension during both regional and general anesthesia and an increased risk of aspiration due to gastroparesis. Although rare, the anesthesiologist should screen women with Type 1 diabetes mellitus for evidence of the "stiff-joint" syndrome by looking for the "prayer sign" (Fig. 8-5). This syndrome may include involvement of the atlanto-occipital joint, resulting in limited movement of the joint, which may lead to difficult direct laryngoscopy and intubation.

Epidural analgesia for labor pain management provides several benefits in the patient with diabetes. It provides excellent analgesia. In addition, it will attenuate the physiologic response to pain, resulting in decreased maternal plasma concentrations of catecholamines. Because uteroplacental blood flow is reduced in diabetic pregnancies, the decrease in catecholamine levels associated with neuraxial analgesia may be especially beneficial in diabetic parturients, leading to improved uteroplacental perfusion. Catecholamines are also counter-regulatory hormones that oppose insulin activity. Although no stud-

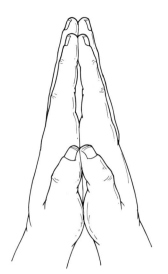

Figure 8-5 The "prayer sign" in diabetic patients with stiff joint syndrome.

ies in pregnant patients with diabetes have been performed, in theory the provision of epidural labor analgesia with associated decreases in plasma catecholamine concentrations could contribute to improved glucose control during labor and delivery.

Certain precautions should be taken when administering epidural analgesia to parturients with diabetes. Patients with pregestational diabetes who have suspected autonomic neuropathy are especially prone to hypotension during the initiation of sympathetic blockade. They should receive vigorous intravenous hydration before proceeding with epidural analgesia. In addition, hypotension related to epidural analgesia may be more likely to lead to fetal compromise in diabetic pregnancies compared to nondiabetic pregnancies because of the reduction in uteroplacental perfusion associated with diabetes. Therefore, efforts to avoid hypotension should be emphasized. These measures include aggressive volume expansion with a non-dextrose-containing solution before the initiation of epidural analgesia and slow dosing of the epidural catheter to accomplish a slower onset of sympathetic blockade. If hypotension does occur, it should be treated promptly and aggressively with ephedrine.

Because of the 35% to 45% reduction in uteroplacental blood flow that occurs in diabetic pregnancies, these patients may be at increased risk for fetal distress during labor, necessitating an emergency cesarean delivery. Therefore, epidural analgesia may be preferable to CSE analgesia in many parturients with diabetes, especially those who have suspicious fetal heart rate tracings, because the epidural catheter remains unproven during the initial intrathecal analgesia component of the CSE. If emergency cesarean delivery is required during this time period, an undetected, nonfunctioning epidural catheter would require the induction of general anesthesia.

Cesarean delivery is performed more frequently in diabetic than in nondiabetic women. As with all parturients, regional anesthesia is preferred over general anesthesia for cesarean delivery whenever possible. Early studies found an association in women with diabetes between spinal and epidural anesthesia for cesarean delivery and umbilical cord and neonatal acidosis. However, these women received intravenous hydration with dextrose-containing fluids. Maternal hyperglycemia and hypotension were believed to be the factors primarily responsible for the acidosis in these studies. Subsequent studies in which non-dextrose-containing solutions for hydration were utilized did not find an increased incidence of acidosis. When providing epidural or spinal anesthesia in a parturient with diabetes, the anesthesiologist should make certain that adequate hydration with a non-dextrose-containing solution is accomplished, maternal glycemic control is satisfactory, and hypotension is aggressively treated with ephedrine. If those conditions are met, the risk of neonatal acidosis is not increased by regional anesthesia.

No studies have compared the maternal or neonatal effects of spinal versus epidural anesthesia for cesarean delivery in women with diabetes. However, when the clinical situation does not require urgent delivery and adequate time is available to initiate epidural anesthesia, it may be preferable to spinal anesthesia. Its slower onset of sympathetic blockade could decrease the risk of anesthesia-induced hypotension compared to spinal anesthesia, and the avoidance of hypotension is especially important to ensure fetal well-being in these patients. When an urgent clinical scenario does not allow time for epidural anesthesia, spinal anesthesia is usually preferred over general anesthesia, despite the risk of hypotension. Spinal anesthesia is a safer technique for the mother. If hypotension does occur, it can quickly be treated with ephedrine, thus avoiding fetal compromise.

Emergency cesarean delivery will sometimes require general anesthesia in a diabetic patient, especially if an epidural catheter has not already been placed for labor analgesia. The same principles used for providing general anesthesia for any parturient should be followed when caring for women with diabetes. Some special considerations also exist, especially in patients with pregestational diabetes. Because those patients are at risk for autonomic neuropathy, the administration of metoclopramide to minimize the risk of aspiration secondary to gastroparesis is recommended. Based on a study in nonpregnant patients with diabetes that found autonomic dysfunction was associated with increased requirements for vasopressors during general anesthesia, the anesthesiologist should be prepared for more frequent and severe hypotension in parturients with autonomic dysfunction. Measures to prevent hypotension, such as vigorous intravenous hydration and left uterine displacement, should be taken preoperatively and intraoperatively. If hypotension does occur, prompt, aggressive therapy is necessary. Finally, if a patient with longstanding, pre-existing diabetes has a positive "prayer sign," the anesthesiologist should carefully assess the risk for difficult intubation and decide if awake intubation is warranted.

MORBID OBESITY

Obesity in the United States has become a national epidemic with more than 60% of the adult population being classified as overweight or obese. As a result, anesthesiologists are confronting the challenges of caring for morbidly obese parturients with increasing frequency. The pathophysiologic changes associated with obesity significantly affect the anesthetic management of these patients. In addition, the incidence of pregnancy complications is increased in obese patients compared to nonobese patients. The anesthesiologist needs a thorough understanding of these issues to provide optimal care to these high-risk patients.

Many of the pathophysiologic changes associated with obesity are similar to the physiologic changes of pregnancy. In fact, some of the physiologic changes of pregnancy may be exaggerated in morbidly obese parturients. The pulmonary, cardiovascular, and gastrointestinal changes that occur in morbidly obese patients contribute significantly to increased anesthetic risk in these patients. Important pulmonary changes associated with morbid obesity are listed in Box 8-8. All these changes can lead to respiratory compromise and hypoxemia in the pregnant, morbidly obese patient.

Like pregnancy, morbid obesity leads to increases in total blood volume and cardiac output. Pulmonary blood volume increases in proportion to these increases in cardiac output and blood volume. In those morbidly obese patients who have developed chronic hypoxemia as a result of the pathophysiologic pulmonary changes, pulmonary vascular resistance is also increased. Therefore, parturients with a long history of morbid obesity may

---

| Box 8-8 | Pulmonary Changes in Morbidly Obese Patients |

Increased oxygen consumption and carbon dioxide production
Increased work of breathing
Decreased tidal volume
Decreased functional residual capacity, expiratory reserve volume, and vital capacity
Airway closure during tidal ventilation
Ventilation-perfusion mismatch

---

be at risk for pulmonary hypertension, which is associated with a high maternal mortality rate. The gastrointestinal changes associated with obesity are similar to the changes that occur in all parturients. Over 80% of nonpregnant obese patients have a gastric pH <2.5 and a gastric volume >25 mL, thus placing these patients at risk for aspiration. It is unclear whether morbid obesity in pregnancy further decreases gastric pH and increases gastric volume compared to nonobese parturients.

Obstetric Concerns

The presence of morbid obesity during pregnancy has significant implications for both mother and fetus. The incidence of several maternal complications is increased among the morbidly obese. Hypertensive disorders, including both chronic hypertension and pre-eclampsia, are increased. These patients are more likely to develop gestational diabetes. They are also at increased risk for thromboembolic disease and infection. Obesity affects the progress and outcome of labor, with some studies suggesting that these patients are more likely to have abnormal labor. Failed induction is more likely to occur in morbidly obese patients, and cesarean delivery for failure-to-progress during labor may be increased. Both the overall cesarean delivery rate and emergency cesarean delivery rate are increased in morbidly obese patients. The causes of these increased rates are multifactorial, with the increased incidences of fetal macrosomia and maternal complications, such as pre-eclampsia and diabetes, being important factors. Soft tissue dystocia that may actually alter the anatomy of the birth canal may be another contributing factor. When a morbidly obese patient requires cesarean delivery, prolonged surgery duration can be expected, and the likelihood of excessive blood loss may be increased.

Especially concerning for both the obstetrician and anesthesiologist is the face that obesity has been found to increase the risk of maternal death. Several factors contribute to increased maternal mortality among morbidly obese parturients. These include the increased incidences of pre-eclampsia, diabetes, pulmonary embolism, and infection. Anesthesia-related maternal mortality is also increased, with airway difficulties being a major cause.

Perinatal outcome is also adversely affected by morbid obesity. An increased incidence of abnormal fetal heart rate tracings during labor has been noted among obese parturients. The increased incidence of macrosomia associated with obesity leads to a greater risk of birth trauma and shoulder dystocia. Meconium aspiration occurs more frequently in infants of obese women. These infants are also at greater risk for neural tube defects and other congenital anomalies. Most important, a recent study reported a higher incidence of antepartum stillbirth and early neonatal death in pregnancies complicated by morbid obesity.

Anesthetic Management

Preanesthetic Evaluation and Preparation

The high incidence of medical diseases and obstetric complications associated with morbid obesity as well as the difficulties encountered solely because of body habitus present the anesthesiologist with significant challenges. A thorough preanesthetic evaluation and careful planning and preparation are essential to provide optimal care to these patients. Whenever possible, antepartum anesthetic evaluation should be utilized to facilitate the appropriate and timely care of these patients. The patient should be encouraged to receive neuraxial labor analgesia early in the course of her labor to decrease the likelihood that general anesthesia would be required should an obstetric emergency occur. The patient should also be counseled that difficulties with both regional and general anesthesia may be encountered.

A thorough airway examination is mandatory in these patients. Equipment necessary for the management of a difficult airway, including a fiber-optic bronchoscope, should be available in the labor and delivery suite. If the anesthesiologist anticipates airway difficulties that would preclude rapid sequence induction of general anesthesia, he should communicate this information to the obstetrician. Careful assessments of the patient's pulmonary and cardiac status are other important components of preanesthetic evaluation. Because functional residual capacity is reduced further in the supine position, baseline pulse oximetry measurements should be obtained in both the sitting and supine position to assess for hypoxemia. Especially in patients with long-standing morbid obesity, the anesthesiologist should also consider obtaining an arterial blood gas reading to assess for CO_2 retention, a sign of the obesity-hypoventilation syndrome. If clinical characteristics suggest the presence of obesity-hypoventilation syndrome, a thorough cardiac evaluation, including ECG and echocardiogram, is necessary to evaluate for the presence of pulmonary hypertension or cor pulmonale.

The anesthesiologist should determine whether the available equipment for noninvasive monitoring of blood pressure is able to accurately measure the morbidly obese parturient's blood pressure. If a blood pressure cuff that appropriately fits the woman's arm is not available, blood pressure measurement with an intra, arterial catheter may be necessary. The anesthesiologist should also have available long needles for performing neuraxial techniques. Finally, labor and delivery personnel must also make certain the labor and operating room beds that are to be used can adequately support the patient's weight.

Labor Analgesia

Epidural analgesia is a reasonable choice for labor analgesia in morbidly obese parturients. It provides superior pain relief compared to systemic opioids and is significantly less likely to cause maternal or neonatal respiratory depression. It also reduces oxygen consumption in these patients who are at risk for hypoxemia. In patients with obesity-related cardiac dysfunction, its ability to attenuate the increase in cardiac output that occurs during labor and delivery may be beneficial. Because morbidly obese women are more likely than nonobese women to require cesarean delivery and the risks of general anesthesia in morbidly obese patients are substantial, one of the greatest advantages of epidural analgesia is the ability to extend the block to achieve surgical anesthesia if necessary.

Although the advantages of epidural analgesia are many, the technical challenge of performing the technique in a morbidly obese parturient is often great. The depth of the epidural space is increased, and special, long needles may be required to reach the space.

CLINICAL CAVEAT: FAILURE OF EPIDURAL LABOR ANALGESIA IN MORBIDLY OBESE PATIENTS

- A 94% success rate has been reported (not significantly different than in nonobese patients).
- However, more attempts to identify the epidural space will likely be required.
- Be prepared to replace the epidural catheter during labor.
- Because a "false" loss of resistance may be felt as the needle is advanced through layers of adipose tissue, as many as 40% of epidural catheters will not function initially.
- An additional 20% of catheters may become dislodged during labor.

CLINICAL CAVEAT: SECURING THE EPIDURAL CATHETER IN MORBIDLY OBESE PATIENTS

- The skin-to-epidural space distance is greater in the lateral compared to sitting position.
- In morbidly obese patients, the epidural catheter will be drawn inward toward the epidural space an average of 1 cm when moving from the sitting, flexed position to the lateral position. In some patients, it moves as much as 4 cm.
- If the catheter is secured while the patient is still sitting, the catheter may be pulled out of the epidural space as the patient assumes the lateral position.
- The epidural catheter should be secured after the patient has assumed the lateral position to decrease the risk of catheter dislodgement.

Especially in obese patients, utilization of the sitting rather than the lateral position will often facilitate successful identification of the epidural space.

Because the failure rate for epidural analgesia is increased in obese parturients, it is essential that the anesthesiologist frequently monitor these patients and promptly replace the epidural catheter if evidence suggests inadequate analgesia. Adopting a particular procedure to secure the epidural catheter may also decrease epidural failure rates due to catheter displacement.

Epidural analgesia should be initiated early in labor to minimize the chance that general anesthesia would be required should emergency cesarean delivery become necessary at any time during labor. The goal of epidural analgesia for all parturients is to provide excellent analgesia while minimizing motor block. This is especially important in morbidly obese parturients because nursing care is very difficult if the patient cannot move adequately during labor and delivery. Therefore, administration of a dilute local anesthetic + opioid is recommended. Bupivacaine or ropivacaine 0.125% to 0.0625% + fentanyl 2 µg/mL will achieve adequate analgesia with minimal motor block in most parturients.

Continuous spinal analgesia is another option for labor analgesia which does provide some advantages over epidural analgesia in morbidly obese patients. Superior labor analgesia can be achieved using intermittent doses of intrathecal opioids during early labor and opioids plus small doses of local anesthetics during the late stage of labor and delivery. Because analgesia can be provided with minimal doses of local anesthetics compared to epidural analgesia, motor block is often nonexistent. This might facilitate vaginal delivery and will certainly make nursing care easier. More importantly, correct placement of the catheter is confirmed by aspiration of cerebrospinal fluid, so initial failure rates should be less than with epidural analgesia. If the catheter becomes dislodged during labor, identification of the problem and replacement of the catheter could occur more promptly compared to epidural analgesia because the loss of ability to aspirate cerebrospinal fluid would confirm the dislodgement before analgesia had dissipated. Identification of a displaced epidural catheter is generally delayed until the patient no longer has adequate pain relief. Because spinal microcatheters are not currently available for clinical use, a large-gauge epidural needle and catheter must be used to administer continuous spinal analgesia. Therefore, the risk of developing a postdural puncture headache is a significant disadvantage of this technique. There have been some anecdotal reports that the incidence of spinal headache is decreased in morbidly obese patients, but this has not been proven, and certainly some patients will develop a headache and require treatment.

CSE analgesia provides excellent pain relief for labor. However, until the initial intrathecal analgesia dissipates, the epidural catheter remains unproven. If emergency cesarean delivery was required during this time interval and epidural anesthesia failed, general anesthesia would be required. Therefore, because the risks of general anesthesia are significant in morbidly obese parturients and the incidence of cesarean delivery is increased in these patients, I do not advocate using CSE analgesia for administering labor analgesia in this patient population.

Anesthesia for Cesarean Delivery

The incidence of cesarean delivery is increased in obese women compared to nonobese women. In one study, nearly 50% of morbidly obese parturients who underwent a trial of labor eventually required cesarean delivery. The anesthesiologist may confront several challenges when caring for these patients. Longer surgery duration and increased blood loss should be anticipated. Particular attention should be paid to positioning of the patient. Left uterine displacement is mandatory, but the anesthesiologist must be certain that the patient is adequately secured to the operating table before tilting the table. The obstetrician frequently requests cephalad retraction of the patient's panniculus so that a Pfannenstiel skin incision can be utilized. If cephalad retraction is performed, the anesthesiologist must be vigilant for hypotension caused by aortocaval compression that could lead to fetal or maternal compromise as well as signs or symptoms of maternal respiratory compromise caused by increased chest wall compliance. The obstetrician must be aware that if the patient experiences adverse effects from the cephalad retraction of the panniculus, this approach will need to be abandoned, and a vertical skin incision may be required. Because these patients are at high risk for aspiration, all patients should receive aspiration prophylaxis preoperatively, even if general anesthesia is not initially planned. Sodium citrate, metoclopramide, and an H_2-receptor antagonist are all recommended. Finally, regardless of the type of anesthesia chosen, the anesthesiologist should realize that technical difficulties are more likely to occur in the morbidly obese parturient.

The risks associated with general anesthesia in pregnant patients (e.g., difficult airway, aspiration) are increased even further in obese parturients. Therefore, regional anesthesia is preferred for cesarean delivery. Epidural anesthesia offers several advantages. The dose of local anesthetic can slowly be titrated. This is especially important in obese patients because studies suggest that the epidural spread of local anesthetic is exaggerated in these patients, leading to higher sensory levels than might be expected. Slow administration of epidural local anesthetic also results in a slower onset of sympathetic blockade, which could decrease the risk of hypotension. An important advantage of epidural anesthesia is the ability to administer additional local anesthetic to maintain surgical anesthesia if surgery is prolonged. Rarely do these patients experience respiratory difficulty associated with the high level of sensory blockade (T4–T6) required for surgery. The choice of local anesthetic drug will be determined by the urgency of surgery and the personal preference of the physician. Some physicians prefer to use 2% lidocaine with epinephrine 1:200,000 for nonemergent situations and 3% 2-chloroprocaine for emergency cesarean deliveries.

Some disadvantages of epidural anesthesia do exist. Compared to spinal anesthesia, the depth of sensory blockade may be less, and the patient may experience discomfort during the surgery. In the morbidly obese parturient, the greatest disadvantage of this technique is the high initial failure rate. However, because the benefits of regional anesthesia for cesarean delivery are so great in morbidly obese patients, an initial failure should not deter the anesthesiologist from making subsequent attempts to perform epidural anesthesia.

Some of the disadvantages of epidural anesthesia can be avoided with continuous spinal anesthesia while maintaining many of the advantages of an epidural technique. Therefore, some anesthesiologists consider it the ideal anesthetic for cesarean delivery in morbidly obese patients. Like epidural anesthesia, this technique allows for slow titration of the local anesthetic dose. Because some studies suggest that obesity results in an exaggerated spread of spinal local anesthetic, thereby increasing the risk of high spinal anesthesia, the ability to titrate the dose of local anesthetic is an important benefit in morbidly obese parturients. Administration of incremental 0.5-mL doses of 0.75% hyperbaric spinal bupivacaine should be continued until a T4–T6 sensory level is achieved. Spinal anesthesia generally produces a denser sensory block compared to epidural anesthesia, and patients undergoing cesarean delivery with spinal anesthesia often seem to experience less intraoperative discomfort than patients receiving epidural anesthesia. Most important, the initial failure rate of the continuous spinal technique should be significantly less than epidural anesthesia because the aspiration of cerebrospinal fluid through the spinal catheter confirms correct placement. Obviously, the major disadvantage of this technique is the high likelihood that the patient will develop a spinal headache.

Single-shot spinal anesthesia is the quickest regional anesthesia technique available for cesarean delivery. When the urgency of the situation does not allow time to perform a continuous neuraxial technique, the administration of spinal anesthesia to a morbidly obese parturient may be preferred over general anesthesia. However, significant disadvantages of single-shot spinal anesthesia in the morbidly obese patient do exist. The dose of local anesthetic cannot be titrated, and exaggerated spread of the local anesthetic could lead to high spinal anesthesia with the use of a conventional spinal dose. However, the spread of local anesthetic cannot be easily predicted, so

if the dose is reduced to avoid a high sensory level, the anesthetic block could be inadequate for surgery. Most important, surgery duration is more likely to be prolonged in morbidly obese patients. If surgery duration extends beyond the duration of spinal anesthesia, induction of general anesthesia would be required, thus exposing the patient to all the risks associated with that anesthetic technique.

CSE anesthesia is another option for cesarean delivery. With this technique, the onset of blockade is achieved more quickly and the sensory block is denser than with epidural anesthesia. However, significant disadvantages exist. The dose of spinal anesthesia cannot be titrated. In addition, the epidural catheter remains untested. If the duration of surgery outlasts the duration of spinal anesthesia and epidural anesthesia must be administered, the possibility exists that the epidural catheter will not function appropriately, thus necessitating general anesthesia. Because technical difficulties with regional anesthesia are more frequently encountered in morbidly obese patients, the likelihood of a nonfunctioning epidural catheter may be increased. Therefore, some physicians do not consider CSE anesthesia a preferred technique for cesarean delivery in morbidly obese women.

Although general anesthesia for cesarean delivery is avoided whenever possible in morbidly obese patients, some clinical scenarios will require its use. Induction of general anesthesia in a morbidly obese parturient is fraught with danger and requires meticulous planning and preparation to avoid disaster. Anesthesia-related mortality during cesarean delivery is increased in obese patients, and many of these deaths are due to aspiration and airway complications during general anesthesia. Careful evaluation of the airway is essential, even in emergency situations. Intubation is known to be more difficult in obstetric patients; the very large breasts and fat deposits in the neck and shoulders often present in obese patients increase the difficulty even further. These anatomic characteristics also make mask ventilation more difficult in the morbidly obese patient. Previous easy intubation does not guarantee success in the pregnant patient. In one study, difficult intubation was encountered in 33% of morbidly obese parturients. In two thirds of those patients, difficulty was not anticipated.

Before proceeding with the induction of general anesthesia, the anesthesiologist must be certain that any airway equipment that might be necessary is immediately available. A variety of laryngoscope blades, small endotracheal tubes, a fiber-optic bronchoscope, and a short-handled laryngoscope, which makes insertion of the laryngoscope easier in patients with large breasts, should all be available. A laryngeal mask airway and equipment for performing percutaneous cricothyrotomy and transtracheal jet ventilation should also be available in the event that both intubation and mask ventilation cannot be successfully performed. Although use of a laryngeal mask airway will not protect against aspiration, it provides the ability to ventilate the patient as well as a conduit for performing fiber-optic intubation. The anesthesiologist should be aware that technical difficulties may be encountered when attempting to perform percutaneous cricothyrotomy in a morbidly obese patient. Regardless of the urgency of the situation, rapid sequence induction of general anesthesia should not proceed if difficult intubation is anticipated. Instead, awake intubation, usually utilizing fiber-optic laryngoscopy, should be performed. Although it may be difficult for the anesthesiologist to insist on this plan when the obstetrician is emphasizing the dire condition of a fetus, the anesthesiologist must realize that neither mother nor fetus will benefit from a situation in which neither intubation or ventilation can be achieved in an apneic patient.

Once the decision has been made to proceed with rapid sequence induction of general anesthesia, the anesthesiologist should make certain that aspiration prophylaxis has been administered. The patient should at minimum receive sodium citrate if time does not allow for the administration of metoclopramide and an H_2-receptor antagonist. Emphasis should be placed on careful positioning of the patient because this can facilitate both mask ventilation and intubation. Towels placed under the shoulders will elevate the shoulders and cause the large breasts to fall away from the chin and neck. Towels should also be used under the head to place the patient in a sniffing position. Because both pregnant and obese patients rapidly become hypoxemic after the onset of apnea, adequate preoxygenation to achieve denitrogenation is essential before proceeding with rapid sequence induction. Three to 5 minutes of tidal ventilation or four vital capacity breaths with 100% oxygen are equally effective at providing preoxygenation. The technique chosen is usually dictated by the urgency with which cesarean delivery is required.

The choice of induction agent is based on the patient's current hemodynamic status and underlying medical conditions. Most commonly, thiopental 4 mg/kg is administered. Succinylcholine is the muscle relaxant of choice for rapid sequence induction. A dose of 1.0 to 1.5 mg/kg should be administered to ensure complete relaxation during laryngoscopy. Identification of the cricoid ring may be difficult in morbidly obese patients. Therefore, it is important that personnel adequately trained in applying cricoid pressure be available during induction of general anesthesia.

Anesthesia is usually maintained before delivery of the infant with N_2O 50% and a volatile halogenated anesthetic agent. After delivery, intravenous opioids can be administered, and the concentration of volatile agent may be decreased to avoid any effects on uterine tone. Some morbidly obese patients may require a high concentration of oxygen to maintain adequate oxygenation in the supine position. In that case, nitrous oxide might need to be eliminated or the concentration reduced. Other maneuvers that can be utilized intraoperatively to improve oxygenation include the use of a large tidal volume and the administration of positive end-expiratory pressure, although some controversy exists concerning the utility of the latter in obese patients. At the end of surgery, the morbidly obese parturient should be fully awake before removing the endotracheal tube in order to decrease the risk of aspiration.

CARDIAC DISEASE

Cardiac disease complicates up to 4% of pregnancies. Depending on the type and severity of the disorder, maternal and fetal outcome may be adversely affected. Over the past several years, advances in medical and surgical treatment have changed the composition of cardiac lesions encountered in parturients. Many patients with congenital heart disease are now reaching childbearing age because of improved surgical treatments. They now constitute an increasing proportion of pregnant cardiac patients. In contrast, the number of pregnant patients with rheumatic heart disease has declined. Regardless of the cause of the heart disease, the cardiovascular changes of pregnancy produce added stress on the already compromised cardiovascular system and may result in cardiac decompensation. These patients require close observation and careful management throughout pregnancy, labor, and delivery. An interdisciplinary approach that includes obstetricians, anesthesiologists, cardiologists, and nurses working closely together optimizes patient care.

Congenital Heart Disease

In the past, few patients with complex congenital heart disease survived into the childbearing years. With the improvements in the diagnosis and surgical treatment of congenital heart defects that have occurred over the past 20 years, a significant proportion of pregnant cardiac patients in contemporary practice have congenital heart disease. Many of these women had successful surgical repair of the defects during childhood and are asymptomatic with normal cardiac function. These patients often require only standard monitoring and anesthetic management during labor and delivery, but they should undergo cardiology evaluation early during pregnancy. Echocardiography is beneficial for evaluating patients for asymptomatic residua of the surgical correction that could be exacerbated by the cardiovascular changes of pregnancy. Some of these patients will require antibiotic prophylaxis for bacterial endocarditis during labor and vaginal delivery. In contrast, other parturients present with uncorrected or partially corrected congenital lesions in which the physiologic changes of pregnancy have resulted in serious cardiac decompensation. The anesthetic management of these patients is quite challenging. The most common congenital heart disorders encountered by the obstetric anesthesiologist include Tetralogy of Fallot, left-to-right shunts, and Eisenmenger's syndrome.

Tetralogy of Fallot

Tetralogy of Fallot includes the following: (1) right ventricular outflow tract obstruction, (2) ventricular septal defect (VSD), (3) right ventricular hypertrophy, and (4) an overriding aorta. This is the most common congenital heart defect that produces a right-to-left shunt and cyanosis. It is rare for these patients to survive to adulthood without surgical correction. Most pregnant patients who have had surgical repair, which includes closure of the VSD and widening of the pulmonary outflow tract, are asymptomatic. A small VSD may occasionally recur, or hypertrophy of the pulmonary outflow tract may develop. Patients with these defects require additional attention during labor and delivery. Symptoms experienced by these patients depend on the size of the VSD, the magnitude of outflow tract obstruction, and the degree of right ventricular dysfunction.

In patients with a recurrence of VSD or pulmonary outflow tract obstruction, epidural analgesia is advantageous for preventing the hemodynamic changes associated with labor pain. However, it is important to maintain systemic vascular resistance (SVR) to prevent an increase in right-to-left shunting. Phenylephrine should be administered to prevent or treat any reductions in SVR that occur secondary to the sympathetic blockade produced by epidural analgesia.

Maintenance of venous return is also important for these patients. Patients with severe right ventricular dysfunction benefit from high filling pressures that improve right ventricular output and pulmonary blood flow.

Left-to-Right Shunts

Parturients with a surgically corrected VSD or atrial septal defect (ASD) are usually asymptomatic and require no special anesthetic care. Patients with small, asymptomatic VSDs and ASDs generally tolerate labor and delivery without difficulty and do not require invasive monitoring. However, the pain of labor increases maternal catecholamine levels, resulting in increased SVR. This increased SVR may produce greater left-to-right shunting that ultimately leads to pulmonary hypertension. Epidural analgesia should be initiated early in labor to prevent these consequences. The mild decrease in SVR associated with epidural analgesia also provides additional benefit by reducing left-to-right shunting through

the defect. Epidural blockade should be achieved slowly to prevent a rapid decrease in SVR that could produce right-to-left shunting and, ultimately, hypoxemia.

Patients with a VSD or ASD are at risk for systemic embolization. All air should be removed from intravenous lines before infusion of fluids. The loss-of-resistance-to-air technique should not be used when performing an epidural procedure. Because even mild hypoxemia can lead to increased pulmonary vascular resistance and subsequent right-to-left shunting, supplemental oxygen should be administered throughout labor and delivery.

Parturients with a large VSD or ASD commonly have chronically increased pulmonary blood flow that produces pulmonary hypertension. These patients require special attention during labor and delivery, including intra-arterial and pulmonary artery pressure monitoring. Increases in heart rate and systemic and pulmonary vascular resistance must be avoided. Marked decreases in systemic and pulmonary vascular resistance are also not well tolerated. Adequate labor analgesia helps to attenuate changes in SVR. Carefully titrated epidural analgesia is an acceptable labor analgesia technique in these patients. However, a CSE technique using primarily spinal opioids may be preferable because decreases in SVR are minimized.

Eisenmenger's Syndrome

Eisenmenger's syndrome results when chronic pulmonary volume overload from an uncorrected left-to-right shunt leads to pulmonary hypertension (Fig. 8-6). Initially, the shunt becomes bidirectional with acute changes in pulmonary vascular resistance or SVR determining the direction of flow. Eventually, the pulmonary hypertension becomes irreversible, and shunt flow

---

> ## CURRENT CONTROVERSIES: USE OF PHENYLEPHRINE IN PREGNANT CARDIAC PATIENTS
>
> - Phenylephrine has traditionally been avoided in obstetric patients because its α-adrenergic effects have the potential to compromise uteroplacental perfusion. Ephedrine has been the vasopressor of choice to treat hypotension during neuraxial anesthesia.
> - In cardiac patients, though, the choice of vasoactive drug should be based primarily on the pathophysiology of the patient's cardiac defect rather than effects on uteroplacental blood flow.
> - Furthermore, a meta-analysis that assessed the use of phenylephrine versus ephedrine in normal pregnancies found no difference in the incidence of fetal acidosis between the two drugs. In fact, the mean umbilical artery pH was higher among neonates whose mothers received phenylephrine.

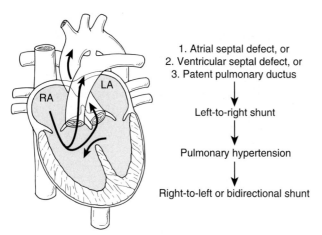

1. Atrial septal defect, or
2. Ventricular septal defect, or
3. Patent pulmonary ductus

↓

Left-to-right shunt

↓

Pulmonary hypertension

↓

Right-to-left or bidirectional shunt

Figure 8-6   Pathophysiology of Eisenmenger's syndrome. RA, right atrium; LA, left atrium (Redrawn from Mangano DT: Anesthesia for the Pregnant Cardiac Patient. In Hughes SC, Levinson G, Rosen MA [eds]: Shnider and Levinson's Anesthesia for Obstetrics, Fourth edition. Philadelphia, Lippincott, Williams & Wilkins, 2002, p 469.)

reverses. Right-to-left shunting occurs when pulmonary artery pressure exceeds systemic pressure.

Patients with Eisenmenger's syndrome do not tolerate pregnancy well. The decreased SVR that occurs during pregnancy may increase the shunt fraction. In addition, respiratory changes of pregnancy, including decreased functional residual capacity and increased oxygen consumption, exacerbate maternal hypoxemia. Maternal mortality is as high as 40% to 50%, with thromboembolic phenomena a leading cause of death. Maternal hypoxemia also compromises oxygen delivery to the fetus. As a result, the incidences of intrauterine growth restriction and fetal demise are increased.

Anesthetic management of the parturient with Eisenmenger's syndrome is extremely challenging. If a vaginal delivery is planned, it is essential that adequate labor analgesia be provided. The significant increase in serum catecholamine levels caused by untreated labor pain contributes to increases in pulmonary vascular resistance and right-to-left shunting. The patient should receive supplemental oxygen throughout labor and delivery, and pulse oximetry monitoring is utilized. Worsening hypoxemia must be treated aggressively to avoid increases in pulmonary vascular resistance. Because prevention of hypotension and decreases in SVR is also essential in the management of these patients, continuous blood pressure monitoring with an intra-arterial catheter is indicated.

Central venous pressure (CVP) monitoring is very beneficial in the management of patients with Eisenmenger's syndrome because maintenance of adequate preload is important. Most experts do not recommend using a pulmonary artery catheter because little useful information is derived from pulmonary artery pressure monitoring in patients with fixed pulmonary hyperten-

sion and a large intracardiac shunt. In addition, insertion of the catheter is difficult, and common complications associated with the procedure, including dysrhythmias and pneumothorax, could be life threatening for these patients who lack cardiac reserve.

Providing adequate labor analgesia to the woman with Eisenmenger's syndrome without producing deleterious hemodynamic effects is a significant challenge for the anesthesiologist. A CSE technique is an excellent choice. Administration of an intrathecal opioid during the first stage of labor provides rapid and profound analgesia without causing a sympathetic block. Small incremental doses of dilute local anesthetic are administered epidurally once the intrathecal analgesia has resolved. Although bupivacaine has been used safely in pregnant cardiac patients, ropivacaine or levobupivacaine might be better choices because these drugs possess less cardiac toxicity. A continuous infusion of very dilute local anesthetic and opioid (such as 0.125% to 0.0625% levobupivacaine plus 2 μg/mL fentanyl) or patient-controlled epidural analgesia is then administered for the duration of labor. Decreases in SVR caused by sympathetic blockade are avoided by slow incremental dosing of the epidural catheter, continuous blood pressure monitoring, and careful intravenous fluid administration. Infusion of intravenous phenylephrine is used to prevent or treat decreases in SVR.

Often an instrument-assisted vaginal delivery is planned in patients with Eisenmenger's syndrome to minimize maternal expulsive efforts. Epidural anesthesia with a higher concentration of local anesthetic than was used for labor analgesia is required to provide adequate anesthesia for a forceps-assisted delivery. Ropivacaine, levobupivacaine, and lidocaine are good local anesthetic choices.

Continuous spinal analgesia and epidural analgesia are other options for providing labor analgesia in parturients with Eisenmenger's syndrome. Intrathecal opioid dosing is repeated as needed during the first stage of labor with continuous spinal analgesia, and very small doses of local anesthetic are added during the second stage of labor. With continuous spinal analgesia, the hemodynamic changes caused by sympathetic blockade could be minimized even further than with a CSE technique. However, a high incidence of postdural puncture headache is a disadvantage of this technique. The need to administer epidural local anesthetics beginning in early labor is the major disadvantage of epidural analgesia. Significant sympathectomy and decreased SVR are more likely to occur compared with CSE and continuous spinal analgesia.

Epidural anesthesia is often the preferred anesthetic technique for cesarean delivery in women with Eisenmenger's syndrome. A sudden drop in SVR during the induction of epidural anesthesia must not be allowed to occur because it will worsen right-to-left shunting.

This problem can be prevented by the slow induction of epidural anesthesia, maintenance of adequate preload with careful monitoring of CVP, and use of a phenylephrine infusion to maintain SVR. Ropivacaine, levobupivacaine, and 2% lidocaine without epinephrine are all acceptable local anesthetic choices. Chloroprocaine should be avoided because of its rapid onset. Anxiolysis with a benzodiazepine may be administered to prevent increases in catecholamine release secondary to maternal anxiety. Continuous spinal anesthesia is another reasonable anesthetic technique for cesarean delivery in these patients. Single-shot spinal anesthesia, however, is not recommended in patients with Eisenmenger's syndrome because of the hypotension and rapid decrease in SVR that could occur.

Some anesthesiologists advocate general anesthesia for cesarean delivery in women with Eisenmenger's syndrome. However, disadvantages of this technique do exist. Decreased venous return associated with positive pressure ventilation is not tolerated well in these patients. In addition, the patient's cardiovascular compromise requires a slow induction of general anesthesia, preferably with a high-dose opioid technique, to maintain cardiovascular stability. However, these parturients are also at risk for pulmonary aspiration. While measures such as pharmacologic aspiration prophylaxis and maintenance of cricoid pressure throughout the induction of anesthesia will lessen aspiration risk, the risk likely remains higher compared to patients undergoing rapid sequence induction. Finally, the use of a high-dose opioid general anesthetic increases the likelihood of neonatal respiratory depression.

The risk of maternal mortality persists into the postpartum period. Therefore, extended hemodynamic monitoring in an intensive-care setting is essential for at least 24 to 48 hours after delivery. Because thromboembolic events are a significant cause of maternal death, prophylactic anticoagulation should be considered when the risk of bleeding has subsided in the postpartum period.

Valvular Heart Disease

Anesthesiologists are caring for fewer patients with rheumatic valvular disease because the incidence of rheumatic fever has markedly decreased in the United States. As more women delay childbearing into their fourth and fifth decades, however, anesthesiologists should anticipate that they will encounter an increasing number of parturients with aortic stenosis and insufficiency caused by a congenital aortic bicuspid valve.

Aortic Stenosis

Aortic stenosis during pregnancy usually results from a congenital bicuspid valve or rheumatic heart disease. Women with mild stenosis generally tolerate pregnancy well. Many of the cardiovascular changes of pregnancy are deleterious to parturients with moderate to severe stenosis, however. Therefore, it is recommended that women with moderate to severe stenosis undergo aortic valve replacement before conception.

The increased cardiac output and oxygen consumption and the decreased SVR that occur during pregnancy are deleterious to the patient with severe aortic stenosis. Because stroke volume is relatively fixed with the stenotic lesion, cardiac output increases primarily by an increase in heart rate. Tachycardia decreases the time available for diastolic coronary perfusion and increases myocardial oxygen demand. The increased left ventricular end-diastolic pressure and left ventricular hypertrophy that are present in severe aortic stenosis also decrease myocardial perfusion. The decreased SVR of pregnancy reduces coronary filling during diastole and decreases perfusion to the hypertrophied left ventricle. These parturients are therefore at risk for myocardial ischemia. Additional increases in cardiac output occur during labor and delivery, thus elevating the risk of ischemia even further.

Some obstetricians perform cesarean delivery in these patients only for obstetric indications and prefer a vaginal delivery. An instrument-assisted vaginal delivery with minimal maternal expulsive efforts is usually planned to avoid the adverse hemodynamic effects of the Valsalva maneuver. Other obstetricians prefer a cesarean delivery to avoid the uncertain duration and course, and the hemodynamic stress of labor. The unique characteristics of each patient are used to determine an anesthetic plan.

Regardless of the anesthetic technique chosen, certain hemodynamic conditions should be maintained when anesthetizing patients with aortic stenosis. A normal heart rate and sinus rhythm are essential. Tachycardia is not well tolerated for the reasons discussed earlier, and bradycardia provides inadequate cardiac output because of the fixed stroke volume. The atrial "kick" contributes 40% to the ventricular filling and cardiac output. Prompt treatment is necessary when dysrhythmias occur. Normal SVR must be maintained to ensure adequate myocardial perfusion. Normal venous return is required to maintain adequate end-diastolic volume and left ventricular stroke volume.

Invasive monitors, including an intra-arterial catheter and a CVP or pulmonary artery catheter, are necessary to optimize management of these parturients. A pulmonary artery catheter is usually preferable over a CVP catheter. The measurements are more indicative of left-sided pressures, and additional information is provided that is not available with a CVP catheter.

Although excellent analgesia for labor and vaginal delivery is an essential component in the anesthetic management of women with aortic stenosis, it can be a challenge to provide analgesia and still maintain the hemodynamic goals of aortic stenosis. At least in the past, some anesthesiologists avoided regional anesthesia in these patients because of the decreases in venous return and SVR associated with the technique. Instead, they utilized intravenous opioids for first-stage labor pain and pudendal nerve block for second-stage labor pain. However, systemic opioids often don't provide adequate analgesia, and the tachycardia that develops when pain is inadequately treated is deleterious to these women. Safe and effective labor analgesia can be achieved with slow and careful titration of epidural analgesia, provided that invasive monitors are utilized to assess and quickly treat any decreases in venous return or SVR. Hypotension is managed with intravenous fluids and phenylephrine; ephedrine is less desirable because of the associated tachycardia.

The administration of intrathecal opioids is another excellent alternative for labor analgesia in women with aortic stenosis. With a CSE technique, excellent analgesia is initially provided with intrathecal opioids, whereas the decreased venous return and SVR associated with epidurally administered local anesthetics are avoided. When the initial intrathecal analgesia resolves, the slow administration of epidural local anesthetics provides pain relief. A continuous spinal catheter technique permits intermittent intrathecal opioid injection throughout the first stage of labor. Small doses of intrathecal local anesthetic can be added to the opioid to provide anesthesia for the second stage of labor and delivery. Hemodynamic stability may be more easily achieved with this technique compared to epidural anesthesia because a local anesthetic-induced sympathectomy is avoided during the majority of the labor process.

Both regional and general anesthesia have been safely used to provide anesthesia for cesarean delivery in parturients with aortic stenosis. A single-shot spinal technique is not an acceptable option because of the rapid hemodynamic changes that may occur. When invasive monitors are used to guide management, the slow administration of either epidural or spinal anesthesia via a continuous catheter technique provides excellent anesthesia and maintains hemodynamic stability. Regional anesthesia avoids the risks of aspiration and difficult intubation that are present in all pregnant women undergoing general anesthesia. The deleterious effects of tachycardia associated with laryngoscopy are also avoided.

The hypotension and reduction in SVR that could occur with regional anesthesia could be catastrophic in a parturient with aortic stenosis. Therefore, some anesthesiologists prefer using general anesthesia for cesarean delivery in these patients. Anesthetic agents that maintain hemodynamic stability should be used. Successful induction of general anesthesia with etomidate, alfentanil, and succinylcholine in a parturient with severe aortic stenosis has been reported. Other anesthesiologists recommend induction with a slow, high-dose opioid technique. Regardless of the particular drugs chosen for induction, the administration of opioids before delivery of the infant is necessary to prevent tachycardia during laryngoscopy. Therefore, a neonatologist should be present at delivery. Volatile agents produce myocardial depression and should either be avoided or used very cautiously. Anesthetic maintenance is best achieved with a high-dose opioid technique.

Patients with moderate to severe aortic stenosis should be monitored closely in the postpartum period. Cardiac decompensation could occur in response to the marked increase in cardiac output that occurs after delivery. Therefore, invasive monitoring should continue for 24 hours after delivery. Excellent postoperative analgesia is also important in the management of postcesarean patients to prevent tachycardia.

Aortic Insufficiency

Rheumatic heart disease is the most common cause of chronic aortic insufficiency in pregnant women. Acute aortic insufficiency may occur in parturients with infective endocarditis. The pathophysiology of aortic insufficiency involves left ventricular volume overload that results from regurgitation of blood into the left ventricle from an incompetent aortic valve. Left ventricular hypertrophy and dilation develop. As end-diastolic volume increases, ventricular function declines, and forward stroke volume decreases. Progressive deterioration of left ventricular function leads to marked increases of left ventricular end-diastolic volume and pressure, ultimately leading to pulmonary edema. These changes occur over many years in patients with chronic insufficiency, so many parturients with aortic insufficiency are asymptomatic. However, as an increasing number of women delay childbearing into their fourth and fifth decades, anesthesiologists may encounter more patients with severe aortic insufficiency.

The physiologic changes of pregnancy are beneficial to the patient with aortic insufficiency. The reduction in SVR decreases the regurgitant fraction and improves forward stroke volume. The small increase in heart rate decreases time in diastole. As a result, there is less time for regurgitation and subsequently a smaller end-diastolic volume. Patients with mild to moderate aortic insufficiency usually tolerate pregnancy well. However, patients with severe aortic insufficiency in whom significant declines in left ventricular function have occurred before pregnancy require intensive management. These patients are often unable to compensate for the increased blood volume of pregnancy. Invasive hemodynamic monitors, including intra-arterial and pulmonary artery catheters, are indicated for these women during labor and delivery.

Labor analgesia plays an important role in the management of parturients with aortic insufficiency. The pain of labor causes an increase in SVR. This increased SVR produces an increase in left ventricular volume overload, which could lead to pulmonary edema. Epidural analgesia is an ideal technique for providing pain management in these patients. Not only does the excellent analgesia attenuate any increases in SVR, but the local anesthetic-induced sympathetic blockade actually decreases SVR, thereby improving forward stroke volume and cardiac output. In parturients with severe disease, the pulmonary artery catheter is helpful in guiding fluid management during the induction and maintenance of epidural analgesia. Maintaining adequate preload and avoiding hypotension are important goals in the anesthetic management of these patients. The vasopressor of choice for treating hypotension is ephedrine. The increase in heart rate associated with this drug is beneficial. In contrast, the bradycardia and increased SVR associated with phenylephrine use could be detrimental.

For the same reasons described for labor analgesia, epidural anesthesia is the preferred technique for cesarean delivery in patients with aortic insufficiency. Slow administration of local anesthetic and the use of invasive monitors to guide fluid and vasopressor management are essential. Cardiac arrest has been reported in a parturient with aortic insufficiency when the epidural block was established too quickly. If the clinical situation requires general anesthesia, the severity of the patient's condition determines the type of anesthetic induction. Asymptomatic women with mild to moderate insufficiency tolerate a rapid sequence induction. A slow induction with high-dose opioids is recommended for patients with severe insufficiency and left ventricular dysfunction. Anesthetic agents that depress myocardial function should be avoided or used cautiously in parturients with severe disease.

Mitral Stenosis

Although the incidence of rheumatic heart disease has declined significantly in the United States, mitral stenosis is the most common cardiac lesion associated with rheumatic heart disease in pregnant women. Therefore, anesthesiologists who care for high-risk obstetric patients are likely to encounter patients with this valvular disorder. In 25% of women with mitral stenosis, the first symptoms occur during pregnancy, precipitated by the cardiovascular changes of pregnancy. The necessary increase in cardiac output during pregnancy is impeded by the stenotic lesion. In addition, the heart rate increase that occurs during pregnancy decreases the diastolic time for left ventricular filling. This leads to increases in left atrial and pulmonary arterial pressures and ultimately to pulmonary edema. Parturients with severe mitral stenosis do not tolerate well the increased demands placed on the cardiovascular system and are likely to experience cardiac decompensation. These patients should be closely monitored by a cardiologist throughout pregnancy.

Careful management by a cardiologist can prevent some complications associated with mitral stenosis in parturients. β-adrenergic blockade is used to maintain a slow heart rate. Some controversy exists concerning the effects of β-blockers on the fetus. However, one study found that the administration of β-blockers to pregnant women with mitral stenosis decreased the incidence of pulmonary edema with no ill effects on the fetus. Atrial fibrillation is detrimental in the parturient with mitral stenosis, resulting in decreased cardiac output and an increased risk of pulmonary edema. Therefore, aggressive therapy is required. Digoxin and β-adrenergic blockers are administered for both the treatment of atrial fibrillation and the maintenance of normal sinus rhythm. If pharmacologic therapy is unsuccessful, cardioversion is performed.

Patients with asymptomatic, mild to moderate mitral stenosis generally tolerate labor and delivery well. It is prudent to observe these patients closely during labor and maintain continuous pulse oximetry monitoring, but invasive monitoring is usually not warranted. Invasive monitoring that includes a pulmonary artery catheter is recommended in patients who either become symptomatic during pregnancy or have severe stenosis. Adequate filling pressures should be maintained in these patients, but fluid overload must also be avoided because they are at significant risk for pulmonary edema, especially in the immediate postpartum period. Maintenance of SVR is necessary to provide adequate perfusion pressure because the ability to increase cardiac output is limited by the stenotic lesion. These patients may not tolerate a sudden increase in venous return associated with the Valsalva maneuver during maternal expulsive efforts. A passive second stage of labor and instrument-assisted vaginal delivery are often planned. Cesarean delivery is usually reserved for obstetric indications.

Excellent analgesia to prevent the undesirable tachycardia associated with labor pain is an important goal in the anesthetic management of parturients with mitral stenosis. In addition, a dense anesthetic block is required during the second stage of labor to prevent the urge to push and to facilitate a forceps- or vacuum-assisted delivery. A CSE anesthesia technique is one reasonable alternative for these patients. Intrathecal opioid can provide initial analgesia during the first stage of labor without producing a significant drop in SVR or requiring a large fluid bolus to maintain adequate preload. As additional labor analgesia and anesthesia for delivery are required, slow incremental dosing of the epidural catheter accompanied by close observation of the hemodynamic monitors will minimize disastrous decreases in SVR and venous return while also preventing inadvertent volume overload. Phenylephrine is preferred over ephedrine to treat anesthesia-induced hypotension because it maintains SVR and avoids maternal tachycardia. Continuous epidural and spinal analgesia are also reasonable options for providing labor analgesia to patients with severe mitral stenosis. Monitoring and hemodynamic management are similar regardless of the regional anesthesia technique chosen.

Epidural anesthesia is often the preferred technique for cesarean delivery in patients with mitral stenosis. Using invasive monitors to guide fluid management, the slow induction of epidural anesthesia is generally well-tolerated with maintenance of hemodynamic stability. A significant sympathectomy does occur with the high sensory level required to provide adequate anesthesia for cesarean delivery. Phenylephrine is administered by slow infusion or small, intermittent doses to prevent a hemodynamically significant reduction in SVR. A single-shot spinal technique is not recommended for parturients with severe mitral stenosis because of the potential for large, rapid declines in venous return and SVR.

Some clinical scenarios will require general anesthesia for cesarean delivery in patients with mitral stenosis. The patient's ventricular function determines if she will tolerate a rapid-sequence induction of general anesthesia, or will require a high-dose opioid technique. A β-adrenergic blocker or a small dose of opioid is administered during rapid-sequence induction to blunt tachycardia and hypertension associated with laryngoscopy. Remifentanil may be a good choice when a high-dose opioid technique is used because its rapid metabolism and very short duration of action could minimize depressant effects in the neonate. In fact, in one case in which remifentanil was used for cesarean delivery in a woman with mitral valve disease, no neonatal depression occurred.

The marked increases in cardiac output and venous return that occur in the immediate postpartum period put patients with severe mitral stenosis at high risk for developing pulmonary edema. Therefore, these patients require close observation and continued hemodynamic monitoring for at least 24 hours postpartum. The anesthesiologist may choose to continue epidural anesthesia for several hours postpartum so that the increased preload associated with resolution of the sympathectomy-induced vasodilation will not coincide with the increased preload that occurs in the immediate postpartum period.

Mitral Insufficiency

The majority of parturients with mitral insufficiency have chronic insufficiency caused by rheumatic heart disease or mitral valve prolapse. Slow dilation of the left atrium develops as left atrial pressure increases. Like parturients with mitral stenosis, the risk of developing atrial fibrillation during pregnancy is increased. The incidence of pulmonary edema and pulmonary hypertension, however, is much lower in pregnant women with mitral insufficiency compared to mitral stenosis. The physio-

logic changes of pregnancy, including decreased SVR and mildly increased heart rate, are advantageous in patients with mitral insufficiency. Most patients tolerate pregnancy well.

Continuous electrocardiographic monitoring is warranted during labor and delivery because of the increased risk for atrial fibrillation. If atrial fibrillation does occur, rapid treatment is essential to maintain adequate cardiac output. No other special monitoring is necessary for asymptomatic patients during labor and delivery. Symptomatic patients and patients with a history of pulmonary edema require invasive monitoring with an intra-arterial catheter and pulmonary artery catheter.

Increased SVR caused by either labor pain or the Valsalva maneuver during expulsive efforts must be avoided. Epidural anesthesia provides excellent labor analgesia and anesthesia for an instrument-assisted delivery while also preventing an undesired increase in SVR. In fact, the technique produces a mild reduction in SVR, which reduces regurgitation, improves forward flow, increases cardiac output, and decreases the likelihood of developing pulmonary edema. Careful attention is given to maintaining adequate venous return and left ventricular filling during epidural anesthesia. CSE analgesia is another acceptable technique for providing labor analgesia to patients with mitral insufficiency. However, the use of epidural local anesthetics is usually preferred over spinal opioids because of the advantageous decrease in SVR that occurs with local anesthetic-induced sympathectomy.

Epidural anesthesia is usually the anesthetic of choice for cesarean delivery in women with mitral insufficiency. A continuous spinal anesthetic also provides cardiovascular effects that are advantageous, but the increased incidence of spinal headache does not justify its use over epidural anesthesia in most patients. Ephedrine is the vasopressor of choice for treating hypotension. Phenylephrine is avoided because the increased SVR and decreased heart rate associated with its use are deleteri-

---

CLINICAL CAVEAT: HEMODYNAMIC GOALS IN PARTURIENTS WITH VALVULAR HEART DISEASE

- Aortic stenosis: Maintain normal heart rate and sinus rhythm; avoid decreases in SVR; maintain normal venous return.
- Aortic insufficiency: Maintain normal to slightly increased heart rate; avoid increases in SVR.
- Mitral stenosis: Maintain slow heart rate and sinus rhythm, maintain normal SVR; maintain normal venous return.
- Mitral insufficiency: Maintain sinus rhythm and normal to slightly increased heart rate; avoid increases in SVR and venous return; maintain normal venous return.

ous to parturients with mitral insufficiency. When general anesthesia is required for cesarean delivery, anesthetic agents that produce decreased afterload and a slightly increased heart rate are chosen. Drugs with myocardial depressant effects are avoided.

Peripartum Cardiomyopathy

Peripartum cardiomyopathy is a rare but life-threatening disease. The currently accepted incidence is approximately 1 per 3000 to 1 per 4000 live births. However, an increasing proportion of maternal deaths in the United States was attributed to peripartum cardiomyopathy in the 1990s. Identified risk factors for peripartum cardiomyopathy include advanced maternal age, multiparity, obesity, multiple gestation, pre-eclampsia, chronic hypertension, and African-American race. Peripartum cardiomyopathy is defined by the presence of four criteria (Box 8-9).

The etiology of peripartum cardiomyopathy remains unknown, despite much investigation that has focused on identifying a cause. Proposed etiologies include myocarditis, abnormal immune response to pregnancy, and maladaptive response to the hemodynamic stresses of pregnancy. There is more evidence to support myocarditis or an autoimmune process as the cause of the disease than for other proposed etiologies. Endomyocardial biopsies in women with peripartum cardiomyopathy have demonstrated myocarditis in many patients, but biopsy results differ markedly among studies.

Patients with peripartum cardiomyopathy present with the typical signs and symptoms of left ventricular failure. The majority of cases occur after delivery and the immediate postpartum period. However, when the disease develops during the last month of pregnancy, the diagnosis of cardiac failure is difficult to make by signs and symptoms alone because some of the symptoms, such as fatigue, orthopnea, and pedal edema, are common among normal parturients during late pregnancy. Further testing is required to establish the presence of cardiac failure. A chest x-ray consistently demonstrates cardiomegaly and pulmonary edema. Echocardiography

confirms ventricular failure with increased left ventricular end-diastolic dimensions and decreased ejection fraction. Once cardiac failure is identified, peripartum cardiomyopathy must be differentiated from other cardiac processes that lead to heart failure.

Maternal mortality from peripartum cardiomyopathy in the United States has been reported to be 25% to 50%. Thromboembolism accounts for approximately 30% of these deaths. Patients who survive the disease have a significantly higher ejection fraction and smaller left ventricular end-diastolic diameter at the time of diagnosis compared with patients who succumb. Normalization of heart size and resolution of congestive heart failure within 6 months after delivery are also good prognostic signs, with mortality rare among these patients.

Medical and Obstetric Management

Medical treatment of peripartum cardiomyopathy is similar to that for other dilated cardiomyopathies. Management goals include preload optimization, afterload reduction, and increased contractility. Anticoagulation is also considered in many patients because of the significant risk of thromboembolism. When the patient develops cardiac failure while still pregnant, some treatment modifications are required. Angiotensin-converting enzyme inhibitors are routinely used for afterload reduction in congestive heart failure. However, these drugs are contraindicated during pregnancy because of adverse fetal effects. Alternative treatments for afterload reduction during pregnancy include amlodipine or a combination of hydralazine and nitroglycerin.

In addition to treatment of the cardiac failure, an obstetric plan of care must also be developed. Collaboration among the obstetrician, cardiologist, and anesthesiologist is essential to optimize care. If the parturient's cardiac status can be stabilized with medical therapy, induction of labor is usually recommended, with cesarean delivery reserved for obstetric indications. However, in parturients who experience acute cardiac decompensation, cesarean delivery may be required because of an inability of the mother to tolerate the prolonged stresses of labor.

Anesthetic Management

Parturients with peripartum cardiomyopathy require special anesthetic care during labor and delivery. Invasive monitoring, including an intra-arterial catheter and pulmonary artery catheter, should be utilized to assess the patient's hemodynamic status and guide management. The cardiovascular stress of labor and delivery may lead to cardiac decompensation. When that situation occurs, the anesthesiologist may need to infuse vasoactive agents, such as nitroglycerin or nitroprusside for preload and afterload reduction and dopamine, dobutamine, or milrinone for inotropic support.

Box 8-9   Definition of Peripartum Cardiomyopathy

Development of cardiac failure in the last month of pregnancy or within 5 months of delivery
Absence of an identifiable cause for cardiac failure
Absence of recognizable heart disease prior to the last month of pregnancy
Left ventricular systolic dysfunction demonstrated by echocardiographic criteria such as depressed ejection fraction

Data from the pulmonary artery catheter is essential to determine the appropriate pharmacologic therapy for each patient.

Early administration of labor analgesia to minimize further cardiac stress associated with pain is paramount in the anesthetic management of these patients. Various analgesic techniques provide unique advantages in the hemodynamic management of the parturient while also providing excellent analgesia. By using invasive monitoring data to guide fluid management and titration of vasoactive drugs, the slow induction of epidural analgesia is a safe and effective analgesic technique in parturients with peripartum cardiomyopathy. In fact, the sympathectomy-induced afterload reduction that occurs with epidural anesthesia can contribute to an improvement in myocardial performance in these patients. CSE analgesia is another excellent analgesic option. Because the initial analgesia can be accomplished with spinal opioids, hemodynamic stability may be more easily maintained compared to epidural analgesia since sympathetic blockade is avoided. When injection of epidural local anesthetics is required later in labor, slow titration of the drug can provide the benefits of afterload reduction while avoiding sudden drops in blood pressure that would be deleterious. In the most fragile patients, continuous spinal analgesia is an excellent alternative. A continuous spinal catheter technique permits intermittent intrathecal opioid injection for analgesia throughout the first stage of labor. Supplementation with a small dose of intrathecal local anesthetic is sometimes needed to provide adequate analgesia for the second stage of labor and delivery. A significant advantage of this technique is that hemodynamic stability is more easily achieved because a local anesthetic-induced sympathectomy is avoided for the majority or all of the labor process.

If cesarean delivery is required, a continuous epidural or spinal anesthetic is usually the best anesthetic option. The patient's hemodynamic status is carefully followed, and fluid management is guided by data from the invasive monitors while the anesthesia level is slowly raised. A single-shot spinal technique is not recommended because the rapid hemodynamic changes associated with this technique may not be well tolerated in these fragile patients. General anesthesia is sometimes required when cesarean delivery is required because of acute fetal distress or maternal decompensation. Anesthetic drugs with myocardial depressant effects should be avoided. Induction and maintenance with a high-dose opioid technique are often preferred. If this technique is utilized, remifentanil is a good choice because its short half-life can minimize effects on the neonate. Trained personnel must be available to manage neonatal depression whenever a high-dose opioid anesthetic is used.

SUGGESTED READING

American College of Obstetricians and Gynecologists: ACOG Committee Opinion: Mode of term singleton breech delivery. Obstet Gynecol 98:1189-1190, 2001.

American College of Obstetricians and Gynecologists: Vaginal birth after previous cesarean delivery. Washington, DC, American College of Obstetricians and Gynecologists, 1999, Practice Bulletin No. 5.

Bucklin BA: Vaginal birth after cesarean delivery. Anesthesiology 99:1444-1448, 2003.

Cedeergren MI: Maternal morbid obesity and the risk of adverse pregnancy outcome. Obstet Gynecol 103:219-224, 2004.

Cherayil G, Feinberg B, Robinson J, Tsen LC: Central neuraxial blockade promotes external cephalic version success after a failed attempt. Anesth Analg 94:1589-1592, 2002.

Crochetiere C: Obstetric emergencies. Anesthesiol Clin North Am 21:111-125, 2003.

Dyer RA, Els I, Farbas J, et al: Prospective, randomized trial comparing general with spinal anesthesia for cesarean delivery in pre-eclamptic patients with a nonreassuring fetal heart trace. Anesthesiology 99:561-569, 2003.

Friedman SA, Schiff E, Lubarsky SL, Sibai BM: Expectant management of severe pre-eclampsia remote from term. Clin Obstet Gynecol 42:470-478, 1999.

Hamilton CL, Riley ET, Cohen SE: Changes in the position of epidural catheters associated with patient movement. Anesthesiology 86:778-784, 1997.

Hannah ME, Hannah WJ, Hewson SA, et al: Planned caesarean section versus planned vaginal birth for breech presentation at term: A randomized multicentre trial. Lancet 356: 1375-1383, 2000.

Hood DD, Curry R: Spinal versus epidural anesthesia for cesarean section in severely pre-eclamptic patients: A retrospective survey. Anesthesiology 90:1276-1282, 1999.

Hood DD, Dewan DM: Anesthetic and obstetric outcome in morbidly obese parturients. Anesthesiology 79:1210-1218, 1993.

Mancuso KM, Yancey MK, Murphy JA, Markenson GR: Epidural analgesia for cephalic version: A randomized trial. Obstet Gynecol 95:648-651, 2000.

O'Brien JM, Shumate SA, Satchwell SL, et al: Maternal benefit of corticosteroid therapy in patients with HELLP (hemolysis, elevated liver enzymes, and low platelet count) syndrome: Impact on the rate of regional anesthesia. Am J Obstet Gynecol 186:475-479, 2002.

Pearson GD, Veille JC, Rahimtoola S, et al: Peripartum cardiomyopathy: National Heart, Lung, and Blood Institute and Office of Rare Diseases (National Institutes of Health) workshop recommendation and review. JAMA 283:1183-1188, 2000.

Pratt SD: Anesthesia for breech presentation and multiple gestation. Clin Obstet Gynecol 46:711-729, 2003.

Smith GC, Pell JP, Cameron AD, Dobbie R: Risk of perinatal death associated with labor after previous cesarean delivery in uncomplicated term pregnancies. JAMA 287:2684–2690, 2002.

Tsen LC: Anesthetic management of the parturient with cardiac and diabetic diseases. Clin Obstet Gynecol 46:700–710, 2003.

Weiss BM, Atanassoff PG: Cyanotic congenital heart disease and pregnancy: Natural selection, pulmonary hypertension, and anesthesia. J Clin Anesth 5:332–341, 1993.

CHAPTER 9

Obstetric Anesthesiology Services

FERNE R. BRAVEMAN

Introduction
Practical Application of the ASA and ACOG Guidelines for
Obstetric Anesthesia Care
Summary

INTRODUCTION

The most recently published manpower data for obstetric anesthesiology services in the United States were published in July 1997, based on data from 1992. In hospitals with greater than 1500 deliveries (stratum I), 62% had full-time anesthesiology (MD or CRNA) coverage specific to labor and delivery. An additional 34% of these hospitals had coverage shared with other duties (i.e., surgical services). In hospitals with fewer than 1500 deliveries, 64% provided obstetric anesthesia care as shared coverage with other duties. Of all hospitals, only 1% did not provide regional anesthesia available for cesarean delivery. Twenty percent of hospitals performing fewer than 500 deliveries (stratum III) did not provide regional labor analgesia.

CLINICAL CAVEAT

Unless contraindicated, women who request epidural labor analgesia should be able to receive it.

Approximately 50% of labor epidural analgesia in 1992 was provided by CRNAs and approximately 2% by obstetricians. Only 4% of obstetric anesthetics (cesarean delivery or labor) were performed by independent CRNAs.

Reimbursement for labor analgesia in 1992 was not significantly changed from 1981. Twenty-five percent of anesthesiologists reported claims denied for labor analgesia. This occurs despite the belief that patient request

should be adequate indication for epidural analgesia. In 1999, the American Society of Anesthesiologists (ASA) and American College of Obstetricians and Gynecologists (ACOG) issued the joint statement that ". . .third party payers. . .who provide reimbursement from obstetric services. . .should not deny reimbursement for epidural anesthesia because of an absence of other 'medical indications.'"[1] Despite this statement, anesthesiologists still report difficulties with reimbursement for labor analgesia.

Obstetric anesthesiology care should be provided in a cost effective manner consistent with ASA and ACOG guidelines that meets the needs of patients. Recommendation to consolidate small obstetric services may be necessary to maintain appropriate care. The ASA and the ACOG have issued guidelines, practice parameters, statements, and standards relating to the practice of obstetric anesthesiology. Standards for basic anesthetic monitoring and for postanesthesia care are also available. In addition, the ASA and ACOG have published joint guidelines for care, "Optimal Goals for Anesthesia Care in Obstetrics" (Box 9-1).

The ASA has two practice guidelines that relate directly to obstetric anesthesia. The first "Practice Guidelines for Obstetric Anesthesia" was developed by the ASA's task force on obstetric anesthesia care and became effective January 1, 1999 (see Box 9-2 for a summary of these guidelines). "Guidelines for Regional Anesthesia in Obstetrics" was originally published in 1988 and last amended October 18, 2000 (Box 9-3).

PRACTICAL APPLICATION OF THE ASA AND ACOG GUIDELINES FOR OBSTETRIC ANESTHESIA CARE

Practice guidelines for obstetric anesthesia are meant to enhance the quality of anesthesia care for obstetric patients

Box 9-1 Optimal Goals for Anesthesia Care in Obstetrics

Availability of practitioner credentialed to administer an anesthetic whenever necessary/requested

Availability of practitioner credentialed to maintain vital functions in an emergency

Availability of personnel to permit the start of cesarean delivery within 30 minutes of the decision to operate

Availability of anesthesiologist to the obstetric unit

Availability of equipment and personnel equal to that provided in the surgical suite, including the availability of facilities for recovery for regional or general anesthesia

Availability of personnel, other than surgical team, to provide neonatal resuscitation

From Optimal Goals for Anesthesia Care in Obstetrics. Approved by the ASA House of Delegates on October 18, 2000.

Box 9-2 Practice Guidelines for Obstetric Anesthesia

Focused history and physical.

Decision to order laboratory tests, including platelet count and type and screen should be individualized.

Oral intake of clear liquids in uncomplicated laboring patients may be allowed.

Anesthesia care is not necessary for labor and/or delivery; but when sufficient manpower (anesthesiology and nursing staff) is available, epidural analgesia should be offered.

Spinal opioids or combined spinal/epidural techniques may also be offered.

Monitored anesthesia care for complicated deliveries should be available when requested by the obstetrician.

From Practice guidelines for obstetrical anesthesiology: A report by the American Society of Anesthesiologists Task Force on Obstetrical Anesthesia. Anesthesiology 90:600-611, 1999.

Box 9-3 Guidelines for Regional Anesthesia in Obstetrics

These guidelines apply whenever regional analgesia/anesthesia is administered during labor and delivery.

Immediate availability of equipment and drugs to manage procedurally related problems.

An anesthesiologist should personally initiate and maintain or medically direct the individual who initiates and maintains the anesthetic/analgesia.

Before administering anesthetic/analgesia, the patient should be examined by her obstetric caregiver, and a physician who can perform operative delivery should be readily available should complications arise.

An IV should be placed and vital signs monitored appropriate to patient's condition.

Regional anesthesia for cesarean delivery requires that the standards for monitoring be applied and an obstetrician be immediately available prior to inducing anesthesia.

Personnel for neonatal resuscitation should be immediately available.

An anesthesiologist should be readily available until the patient is stable postoperatively.

All patients recovering from extensive regional blockade must receive care in a manner which meets the standards for postanesthesia recovery.

From Guidelines for Regional Anesthesia in Obstetrics. Approved by the ASA House of Delegates, October 12, 1988, amended October 18, 2000.

unit (PACU) must be available to receive patients following intraoperative anesthesia care having been transported to the PACU by a member of the anesthesia care team. This PACU must meet all requirements for PACU equipment and staffing as designated by the Joint Commission on Accreditation of Healthcare Organization (JCAHO). A PACU nurse responsible for the patient must continually evaluate the patient's condition while she is in the PACU, and the patient will be discharged from the PACU only when discharge criteria are met and documented. These are the minimum requirements related to anesthesia care of patients in labor and delivery.

The ACOG Practice Bulletin Number 36 published in July 2002 covers management guidelines for obstetric analgesia and anesthesia, some of which relate specifically to anesthesia/analgesia care administered by the anesthesiologist. Box 9-4 summarizes the recommendations from this practice bulletin. ACOG Practice Bulletin Number 5 (July 1999) provides clinical management guidelines for vaginal birth after cesarean (VBAC) delivery.

Obstetric anesthesia coverage in hospitals with busy obstetric services is ideally with full-time coverage; that is, the in-house presence of an anesthesiologist and/or nurse anesthetist whose only responsibility is to patients on the labor and delivery floor. In fact, in hospitals with

and increase patient satisfaction. The guidelines defined by the ASA focus on management of pregnant patients during labor, nonoperative delivery as well as operative delivery; and, when necessary, postpartum care. Box 9-2 summarizes the guidelines for obstetric anesthesia care.

To meet standards for anesthesia care of patients on the labor and delivery unit, the Department of Anesthesiology and the hospital must be able to provide qualified anesthesia personnel to administer anesthesia for the intraoperative care of the patient undergoing operative delivery. These patients must be monitored for oxygenation, ventilation, and vital signs in a manner consistent with the care in other anesthetizing locations within the institution. In addition, a postanesthesia care

Box 9-4 ACOG Recommendations Regarding Obstetric Analgesia

Regional analgesia provides superior pain relief and should be available to all parturients.
Parenteral analgesics decrease fetal heart rate (FHR) variability.
Decision of when to place epidural analgesia should be made individually.
Women should not be required to reach a pre-determined degree of cervical dilation.

From ACOG Practice Bulletin Number 36, July 2002.

Box 9-5 Vaginal Birth After Previous Cesarean Delivery

Physician immediately available throughout labor capable of monitoring labor and performing an emergency cesarean delivery
Availability of anesthesiologist and other personnel for emergency cesarean delivery
VBAC contraindicated if above requirements are not met
Epidural analgesia may be used

From ACOG Practice Bulletin Number 5, July 1999.

perinatal fellowships, ACOG guidelines for services include the presence of a dedicated obstetric anesthesiologist. Reimbursement for obstetric anesthesia services has plateaued and in many areas decreased. Thus, many hospitals, even larger community hospitals, do not have dedicated obstetric anesthesia services; and based on guidelines for care, this level of service is not required. In institutions without dedicated in-house obstetric anesthesia care, the following options have been used to provide laboring patients with analgesia. First, obstetricians administer (and are reimbursed for) obstetric labor epidurals (<2% in 1992). Secondly, the anesthesiologist who takes calls out of the hospital administers a single intrathecal injection of an opioid, monitors the patient until it is determined that she is stable, and then leaves the hospital (an option used primarily in stratum III facilities). Third, anesthesiologists/CRNAs who are present in the hospital but not dedicated to the labor and delivery floor will place an epidural for analgesia, monitor the patient until stable, and then return to duties elsewhere in the hospital (an option used in 34% of stratum I and 64% of stratum II and III facilities). In this scenario, a second anesthesia care provider must be present in the hospital if a surgical case, either cesarean delivery or surgical suite procedure, is undertaken. Once the epidural is placed in a laboring patient, the anesthesiologist/CRNA must be readily available to manage complications and, thus, cannot be in continuous attendance in an operative case.

CLINICAL CAVEAT

Regional anesthesia/analgesia in obstetrics should be initiated and maintained by personnel approved to administer obstetric anesthesia. This individual must be qualified to manage related complications.

Institutions with busy obstetric and surgical services often have more than one anesthesia care provider present continuously in the hospital to manage surgical and labor and delivery patients. However, the presence of a dedicated anesthesiologist or CRNA in the

labor and delivery suite even in hospitals with busy obstetric services continues to be uncommon except in stratum I hospitals.

Specific to VBAC delivery, ACOG practice guidelines have been clear in the recommendation that VBAC be attempted only with personnel immediately available for emergency cesarean delivery (Box 9-5). Although not the standard of care, this has been interpreted by most institutions as warranting the presence of the patient's obstetrician and an anesthesia care provider in the hospital while the patient is in labor. Thus, VBACs should be attempted primarily in institutions with busy obstetric/surgical services where this level of staffing is available. This would be in stratum I facilities, and many, but not all stratum II facilities.

SUMMARY

Anesthesia care for intrapartum patients should be available at all institutions that provide obstetric services. The equipment available for care of these patients should be comparable to that used for surgical patients, and intraoperative and postoperative care must meet the same standards as for surgical patients. VBACs should be undertaken only in institutions with personnel immediately available to provide emergency care for the patient and infant and the facilities to accommodate this care (Boxes 9-6 and 9-7). As with any surgical patient, the need for antepartum consultative assessment by the anesthesiologist must be recognized and

Box 9-6 Availability of Resources for Obstetric and/or Anesthetic Emergencies

Ability to manage massive hemorrhage
Availability of equipment for management of airway emergencies
Resources for utilization of central venous pressure (CVP) or pulmonary artery (PA) catheters

Box 9-7   Need for Postpartum ICU Care

Complications from pre-eclampsia
   Pulmonary edema
   Seizures
Hemorrhage
Comorbid disease
   Cardiac
   Asthma

Box 9-8   Factors Prompting Anesthetic Consultation

Morbid obesity
Severe facial/neck/spinal abnormalities
Serious maternal medical disease
   Cardiac
   Pulmonary
   Neurologic

requested by the patient's obstetrician, to allow the safest care for patients with significant comorbid disease (Box 9-8).

REFERENCE

1. American Society of Anesthesiology/American College of Obstetrics and Gynecology: Statement on Pain Relief During Labor. Approved October 13, 1999.

SUGGESTED READING

American College of Obstetrics and Gynecology Practice Bulletin. Clinical management guidelines for obstetrician-gynecologists. Vaginal Birth After Previous Cesarean Delivery. Number 5, July 1999.

American College of Obstetrics and Gynecology Practice Bulletin. Clinical management guidelines for obstetrician-gynecologists. Obstetric Analgesia and Anesthesia. Number 36, July 2002.

American Society of Anesthesiologists Task Force on Obstetrical Anesthesia: Practice guidelines for obstetrical anesthesia: A report by the American Society of Anesthesiologists Task Force on Obstetrical Anesthesia. Anesthesiology 90:600–611, 1999.

American Society of Anesthesiologists Task Force on Postanesthetic Care: Practice guidelines for postanesthetic care: A report by the American Society of Anesthesiologists Task Force on Postanesthetic Care. Anesthesiology 96:742–752, 2002.

Hawkins JL, Gibbs CP, Orleans M, et al: Obstetric anesthesia work force survey, 1981 versus 1992. Anesthesiology 87(1): 135–143, 1997.

CHAPTER 10

Complication and Risk Management in Obstetrics and Gynecologic Anesthesia

NALINI VADIVELU

INTRODUCTION

In 1847 James Simpson, a Scottish obstetrician, first administered ether to a woman during labor to treat the pain of childbirth. Since then, the maternal and fetal effects of analgesia continue to intrigue anesthesiologists, obstetric caregivers, and patients. Obstetric anesthesia is considered by many to be a difficult, high-risk practice that exposes the anesthesiologist to increased medicolegal liability. Obstetric patients are at greater risk of developing complications following difficult tracheal intubation, especially aspiration of gastric contents, because of altered physiology of pregnancy and labor. Perhaps for this reason regional anesthesia is preferred for the obstetric patient.

REGIONAL ANESTHESIA FOR VAGINAL DELIVERY

Controversies exist in obstetric anesthesiology over the effects of regional anesthesia on the progress and outcome of labor as well as its effects on the neonate. A number of randomized trials have sought to address the effects of various techniques for labor analgesia. This review will provide an overview of the complications, risks, and benefits of the presently utilized techniques.

Approximately 60% of parturients in the United States, or 2.4 million each year, select epidural or combined spinal-epidural (CSE) analgesia for pain relief during labor. The use of a subarachnoid bolus of opioids results in the rapid onset of profound relief of pain with virtually no motor blockade. In contrast to epidural local anesthetics, spinal opioids do not cause impairment of balance, giving the parturient woman the option to continue ambulation. CSE is associated with a higher degree of satisfaction among parturient women than conventional epidural analgesia. However, some studies have suggested that there may be an increase in the frequency of nonreassuring patterns in the fetal heart rate, particularly bradycardia, when CSE analgesia is used. Other studies show no difference in the fetal heart rate and no increase in the rate of cesarean deliveries necessitated by fetal bradycardia. Risk management studies have shown that the use of epidural analgesia is associated with better pain relief than systemic opioids, as assessed by the verbal analog score. However, a major concern regarding epidural analgesia is its effect on the progress of labor, leading to increased incidence of cesarean delivery, vaginal delivery requiring the use of forceps or vacuum extraction, or prolongation of labor. Instrument-assisted deliveries and cesarean deliveries may be associated with a greater incidence of maternal complications than unassisted vaginal deliveries. The rate of instrument-assisted vaginal deliveries is associated with a higher rate of serious perineal lacerations, which has been implicated as a risk factor for later fecal incontinence. Instrument-assisted vaginal deliveries have also been linked to higher rates of neonatal birth injuries.

A recent prospective, randomized meta-analysis represents the experience of nearly 2400 patients randomly assigned to receive either epidural analgesia or parenteral opioid analgesia. Epidural analgesia was associated with a prolongation of the second stage of labor by an average of 14 minutes. No significant difference between groups in the rate of cesarean delivery could be demonstrated by intention to treat analysis (8.2% of women in the epidural group had cesarean deliveries as compared with 5.6% in the parenteral opioid group).

It is important to realize that the effect of epidural analgesia on the likelihood of cesarean delivery may vary according to obstetric practice and the population studied and that such variations may influence the differences observed in various studies. Studies have clearly demonstrated great variations in physician-specific rates of cesarean delivery, suggesting that management practices are certainly a confounding variable. In a study by Goyert et al.[1] of 1533 parturient women who were cared for by 11 obstetricians, the rate of cesarean delivery varied from 19% to 41% depending on the caregiver. An additional variable that may account for the varying cesarean section rates among study participants is that women enrolled in many of the randomized trials were much younger than the general population of women delivering babies in the United States. Studies have also consistently demonstrated an increase in the rate of cesarean delivery with an increase in age. Therefore, there is no definite conclusion whether epidural analgesia is an independent variable with respect to increases in the rate of cesarean deliveries.

There seems to be a clearer association between instrument-assisted delivery and epidural analgesia; there is a consistent increase in the rates of deliveries involving forceps and vacuum extraction in patients receiving epidural analgesia. A meta-analysis of randomized trials found a doubling of the rate of instrument-assisted vaginal deliveries. A recent randomized trial found an increase in the rate of deliveries involving forceps from 3% in the opioid group to 12% in the epidural analgesia group. The exact reason for this increase seen with

epidural analgesia remains unclear. Several hypotheses have been developed to explain this. One hypothesis is that the motor blockade in association with epidural analgesia may prevent the mother from pushing, thereby necessitating the use of instruments. Epidural analgesia is also associated with a higher frequency of the occiput posterior position of the fetus at delivery, which could also represent a mechanism by which epidural analgesia contributes to the higher rate of instrument-assisted delivery. In addition, it is possible that the presence of an epidural block may decrease the obstetrician's threshold for performing instrument-assisted deliveries as well as allowing instrument-assisted delivery for the purpose of teaching residents.

Studies of sentinel events have shown that epidural analgesia may prolong labor by approximately 1 hour on average. Most observational studies demonstrate higher rates of cesarean delivery with early administration of epidural analgesia. There is, however, insufficient evidence to determine the impact of waiting until a certain degree of cervical dilatation or a certain fetal station is reached before instituting epidural analgesia (Box 10-1).

COMPLICATIONS OF REGIONAL ANESTHESIA

Maternal Fever

The association between the use of epidural analgesia and maternal fever is complex. Some authors assert that the increase in the frequency of fever is the result of placental infection, as assessed by neutrophilic infiltration of the placenta, possibly associated with the longer duration of labor among women who receive epidural analgesia. This explanation seems unlikely because women with long labors but no epidural analgesia do not tend to have higher incidents of fever. The rate of sepsis among term infants is equally low, whether or not the mother receives epidural analgesia.

Back Pain

There is a concern among many parturients that epidural analgesia may lead to back pain. Howell et al.[2]

Box 10-1   Adverse Events That Have Been Associated With Regional Labor Analgesia

Increase in instrumented vaginal deliveries
Increase in cesarean deliveries
Prolonged duration of labor
Fetal occiput posterior presentation

studied 385 nulliparous parturient women for 12 months after delivery and demonstrated no difference in the incidence of backache between women who were randomly assigned to receive epidural analgesia and those who were not. The results of other nonrandomized trials are consistent with these findings. In contrast, studies have provided evidence that postpartum back pain is most likely to be a continuation of antepartum pain. In a study by Breen[3] in 1994, new onset back pain was associated with greater weight and short stature and not with the number of attempts at epidural placement.

Neurologic Complications After Regional Anesthesia

A recent survey conducted in the United Kingdom that included 42,000 neuroaxial blocks in pregnant patients reported no differences between the incidence of epidural abscess and spinal hematoma associated with CSE versus single-shot spinal anesthesia. In obstetrics, although neurologic complications may be secondary to the labor and delivery processes, the neural block is usually considered to be causative until proven otherwise. It is important to recognize that spontaneous neurologic complications may occur unrelated to regional anesthesia; spontaneous epidural abscesses of unknown etiology have been seen in obstetric patients. Monitoring, early diagnosis, and prompt treatment of neurologic complications will usually lead to complete resolution of neurologic deficit in cases of epidural abscess and epidural hematoma.

Postdural Puncture Headache

Techniques that lead to puncture of the dura have a small but clinically significant risk for headache in the parturient (Box 10-2). Norris et al.[4] have shown that inadvertent puncture of the dura mater during placement of an epidural catheter occurs in about 3% of parturients, and a severe headache occurs in up to 70% of women with such a puncture. Dural puncture rates have been shown to be inversely proportionate to the number of epidurals performed. The effectiveness of an epidural blood patch to treat postdural puncture headache is well recognized. More than 75% of women with postdural puncture headache managed with an epidural blood patch as a secondary treatment were effectively treated. A second blood patch produced complete relief in approximately 95% of patients. If the headache does not have the pathognomonic postural characteristics or persists despite treatment with an epidural blood patch, other diagnoses must be considered and appropriate testing performed.

Short- and long-term symptoms, particularly headache, have been attributed to dural puncture for spinal anesthesia. The improved needle design with pencil-pointed tips has resulted in a decrease in the incidence of postdural puncture headache (PDPH) and the increase in the popularity of spinal anesthesia in obstetric practice. The incidence of postdural puncture headache using a 25-gauge Whitacre needle or a smaller needle for spinal anesthesia is lower than when a larger diameter needle is used for the administration of spinal anesthesia.

Not every headache occurring after childbirth in patients with a history of neuraxial block is secondary to dural puncture. The differential diagnoses of persistent headache that occurs in the puerperium include spinal headache after regional anesthesia, nonspecific headache, migraine, meningitis, pregnancy-induced hypertension associated with headache, cerebral tumor subarachnoid hemorrhage, subdural hematoma, and cerebral vein thrombosis. There are contradictory reports on long-term headaches following dural puncture.

Neonatal Effects

It has been demonstrated that women who receive epidural analgesia are more likely to have a fetus in the occiput posterior position at delivery. It is not clear, however, whether the use of epidural analgesia contributes to the persistence of this position or whether women with a fetus in this position are more likely to request epidural analgesia secondary to painful labors. Other neonatal effects that have been reported in connection with epidural analgesia include effects for which inadequate data are available to draw definitive conclusions.

Hypotension

Hypotension in the parturient is defined as a systolic blood pressure <100 mm Hg. Hypotension is the most common potential serious adverse effect of spinal anesthesia for cesarean section. An incidence of up to 90% has been reported. A number of strategies have been suggested to prevent hypotension with regional anesthesia, including the use of intravenous crystalloid, colloid, as well as prophylactic intramuscular (IM) or intravenous (IV) administration of vasopressors.

Box 10-2 Complications Associated With Regional Anesthesia

Hypotension
Maternal fever
Back pain
Headache (PDPH)
Inadequate analgesia
Epidural infection
Epidural hematoma

The use of crystalloid for fluid preload has not been totally effective in preventing spinal hypotension. Several authors have reported a lack of clinically significant reduction in spinal hypotension following fluid preload. No clinical advantage of warmed crystalloid preload as compared with cold infusions with regard to incidence of hypotension has been detected so far, although it can be argued that comfort of the patient favors the use of warmed infusions.

There is controversy regarding the use of colloids to prevent hypotension with spinal anesthesia in the parturient. Several reports highlighted advantages of colloid preload. Hydroxyethyl starch has been suggested for use in the prevention of spinal hypotension.

When comparing therapies, the costs and side effects of colloid solutions must be balanced against any improved outcome and against the costs and clinical value of prophylactic administration of vasopressors. Ephedrine is the preferred agent for normalizing blood pressure, although some data suggests phenylephrine may be a better choice. There is a lack of consensus regarding the appropriate route, dosage, and timing of ephedrine and/or phenylephrine administration.

MATERNAL MORTALITY AND GENERAL ANESTHESIA

Maternal death has been defined by the Bureau of Vital Statistics as the death of a woman while pregnant or within 42 days of termination of pregnancy, despite duration and the site of pregnancy, from any cause related to or aggravated by the pregnancy or its management but not from accidental or incidental causes. The American College of Obstetrics and Gynecologists (ACOG) has defined maternal death as the death of any woman that was caused or contributed to by pregnancy, occurring during pregnancy, or within 1 year after the end of pregnancy. A retrospective analysis in 2001 using a Maryland State database attributed 5.2% of maternal deaths to anesthesia-related complications. The death of a woman during pregnancy or in the period after pregnancy presents a wide array of problems for her family and the community. Maternal death is a particularly tragic event because pregnant women are usually young and healthy. The Centers for Disease Control and Prevention (CDC) has estimated that current overall maternal mortality ratio (MMR), defined as the number of deaths per 100,000 live births, to be 7.5. The goal of the United States Public Health Service 2000 Project was to achieve a 50% reduction in the MMR (6.7). In the United States, there are five main sources for identifying maternal deaths. These include published vital records, manual review of death certificates, vital records linkage, review of autopsy reports, and review of medical records.

There are several studies in which maternal death certificates have been reviewed to assess maternal mortality rates. Often, death certificates do not provide enough detail to accurately classify the pathophysiology leading to maternal death or to determine contributing risk factors. The degree of underreporting of maternal death rates by routine vital statistics has been estimated to be 20% to75%.

Anesthesia-associated maternal mortality is between 4.3 and 1.7 per 1 million live births in the United States. This is the sixth leading cause of pregnancy-related deaths in the United States. General anesthesia is associated with a higher risk of airway problems in women undergoing cesarean delivery when compared to nonobstetric patients. Studies have shown that the risk of failed intubation is estimated as 1 in 200 to 1 in 300 cases, about 10 times higher than that seen in nonobstetric patients. Most anesthesia-related deaths occur during general anesthesia for cesarean delivery. The risk of maternal deaths resulting from complications of general anesthesia is 17 times higher than that associated with all types of regional anesthesia. In addition to failed intubation, pulmonary aspiration related to general anesthesia and subsequent respiratory failure may also lead to maternal death.

CLINICAL CAVEAT

General anesthesia is associated with a higher risk of airway problems in the obstetric patient versus the general surgical patient.

Regional anesthesia may be preferable to general anesthesia even when the status of the fetus is not reassuring, as it may be safer for the mother. Recognition of the risks to the mother associated with general anesthesia has resulted in an increase in the use of spinal or epidural anesthesia for both elective and emergency cesarean deliveries. This shift in practice over the last decade has led to a decrease in maternal mortality rates.

The Committee on Obstetric Practice of the American College of Obstetricians and Gynecologists has recommended that a management plan be developed jointly by obstetricians and anesthesiologists if risk factors and signs predicting a difficult intubation are present.

INFORMED CONSENT REGARDING RISKS AND COMPLICATIONS OF OBSTETRIC ANESTHESIA

Informing patients of the possible risks and complications of obstetric anesthesia is essential to their care. It is best done in advance of labor. Detailed and accurate explanations of any and all potential risks, combined with written documentation of this discussion are preferred.

A study done by Jackson et al.[5] on 60 laboring women showed that laboring women wanted to hear about all potential epidural complications, but the majority did not want specific incidences quoted. In the majority of cases, no side effect disclosed during the consent process dissuaded a parturient once the request for an epidural was made. It seemed that laboring women were indeed capable of giving informed consent.

ASA CLOSED CLAIMS FOCUSING ON OBSTETRIC COMPLICATIONS

The ASA closed claims project is an in-depth study of claims against anesthesiologists based upon data collected from the files of 35 professional liability insurance carriers in the United States. The project is conducted under the auspices of the ASA Committee on Professional Liability. Much has been learned from the Obstetrical Anesthesia Closed Claims about liability and anesthesia risk since 1984, when the Committee on Professional Liability of the American Society of Anesthesiologists began this ongoing study. The outcome of this project has been the issuance and revision of standards and procedures for anesthesia care to avoid further morbidity and/or mortality.

In the offices of professional liability insurance carriers, practicing anesthesiologists reviewed files of claims that were no longer active ("close claims"). A standardized data-collection instrument was completed according to a set of instructions provided to each reviewer for claims in which there was enough information to reconstruct the sequence of events leading to injury and the nature of injury. Claims for dental damage were not included. Typical files that were reviewed included hospital and anesthesia records, narrative statements from the personnel involved, expert and peer reviews. Deposition summaries, outcome reports, and data concerning cost of settlement or award were also examined. The data collection instrument consisted of several items, including the ASA physical status and description of the patient, date and time of incident, type of procedure, type of anesthesia personnel, the anesthetic technique and agents, complications or injuries, and whether the complaint was related to the anesthetic in any way. For each claim in which sufficient information was available, reviewers were asked to judge the quality of anesthetic care based on the standard of care that a reasonable and prudent anesthesiologist would have exercised at the time of the event. The outcome of this project was the issuance of recommendations is for care directed at injury avoidance. The uniqueness of the ASA Closed Claims database is that it also reflects the consumer's perspective. It provides a valuable insight into the types and patterns of injury associated with malpractice claims.

OBSTETRIC ANESTHESIA CLOSED CLAIMS

There have been changes in patterns of claims in obstetric anesthesia recently because of the changes in anesthesia practice in the last three decades. Over the past 33 years, there has been a decrease in cesarean deliveries performed under general anesthesia and an increase in cesarean deliveries performed under regional anesthesia. A paper by Davies et al.[6] in 2004 indicated that approximately 12% (792) of the 6449 claims in the ASA Closed Claims Project database involved obstetric anesthesia care. Of these obstetric claims, about two thirds involved claims related to cesarean section, and 33% of the claims involved vaginal deliveries. Concomitant with the increase in the proportion of cesarean sections done under regional anesthesia is an increase in the proportion of claims associated with regional anesthesia along with a decline in claims associated with general anesthesia since the anesthesia work force survey was done in 1981.

Aspiration Pneumonitis

An analysis of obstetric anesthesia cases from the ASA Closed Claims Project database 1996 showed that almost all the obstetric claims in which pulmonary aspiration was identified as the primary damaging event occurred in association with general anesthesia. Aspiration accounted for only 31% of obstetric files but 76% of nonobstetric files. Pulmonary aspiration was noted in 7% of the obstetric files but was not always considered the primary damaging event. In 25 of these cases, the primary anesthetic technique was general anesthesia. In 10 cases, aspiration occurred during difficult intubation or following esophageal intubation; and in seven cases, mask general anesthesia was being used. In three cases, vomiting and aspiration occurred at the time of induction without cricoid pressure. Two cases of aspiration were associated with cricoid pressure. Two cases of aspiration associated with regional anesthesia occurred during resuscitation and intubation following high spinal blocks. In two other cases, heavy sedation was implicated. The Obstetric Closed Claims files from 1996 indicate that damaging events related to the respiratory system were significantly more common among obese (32%) than nonobese (7%) parturients. However, the overall number of claims for aspiration pneumonitis has decreased from 9% in 1970s to 1% in 1990s.

Maternal Death

In the past, maternal death and newborn brain damage were the most common of the anesthesia-related injuries, and maternal death was the leading reason for the claim to be opened. Maternal death was more commonly associated with general anesthesia and cesarean delivery. In the 1980s and 1990s, the number of maternal deaths decreased by more than half that seen in 1970s, when maternal death accounted for the highest proportion of obstetric anesthesia claims (30%). The highest proportion of obstetric anesthesia claims in the 1990s is related to maternal nerve damage.

Newborn Brain Damage

The incidence of claims for newborn brain damage has decreased from 22% in the 1970s to 14% in the 1990s. Because the etiology of newborn brain damage is difficult to determine, it is usually not clear to what extent anesthesia care was causally involved. It appears that anesthesiologists are sometimes unfairly named in a claim for a newborn nerve injury.

Maternal Nerve Injury

With the increase in regional anesthesia use for administering anesthesia for obstetric cases, the incidence of claims for maternal nerve damage has increased from 11% in 1970 to 20% in the 1990s. Nerve injury in the majority of these cases appeared to be a result of direct trauma to neural tissue. Severe pain or paresthesia during needle or catheter placement or during local anesthetic injection was a prominent feature in these claims. Other mechanisms of injury, such as neurotoxicity and ischemic causes such as epidural abscess, hypotension, or vascular insufficiency, were implicated less commonly.

Back Pain

Obstetric claims for back pain increased from 3% in the 1970s to 10% in the 1990s. The greater number of back pain claims may be related to the higher rate of regional anesthesia. Additionally, the back pain may be associated with the pregnancy itself.

Headache

The percentage of headache claims has increased from 12% in the 1970s to 14% in the 1990s. The popularity of regional anesthesia techniques in obstetrics combined with the greater incidence of postlumbar puncture headaches in the young female population likely account for the increased number of headache claims in the obstetric population.

Maternal Brain Damage

The incidence of claims for maternal brain damage in which the mother survived has decreased from 10% in the 1970s to 6% in the 1990s. Reasons for this may include the decreased utilization of general anesthesia over the decades and the subsequent decrease in risk of aspiration pneumonitis, hypoxia, and associated brain damage. Claims from use of general anesthesia for vaginal delivery decreased from 29% in the 1970s to 1% in the 1990s. For cesarean deliveries, claims from the use of general anesthesia decreased from 57 to 28%.

Pain During Surgery

The claims for pain during surgery increased from 4% in the 1970s to 7% in the 1990s. Almost all claims for pain during surgery were associated with cesarean delivery. Claims for pain during cesarean delivery were almost always made by patients who received regional anesthesia. Apparently, inadequate analgesia for labor and vaginal delivery is seldom a source of liability risk, but claims for pain during cesarean delivery is a cause for concern. Some of these claims may result from reluctance on the part of anesthesia personnel to convert to general anesthesia during cesarean delivery, fearing the risk of airway difficulties and /or pulmonary aspiration. Claims for "pain under anesthesia" are less likely with spinals and CSEs, in which a denser and a more reliable block, as compared to epidural anesthesia, is established.

Emotional Distress/Fright

The incidence of claims for emotional distress and fright increased from 6% in the 1970s to 8% in the 1990s. Anesthesiologists must pay more attention to the liability risk associated with less significant outcomes such as emotional distress. It is important to note that in many of the claims patients believed they were ignored, mistreated, or assaulted. Answering all questions to the patients' satisfaction, providing emotional support, and paying heed to their requests and concerns should decrease the incidence of claims for emotional distress in the future.

Newborn Death

Anesthesiologists must be aware that they can be implicated in newborn death, even if the cause is obstetric. Claims for newborn deaths have risen from 1% in the 1970s to 6% in the 1990s.

Regional Techniques and Obstetric Claims

The proportion of lumbar epidural claims has increased for vaginal delivery from 41% in 1970s to 97% in the 1990s and for cesarean deliveries from 17% in the 1970s to 41% in the 1990s. The proportion of claims related to spinal anesthesia has remained about 25% over the last three decades. There has been a decrease in the percentage of obstetric claims from caudal anesthesia from 15% in the 1970s to 1% in the 1990s. This is likely related to the decreased use of caudal anesthesia for childbirth.

Informed Consent

Examination of the database revealed two basic features related to informed consent. First, informed consent was rarely a liability issue; and second, when the quality of informed consent can be assessed in the claim file, it is usually considered appropriate. Informed consent was a liability issue in just 1% of the overall database. When the consent was considered appropriated, two specific patterns of liability were identifiable. The first involved claims when a specific patient request was ignored by the anesthesiologist. These cases serve as a reminder that failure to honor a patient's request can provide an important stimulus for litigation. The second pattern involved cases in which the patient was not informed of a specific complication, or there was an unexpected change in the conduct of anesthesia or surgery. These cases underscore the importance of explicitly mentioning and documenting the range of risks and educating the patient about the unpredictable course of perioperative events and the possibility that alternative approaches may be required (Box 10-3).

Obstetric and Nonobstetric Claims

Liability risk in obstetric anesthesia differs considerably from that in nonobstetric practice. Complications involving the respiratory system account for the largest proportion of damaging events in both groups, and prob-

---

Box 10-3 Anesthesia-Related Maternal Morbidity/Mortality Associated With Malpractice Claims

Aspiration pneumonitis
Maternal death (GA > RA)
Back pain
Headache
Maternal brain damage
Pain during surgery
Emotional distress

---

lems with difficult intubation and pulmonary aspiration are disproportionately represented in obstetric files. These findings agree with most anesthesiologists' belief that the pregnant patient's airway demands additional attention and care.

There was a trend for more problems to occur related to difficult intubation and pulmonary aspiration in obstetric than in nonobstetric patients. However, the most surprising difference between obstetric and nonobstetric claims is the large proportion of claims for relatively minor injuries in the obstetric files. While reducing major adverse anesthetic outcomes in obstetrics is important, attention must be paid to limiting liability risk associated with less severe outcomes such as headache, pain during anesthesia, and emotional distress. To some extent, the large proportion of relatively minor injuries in the obstetric files may be due to a greater incidence of such problems in these patients as well as heightened patient expectations.

PREVENTION OF LAWSUITS FOR UNEXPECTED OUTCOMES

Malpractice litigation may serve the purpose of not only reparation for injury and deterrence of substandard care, but also of emotional vindication. It is again important to note that there is a large proportion of minor injuries in obstetric claims. To avoid lawsuits for unexpected outcomes, obstetricians, obstetric nurses, and anesthesia care providers should develop a rapport with patients and their families.

A lawsuit does not necessarily signify injury or substandard care. It has been suggested that the number of patients harmed by negligent care who file a claim may be <2%. In contrast, lawsuits are usually not filed unless people perceive that they or a family member has been wronged by the system. Patients are not necessarily motivated to bring suit for an unexpected outcome. Suggestions to avoid obstetric claims include careful personal conduct, involvement in prenatal education, early preanesthetic evaluation as well as providing realistic expectations, and, of course, practicing at or above the standard of care.

REFERENCES

1. Goyert GL, Bottoms SF, Treadwell MC, Nehra PC: The physician factor in cesarean birth rates. N Engl J Med 320(11): 706–709, 1989.

2. Howell CJ, Kidd C, Roberts W, et al: A randomised controlled trial of epidural compared with nonepidural analgesia in labour. Br J Obstet Gynaecol 108(1):27–33, 2001.

3. Breen AO: Back pain. J R Soc Med 87(3):184, 1994.

4. Norris MC, Joseph J, Leighton BL: Anesthesia for perinatal surgery. Am J Perinatol 6(1):39-40, 1989.

5. Jackson A, Henry R, Avery N, et al: Informed consent for labour epidural: What labouring women want to know. Can J Anesth 47(11):1068-1073, 2000.

6. Davies J: Obstetric anesthesia closed claims—trends over the last three decades. ASA Newsletter, June 2004.

SUGGESTED READING

Atrash HK, Alexander S, Berg CJ: Maternal mortality in developed countries: Not just a concern of the past. Obstet Gynecol 86(4 Pt 2):700-705, 1995.

Berg CJ, Atrash HK, Koonin LM, Tucker M: Pregnancy-related mortality in the United States, 1987-1990. Obstet Gynecol 88(2):161-167, 1996.

Chadwick HS, Posner K, Caplan RA, et al: A comparison of obstetric and nonobstetric anesthesia malpractice claims. Anesthesiology 74(2):242-249, 1991.

Halpern SH, Leighton BL, Ohlsson A, et al: Effect of epidural vs parenteral opioid analgesia on the progress of labor: A meta-analysis. JAMA 280(24):2105-2110, 1998.

Hawkins JL, Koonin LM, Palmer SK, Gibbs CP: Anesthesia-related deaths during obstetric delivery in the United States, 1979-1990. Anesthesiology 86(2):277-284, 1997.

Hawkins JL, Gibbs CP, Orleans M, et al: Obstetric anesthesia work force survey, 1981 versus 1992. Anesthesiology 87(1):135-143, 1997.

Hickson GB, Clayton EW, Githens PB, Sloan FA: Factors that prompted families to file medical malpractice claims following perinatal injuries. JAMA 267(10):1359-1363, 1992.

Khor LJ, Jeskins G, Cooper GM, Paterson-Brown S: National obstetric anaesthetic practice in the UK 1997/1998. Anaesthesia 55(12):1168-1172, 2000.

Kubli M, Scrutton MJ, Seed PT, O'Sullivan G: An evaluation of isotonic "sport drinks" during labor. Anesth Analg 94(2):404-408, 2002.

Towner D, Castro MA, Eby-Wilkens E, Gilbert WM: Effect of mode of delivery in nulliparous women on neonatal intracranial injury. N Engl J Med 341(23):1709-1714, 1999.

Wong CA, Scavone BM, Peaceman AM, et al: The risk of cesarean delivery with neuroaxial analgesia given early vs late in labor. N Eng J Med 352(7):655-665, 2005.

CHAPTER 11

Pharmacology and Physiologic Issues Specific to the Care of the Gynecologic Patient

MIRJANA LOVRINCEVIC

SURGICAL ANATOMY OF THE FEMALE PELVIS

The organs of the female pelvis are the bladder, ureters, urethra, uterus, fallopian (uterine) tubes, ovaries, vagina, and rectum. These organs do not completely fill the cavity—the remaining space is occupied by ileum and sigmoid colon. The uterus, fallopian tubes, and ovaries are almost completely covered with peritoneum, while the rest of the organs in the pelvis are partially covered.

The blood supply to pelvic organs is primarily from the internal iliac (hypogastric) artery and its visceral branches: uterine artery; superior, middle, and inferior vesical arteries supplying the bladder; the middle and inferior hemorrhoidal artery; and the vaginal artery. However, collateral circulation is rather generous and arises from the aorta in the form of the ovarian artery, from the external iliac artery and from the femoral artery. The veins form extensive plexus that drains into the hypogastric trunk. The lymphatic channels of the female reproductive organs drain predominantly into the pelvic and para-aortic lymph nodes.

The pelvic organs are innervated by both sympathetic and parasympathetic nerves. The superior hypogastric plexus carries the majority of sympathetic fibers. They originate in the first, second, third, and fourth lumbar nerves and are responsible for the innervation of the fundus uteri, cervix, and vagina. The inferior hypogastric plexus is divided into three portions, representing distribution of innervation to the viscera: the vesical plexus, which innervates the bladder and urethra; hemorrhoidal plexus, which innervates the rectum; and uterovaginal plexus (Frankenhäuser's ganglion), which provides innervation to the uterus, vagina, clitoris, and vestibular bulbs. Parasympathetic innervation comes from the second, third, and fourth sacral nerves in the form of nervi erigentes. Pelvic viscera also have nociceptive synapses from T10 to L1 spinal levels and the celiac plexus.

The lumbosacral plexus and its branches provide motor and sensory somatic innervation to the lower abdominal wall, the pelvic and urogenital diaphragms, the perineum, and the hip and lower extremity. A visceral component, the pelvic splanchnic nerve, is also included (Table 11-1).

PHYSIOLOGY OF THE OVARIAN HORMONES

Unlike the reproductive system of men, the reproductive system in women undergoes regular cyclic changes under the influence of female hormones: estrogens and progesterone.

Estrogens

The naturally occurring estrogens are 17β-estradiol, estrone, and estriol. They are secreted primarily by the granulosa and the thecal cells of the ovarian follicles, the corpus luteum, and the placenta, although they are also formed from androgens by biotransformation.

17β-estradiol is the primarily secreted estrogen and the most potent. It is 98% protein bound, with 2% circulating free. Estrone is in equilibrium in the circulation with 17β-estradiol and is metabolized in the liver to estriol, the least potent estrogen.

Table 11-1	Somatic Innervation of Gynecologic Organs	

Nerve	Spinal Segment	Innervation
Iliohypogastric	T12, L1	Sensory—skin near iliac crest, just above symphysis pubis
Ilioinguinal	L1	Sensory—upper medial thigh, mons, labia major
Lateral femoral cutaneous	L2, L3	Sensory—lateral thigh to level of knee
Femoral	L2, L3, L4	Sensory—anterior and medial thigh, medial leg and foot, hip, and knee joints
		Motor—iliacus, anterior thigh muscles
Genitofemoral	L1, L2	Sensory—anterior vulva (genital branch), middle and upper anterior thigh (femoral branch)
Obturator	L2, L3, L4	Sensory—medial thigh and leg, hip, and knee joints
		Motor—adductor muscles of thigh
Superior gluteal	L4, L5, S1	Motor—gluteal muscles
Inferior gluteal	L4, L5, S1, S2	Motor—gluteal muscles
Posterior femoral cutaneous	S2, S3	Sensory—vulva, perineum
Sciatic	L4, L5, S1, S2, S3	Sensory—most of leg, foot, lower extremity joints
		Motor—posterior thigh muscle, leg, and foot muscles
Pudendal	S2, S3, S4	Sensory—Perianal skin, vulva, perineum, clitoris, urethra, vaginal vestibule
		Motor—external anal sphincter, perineal muscles, urogenital diaphragm

Estrogens undergo oxidation in the liver, and then conversion to glucuronide and sulphate conjugates. Significant amounts are secreted in the bile and reabsorbed in the bloodstream (Box 11-1).

Estrogens act by multiple mechanisms in many different tissues:

1. On female genitalia: Estrogens stimulate proliferation of endometrial mucosa, facilitate the growth of the ovarian follicles, increase uterine blood flow, and increase the amount of uterine muscle.

2. On endocrine organs: Estrogens decrease FSH secretion, increase the size of the pituitary, cause epiphyseal closure, and increase secretion of angiotensinogen and thyroid-binding globulin.

3. On central nervous system (CNS): Increase in libido is observed and attributed to direct effect of estrogens on certain neurons in the hypothalamus. In neurons of the hippocampus, an area involved in memory, estrogens increase neuronal sensitivity. Some data suggest that the decline in cognitive function in postmenopausal women is related to estrogen deficiency. Reports have indicated the beneficial role of estrogens in the slowing progression of Alzheimer's disease, although in a randomized trial, estrogen administration had no beneficial effect in already-established disease.

4. On breasts and female secondary sex characteristics: Estrogens cause breast duct growth and differentiation, stimulate the growth of connective tissue, and cause pigmentation of the areolas. The body configuration, female distribution of fat in the breasts and buttocks, and body hair distribution are also influenced by estrogens.

5. On metabolism: Estrogens cause salt and water retention, which is one of the reasons women gain weight just prior to menstruation. (Another one is increased aldosterone levels in the luteal phase of the cycle.) Estrogens also have a cholesterol-lowering effect.

6. On bones: Estrogens directly inhibit the function of osteoclasts. Estrogen deficiency is known to accelerate bone loss and increase susceptibility to fractures. Estrogen therapy diminishes bone loss and reduces the risk of fracture in women with osteoporosis and in those without this condition for the duration of therapy.

7. Vascular effects: Estrogens cause short-term vasodilation by increasing the formation and release of nitric oxide and prostacyclin in endothelial cells. They also reduce vascular smooth-muscle tone by opening calcium channels through a mechanism that is dependent on cyclic guanosine monophosphate (c-gmp).

Synthetic estrogens are indicated for the prevention of osteoporosis and the reduction of hot flashes and other symptoms of menopause. They also stimulate the growth of endometrium and breasts, probably increasing the risk

Box 11-1 Estrogens

Naturally occurring estrogens
  Estrone
  Estriol
  17β-Estradiol
Synthetic estrogens
  Tamoxifen
  Raloxifene

of the endometrial and breast cancer. Two newer products, tamoxifen and raloxifene, show certain selectivity in this regard. Tamoxifen does not stimulate the breast. Raloxifene has estrogen-like effects on bone tissues and on serum lipid concentrations, but not on breast and endometrial tissue. In the brain, however, raloxifene is more of an estrogen antagonist, because it increases the vasomotor symptoms of estrogen deficiency.

It is believed that the effects of estrogens are mediated via increased expression of mRNA. Estrogens combine with protein receptors in the nucleus, and the complexes bind to deoxyribonucleic acid (DNA), promoting formation of mRNA that, in turn, directs the formation of new proteins that modify cell function. So far, two estrogen receptors have been cloned: estrogen receptor α (ER α) and estrogen receptor β (ER β). The former is found primarily in the uterus, testis, pituitary, kidney, epididymis, and adrenals, whereas the latter is commonly present in the ovary, prostate, lung, bladder, brain, and bone. Most of the estrogenic actions are genomic and mediated via receptors α and β. However, there are nongenomic effects of estrogens as well, such as effects on neuronal discharge in the brain and possible feedback effects on gonadotropin secretion, which are presumably mediated by membrane receptors.

CURRENT CONTROVERSY: HORMONE REPLACEMENT THERAPY

- Initial studies showed benefits in treating vasomotor symptoms of menopause, prevention of osteoporosis by decreasing bone resorption and loss, improvement in plasma lipoprotein profiles, and possible delay of the onset of Alzheimer's disease by improving cognitive function and increasing cerebral blood flow.
- Estrogen/Progestin Replacement Study results failed to show benefit in women with coronary vascular disease. The Women's Health Initiative Studies stopped prematurely in 2002 due to overall risks of HRT that outweighed the benefits (increased risk for the ischemic stroke). Last studies suggest that use of combined hormone replacement therapy is associated with an increased risk of breast cancer, particularly invasive lobular tumors.

Progesterone

Progesterone is secreted in large amounts by the corpus luteum and the placenta, 98% of progesterone is protein bound (80% to albumin and 18% to corticosteroid-binding globulin), while 2% is circulating free. Progesterone undergoes metabolism in the liver, where it is converted to pregnanediol. Pregnanediol is conjugated to glucuronic acid and then excreted in the urine (Box 11-2).

Box 11-2   Progesterone

Naturally occurring progesterone
Synthetic progestins (gestagens)
　Medroxyprogesterone acetate
　Chlormadinone acetate

Effects of progesterone:
1. On breasts: Progesterone stimulates the development of lobules and alveoli, and supports the secretory function of the breasts during lactation.
2. On uterus: Myometrial cells are less excitable, less responsive to oxytocin, and show less spontaneous electric activity while influenced by progesterone.
3. On pituitary and hypothalamus: Ovulation is prevented by inhibition of LH secretion as a result of large doses of progesterone.
4. On metabolism: Progesterone is responsible for the rise in the basal body temperature at the time of the ovulation. Large doses of progesterone produce natriuresis, probably by blocking the action of aldosterone on the kidney.
5. On breathing: The stimulatory effect on breathing of endogenous progesterone and the synthetic medroxyprogesterone acetate are established by several studies. Other endogenous progestins such as pregnenolone, have not been studied. Increased secretion of progesterone explains hyperventilation and low carbon dioxide (CO_2) during pregnancy, and also during the luteal phase of the menstrual cycle.

Mechanism of action: The progesterone receptor is bound to a heat-shock protein in the complex process in which DNA initiates synthesis of new mRNA. There are two isoforms of progesterone receptors: progesterone receptor A (PRa) and progesterone receptor B (PRb). Although their physiologic significance is still under investigation, it is known that they play a pivotal role in the maintenance of early pregnancy by stimulating endometrial growth and inhibiting uterine contractility.

Synthetic progesterone-like substances are called progestins or gestagens, and they are clinically used along with estrogens as oral contraceptive agents. Despite the initial enthusiasm for progesterone in the treatment of premenstrual syndrome (PMS) and postnatal depression, there is a lack of evidence for its use in either condition. In fact, the addition of sequential progesterone to estrogen replacement therapy in postmenopausal women is often accompanied by negative mood symptoms, particularly in women who suffered from PMS before menopause. Synthetic progestins (medroxyprogesterone acetate and chlormadinone acetate) have been used for respiratory stimulation with variable success. A few studies have reported some improvement in sleepiness, blood gas levels, and in the number or duration of apneic and hypopneic events.

PSYCHOLOGY OF THE GYNECOLOGIC PATIENT

There have always been numerous reports of differences between the sexes in rates of illnesses and course of illnesses such as schizophrenia, alcoholism, mood and anxiety disorders, and Alzheimer's disease. Why are women and men so different when it comes to certain psychiatric disorders? Why are women disadvantaged with respect to men in Alzheimer's disease, and relatively advantaged when it comes to schizophrenia? It is generally agreed that most of the relative disadvantages that accrue to women do not take place until after puberty. The marked sex difference in rates of illness that begin with the reproductive years suggests that that the brain's hormonal environment during adulthood may be an important point of departure in the search for an explanation.

Results from the National Comorbidity Survey have revealed that lifetime prevalence for major depression is 21.3% for women compared with 12.7% for men. Women are twice as likely as men to experience major depression during their lifetime and seem to be particularly vulnerable at transitions across their reproductive life cycle (premenstruum, puerperium, and perimenopause).

With respect to female-specific mood disorders, about 5% of menstruating women develop premenstrual dysphoric disorder (PMDD); 10% of childbearing women experience postpartum onset of nonpsychotic major depressive disorder, commonly referred to as postpartum depression (PPD); and 0.2% suffer a psychotic mood disorder (most often manic in type). Community-based survey findings suggest that perimenopause, but not postmenopause, is accompanied by depressive symptoms.

Although there is no sex difference in the lifetime prevalence of schizophrenia, women develop the illness later, experience fewer and briefer hospitalizations, and are less likely to abuse substances. Women with schizophrenia enjoy better psychosocial functioning and greater work competence than their male counterparts. In addition, women with schizophrenia perform better on neuropsychological tests. Women suffering from schizophrenia require lower doses of antipsychotic medications than men and respond better to both psychosocial and pharmacologic treatments.

Women are disproportionally prone to Alzheimer's disease, even after adjustment for their longer survival: as many as 30% to 50% of women older than 85 years suffer from a dementing process. Women's cognitive impairments may also be more severe than men's. Part of the increased understanding of Alzheimer's disease lies in the clarification of the effects of estrogens on neurotrophins. Neurotrophins are proteins that play an important role in the growth of new nerve cells. This hormonal modulation of neurotrophins increases the connections among neuronal branches and maintains a complex system of communication in the brain. When estrogen levels drop in menopause, brain cells of women begin to degenerate at a faster pace than those of men. Men are relatively spared because the testosterone is continuously being converted to estradiol in the brain (Box 11-3).

GYNECOLOGIC MALIGNANCIES

There were over 600,000 women diagnosed with cancer in the United States in 2000. Endometrial cancer and ovarian cancer are the fourth and fifth most common sites of cancer in American women. The trends in gynecologic cancers have changed over the past decade: the incidence of invasive cervical cancer has decreased 70%, while preinvasive forms of cancer are increasing. Ovarian cancer incidence shows no changes since 1973, and endometrial cancer has decreased only very slightly.

As more women survive the acute phases of gynecologic cancer, they will be seen more often as chronic patients in a variety of medical settings, including the operating room. The care of such patients needs to take into consideration previous medical interventions because prior surgical history, radiation therapy, and administration of chemotherapeutics will affect clinical decision making and adequate preparation for surgery (Box 11-4).

Chemotherapeutic agents used most commonly in treatment of patients with gynecologic malignancies include Cisplatin, Bleomycin, Doxorubicin, and Methotrexate. Cisplatin is the most effective single agent against ovarian cancer; it is also often accompanied by doxorubicin and/or cyclophosphamide. The major dose-limiting toxicity is renal toxicity: cisplatin is a direct tubular toxin, preferentially affecting the proximal straight tubule and the distal and collecting tubules. Other toxicities include ototoxicity (tinnitus, high-frequency hearing loss), peripheral neuropathy (in the form of stocking-glove distribution paresthesias), and nausea and vomiting. Preoperative evaluation as well as intraoperative manage-

---

Box 11-3   Affective Disorders Highly Influenced by Gonadal Steroids

Major depression
Premenstrual syndrome
Postpartum affective disorders
Menopausal depression

Box 11-4 Chemotherapeutic Agents used in Treatment of Gynecologic Malignancies

Cisplatin
Bleomycin
Doxorubicin
Methotrexate

---

ment of these patients should focus on fluid and electrolyte balance as well as optimizing renal perfusion. Anesthetic agents that have nephrotoxic potential should be avoided. Recently, there were reports of hypersensitivity reactions to intravenous cisplatin during concomitant pelvic radiation. The reaction, which is characterized by fever, anxiety, pruritus, cough, dyspnea, diaphoresis, angioedema, vomiting, bronchospasm, rash, and pruritus, is most likely the result of increased release of cytokines from the tumor. It is important to recognize the patophysiology behind these reactions to provide patients with adequate premedications and to treat those episodes adequately.

DRUG INTERACTION: CHEMOTHERAPEUTIC DRUGS TOXICITY AND CLINICAL IMPLICATIONS

- Cisplatin: Renal toxicity, ototoxicity, peripheral neuropathy, gastrointestinal toxicity.
- Bleomycin: Acute interstitial pneumonia, chronic fibrotic changes in the lung, sensitization of the lung to the toxic effect of oxygen and OH radicals.
- Doxorubicin: Dose-related cardiomyopathy.
- Methotrexate: Gastrointestinal toxicity, impaired liver function, renal tubular injury.

Bleomycin, used to treat cervical cancer and germ cell tumors of the ovary, is known to produce acute interstitial pneumonia and chronic fibrotic changes in the lung. In addition, it appears that bleomycin sensitizes the lung to the toxic effect of oxygen and OH radicals, especially if FiO_2 is kept at >0.3. Baseline pulmonary function tests and arterial blood gas analysis are helpful in defining the patient's pulmonary status after bleomycin therapy. FiO_2 needs to be maintained at the lowest level compatible with adequate oxygenation.

Doxorubicin has been useful in treatment of endometrial and ovarian carcinomas. Its major side effect is a dose-related cardiomyopathy, which might exist in an acute and chronic form. An acute form is characterized by relatively benign electrocardiogram (ECG) changes that include ST-T changes and decreased voltage. The chronic form is characterized by progressive cardiac failure unresponsive to inotropic drugs that may be diagnosed with serial ECHO

studies. It is also important to be aware of the increased risk of doxorubicin-induced cardiotoxicity in the presence of other cardiac insults, such as prior mediastinal irritation, systemic hypertension, or the coadministration of cyclophosphamide or mitomycin C. Newer agents such as epirubicin and pegylated liposomal doxorubicin are associated with a more favorable toxicity profile. Clinical trials are underway to explore their role as first-line or salvage treatment in gynecologic malignancies.

Methotrexate is used in treatment of ovarian cancer and gestational trophoblastic carcinoma. The major toxic complications associated with this agent are gastrointestinal toxicity, impaired liver function manifested by elevated transaminases, and renal tubular injury characterized by a rising BUN and serum creatinine with a decreasing urinary volume. It is important to appreciate that elimination of methotrexate, which occurs by the kidneys, can be inhibited by the coadministration of weak acids, such as aspirin or penicillin. Aspirin can further compound methotrexate's toxicity by displacing the drug from its binding site on albumin, increasing the concentration of the free drug.

CASE STUDY: PERIOPERATIVE CARE OF THE BLEOMYCIN-TREATED PATIENT

A 77-year-old woman with a history of ovarian cancer, status postsurgical excision of the tumor, status postradiation therapy, and status post-one round of Bleomycin treatment is presenting for emergency cholecystectomy. She also has a history of COPD for which she is using metered-dose inhalers, and severe osteoarthritis that is preventing her from taking care of regular house chores.

Perioperative Concerns and Plan of Action

1. Pulmonary function: 5% to 10% of patients treated with bleomycin develop pulmonary toxicity. The likelihood of developing pulmonary toxicity is greater when the total dose of Bleomycin is more than 400 U administered in patients older than 70 years of age with underlying pulmonary disease. Prior radiotherapy may also predispose the patient to pulmonary toxicity.
2. Use of oxygen in the operating room: There is a theory that acutely increased inhaled concentrations of oxygen facilitate production of superoxide and other free radicals in the presence of bleomycin. It has been recommended that inhaled concentrations of oxygen during surgery be maintained below 30% in bleomycin-treated patients.
3. Fluid replacement: To prevent pulmonary interstitial edema in bleomycin-treated patients undergoing surgery, it is prudent to use colloids instead of crystalloids. It is suspected that impaired lymphatic function causes accumulation of the interstitial fluid.

SUGGESTED READING

Ansbacher R: The pharmacokinetics and efficacy of different estrogens are not equivalent. Am J Obstet Gynecol 184(3): 255-263, 2001.

Croce MA, Fabian TC, Malhotra AK, et al: Does gender difference influence outcome? J Trauma Injury Infect Crit Care 53(5): 889-894, 2002.

Desiderio DP: Anesthetic-antineoplastic drug interactions. Semin Anesth 12(2):74-78, 1993.

Epperson CN, Wisner KL, Yamamoto B: Gonadal steroids in the treatment of mood disorders. Psychosom Med 61(5): 676-697, 1999.

Gruber CJ, Tschugguel W, Schneeberger C, Huber JC: Mechanisms of disease: Production and actions of estrogens. N Engl J Med 346(5):340-352, 2002.

Hulley S, Grady D, Bush T, et al: Randomized trial of estrogen plus progestin for secondary prevention of coronary heart disease in postmenopausal women. Heart and Estrogen/ Progestin Replacement Study (HERS) Research Group. JAMA 280(7):605-613, 1998.

Li CI, Malone KE, Porter PL, et al: Relationship between long durations and different regimens of hormone therapy and risk of breast cancer. JAMA 289(24):3254-3263, 2003.

Peppriell JE, Lema MJ: Preanesthetic Considerations for The Patient With Cancer Receiving Cancer Treatment. Problems in Anesthesia 7(4):349-364, 1993.

Rapp SR, Espeland MA, Shumaker SA, et al: Effect of estrogen plus progestin on global cognitive function in postmenopausal women. The Women's Health Initiative Memory Study: A randomized controlled trial. JAMA 289:2663-2672, 2003.

Roberts JA, Brown D, Elkins T, Larson DB: Factors influencing views of patients with gynecologic cancer about end-of-life decisions. Am J Obstet Gynecol 176(1):166-172, 1997.

Saaresranta T, Polo O: Hormones and breathing. Chest 122(6): 2165-2182, 2002.

Schumaker SA, Legault C, Rapp SR, et al: Estrogen plus progestin and the incidence of dementia and mild cognitive impairment in postmenopausal women. The Women's Health Initiative Memory Study: A randomized controlled trial. JAMA 289:2651-2662, 2003.

Seeman MV: Psychopathology in women and men: Focus on female hormones. Am J Psychiatry 154(12):1641-1647, 1997.

Stoelting RK: Chemotherapeutic Drugs. In Stoelting RK, Hillier SC (eds): Pharmacology & Physiology in Anesthetic Practice, 4th edition. Philadelphia, Lippincott, Williams and Wilkins, 2006, pp 551-568.

Taylor M: Unconventional estrogens. Clin Obstet Gynecol 44(4):864-879, 2001.

CHAPTER 12

Anesthesia for Gynecologic/ Oncologic Procedures

MIRJANA LOVRINCEVIC

INTRODUCTION

Providing anesthesia for the gynecologic patient has always been a special mission. While the development of new techniques and equipment has made the surgeon's job a bit easier, the anesthesiologist still has to deal with same issues.

The anesthesiologist must recognize and appreciate a strong emotional component in administering anesthesia to a gynecologic patient, because that influences the perioperative anesthetic plan. The patient must also be evaluated for coexisting medical problems, previous anesthetic complications, potential airway difficulties, and considerations related to intraoperative positioning. This evaluation coupled with the appreciation of the surgeon's needs is used to formulate the anesthetic plan.

PREOPERATIVE CONSIDERATIONS

General Considerations

Preoperative anxiety is universal. It is fear of the unknown or of what the patient imagines she will be forced to endure during the surgery. In the gynecologic patient, however, these issues are compounded by the emotional context of the procedures. Whether having a surgical procedure to treat infertility, to terminate desired or undesired pregnancy, or to remove tumor masses, patients often bear strong feelings of anger, guilt, embarrassment, or inadequacy. It is important for the anesthesiologist to appreciate these issues, because the perioperative course might be significantly influenced. It has been shown that increased baseline anxiety is associated with autonomic dysfunction, arrhythmias, hypertension, decreased gastric motility, and increased intraoperative anesthetic requirements. Preoperative visits are helpful in alleviating anxiety and should be done whenever possible. In addition to psychological preparation, patients also benefit from premedication. Traditionally, goals for premedication are relief of apprehension, sedation, analgesia, amnesia, reduction of gastric fluid volume and acidity, prevention of nausea and vomiting, prevention of autonomic reflex responses, decrease of monitored anesthesia care (MAC), and so on.

Premedication should fit the requirements of the individual patient in the same way that anesthetic techniques do.

Pre-emptive Analgesia

Studies have shown that pre-emptive analgesia can be achieved by different means. While blocking noxious input using epidural opioids and local anesthetics before the incision reduces the rate and amount of morphine consumption, pain on movement, and secondary hyperalgesia compared with intraoperative epidural use in patients undergoing major gynecologic procedure via laparotomy, preoperative wound infiltration with local anesthetic does not reduce postoperative opioid consumption. The new class of nonsteroidal anti-inflammatory medications specific to the COX-2 receptor, COX-2 inhibitors, have been proved to be useful in reducing perioperative opioid consumption for abdominal hysterectomy.

Prevention of Nausea and Vomiting

Patients undergoing gynecologic procedures, especially via the laparoscopic approach, are at high risk of postoperative nausea and vomiting. The optimal strategy for prevention and management of postoperative nausea and vomiting is still controversial. Even though many drugs with different sites of action are available, success is not guaranteed. The combination of antiemetics seems to be superior to a single-agent treatment: 5-hydroxytryptamine antagonists and metoclopramide and 5-hydroxytryptamine antagonists and dexamethasone are most thoroughly investigated and efficacious in clinical studies (Box 12-1).

GYNECOLOGIC PATIENT WITH COEXISTING DISEASES

Patient with Cardiovascular Disease

When assessing a patient's risk for major cardiac events during or after any noncardiac surgery, clinical evaluation is used to determine the risk for fatal and nonfatal cardiac events. Clinical data collection should concentrate on variables that will be most helpful in classifying the patient as low risk, intermediate risk, or high risk.

Box 12-1 Preoperative Considerations

Anxiolysis
Pre-emptive analgesia
Prevention of nausea and vomiting

CURRENT CONTROVERSY: SINGLE AGENT OR A COMBINATION FOR THE PROPHYLAXIS OF POSTOPERATIVE NAUSEA AND VOMITING?

- 5-Hydroxytryptamine 3 antagonists in combination with dexamethasone found to be more effective than either agent alone in several studies
- 5-Hydroxytryptamine 3 antagonists in combination with metoclopramide found to be more effective than metoclopramide alone
- Droperidol's arrhythmogenic potential overshadows its undeniable efficacy even as a single agent

---

Class II or III on the modified Cardiac Risk Index predicts a high risk for perioperative cardiac events. Class I is identified as low risk, and those patients may proceed directly to surgery without further noninvasive testing.

It has been demonstrated that antihypertensives should be continued throughout the perioperative period to avoid abrupt hemodynamic changes. The incidence of intraoperative hypotension and evidence of myocardial ischemia on the electrocardiogram (ECG) are increased in patients who remain hypertensive before the induction of anesthesia. Tachycardia that usually accompanies blood pressure fluctuations should be particularly avoided because it further increases myocardial oxygen consumption. Patients who are already medically treated with β-blockers and whose heart rate is kept within normal limits perioperatively have been shown to have significant reduction of ischemic events related to surgery. Indeed, it has been suggested that such therapy should be started in patients at risk prior to surgery when such patients are not already receiving this type of medication. Postoperative pain control requires special care to avoid additional stress to the cardiovascular system, because some of the gynecologic surgical procedures are associated with more pain than others (e.g., abdominal hysterectomy versus vaginal hysterectomy).

Patient with Respiratory Disease

These patients are also vulnerable in the perioperative period, and continuation/optimization of their existing treatment is important. Certain anesthetic agents are known to interfere with the normal breathing process, and it is crucial to appreciate the particular vulnerability of the patient with respiratory problems. Respiratory center depression due to opioid analgesics is particularly dangerous in patients with obstructive sleep apnea (OSA); failure to reverse neuromuscular blocking agents completely may quickly result in hypercapnic respiratory failure in patients with chronic obstructive pulmonary disease (COPD);

histamine-releasing agents should not be used in patients prone to bronchospasm and asthma.

Patients with Diabetes Mellitus

Preoperative management of the patient with diabetes mellitus should focus on blood glucose control; avoiding hypoglycemia and ensuring long-term complications of this disease are not adversely affected by surgery. Diabetes-related autonomic neuropathy may cause orthostatic hypotension, resting tachycardia, gastroparesis with vomiting, diarrhea, abdominal distention, and bladder atony.

Diabetic patients with poorly controlled insulin-dependent diabetes will probably need to be admitted into the hospital before the surgery and closely monitored. The traditional approaches have been to either administer one half of the dose of the intermediate-acting insulin the morning of surgery and initiate the intravenous infusion of 5% glucose to reduce the risk of hypoglycemia, or to omit the insulin the morning of surgery altogether.

Patient with Gynecologic Malignancies

The type and extent of malignancy play a major role in determining the extent of preoperative preparation and intraoperative monitoring the patient will require. The treatment history must be thoroughly evaluated. Most likely, these patients have had radiation therapy and chemotherapy and, perhaps, numerous surgical procedures. Depending on the type of adjunctive treatment, the patient may come to surgery in poor physical condition from malnutrition or suffering effects of toxicity from chemotherapy. Vascular access may be difficult to obtain, due to sclerosis or thrombosis of peripheral veins.

Pulmonary function may be impaired by some chemotherapeutic agents, most commonly bleomycin, while combination therapy, especially with vincristine or cisplatin increases pulmonary toxicity. A preoperative chest x-ray is mandatory to assess the presence of lung injury. Severe lung disease is an indication for neuraxial anesthesia whenever possible, or postoperative mechanical ventilation may be necessary.

Patients who have been treated with cardiotoxic chemotherapeutic agents such as daunorubicin and doxorubicin are usually monitored for cardiomyopathy, which might be of early or late onset. Although the early form is apparent, because it is manifested by acute ST segment and T wave changes and dysrhythmias, the late form is insidious in onset and usually presents as congestive heart failure. Cardiology consultation is sought for the latter to optimize the medical condition of these patients.

Peripheral neuropathies occur commonly in patients treated with vincristine, cyclophosphamide, and paclitaxel.

It is important to document the presence of neurologic deficits preoperatively for subsequent comparisons.

Chemotherapeutic agents are frequently used together with corticosteroids. A stress dose of steroids should be given perioperatively to avoid Addisonian crisis in patients who have histories of such a treatment combination within the past year.

Bleeding and fluid shifts should be anticipated for any patient undergoing a definitive operation for cancer, whether it be for potential cure, debulking, or palliation. In that respect, the need for blood and blood products should be anticipated and the blood bank notified accordingly.

CLINICAL CAVEAT: PERIOPERATIVE CARE FOR THE PATIENT WITH COEXISTING DISEASE

- Patient with cardiovascular diseases
  - Identify patients as Cardiac Risk Index Class I, II, or III.
  - Continue antihypertensives.
  - Consider starting β-adrenergic blocker, if the patient is not already on it.
  - Pay special attention to postoperative pain control.
- Patient with respiratory diseases
  - Continue/optimize of the current treatment.
  - Exercise caution using respiratory center depressants (e.g., opioids).
  - Assure adequate reversal of neuromuscular blockade.
- Patient with diabetes mellitus
  - Avoid hypoglycemia.
  - Assure that long-term complications of diabetes are not adversely affected by surgery.
- Patient with gynecologic malignancies
  - Consider implications of prior treatments (surgery, radiation therapy, chemotherapy).
  - Assess the need for good vascular access in presence of malnutrition, dehydration, ascites, and blood loss.

ADDITIONAL STUDIES

Laboratory Studies

The laboratory investigation of a patient needs to be limited to those diagnostic procedures that are appropriate to the findings elicited during the history and physical examination. The decision to order electrolyte, creatinine, coagulation studies, chemistry panels, ECG, and chest x-ray films should be based on the evaluation of the patient. Patients with medical illnesses such as diabetes, hypertension, and asthma need to be in optimal control before surgery. Specialty consultation is generally necessary for patients with pulmonary or cardiac disease, to be sure that the best preoperative condition is achieved and that the operative risk is acceptable.

Blood Transfusion

A blood sample should be sent to the blood bank well in advance of the planned operative procedure so that the blood bank will have time to overcome any difficulty encountered in performing the intended crossmatch. For procedures in which blood loss is not anticipated, a type and screen are sufficient. Autologous blood use should be encouraged if the patient is in good general health, whereas epoetin alfa might be considered in patients with low preoperative hemoglobin. Extensive clinical experience with epoetin alfa in anemic patients undergoing major elective orthopedic surgery or those with gynecologic cancers provides a strong basis for its use in gynecologic surgery.

Prophylactic Antibiotics

The goals of antibacterial prophylaxis during gynecologic surgery are similar to those of prophylaxis during intra-abdominal surgery. Prophylactic antibiotics are recommended for vaginal or abdominal hysterectomy. They are not considered necessary for adnexal surgery when there is no evidence of previous pelvic infection. The American College of Obstetricians and Gynecologists has recommended single-dose prophylactic protocols using a variety of agents (penicillins, cephalosporins, and clindamycin). Patients with a valvular heart disease, history of endocarditis, vascular graft, or implanted devices may require special antibiotic coverage (Box 12-2).

INTRAOPERATIVE CONSIDERATIONS

Positioning the Patient

Lithotomy position is used frequently in gynecologic surgery. The patient lies supine with each lower extremity flexed at the hip and knee, and both limbs are simultaneously elevated and separated so that the perineum becomes accessible to the surgeon. Hemodynamic changes can sometimes occur on elevation of legs into the

stirrups, as this increases venous return to the heart. Similarly, problems with hypotension on lowering legs postoperatively are common. When the legs are to be lowered to the original supine position at the end of the procedure, they should first be brought together at the knees and ankles in the sagittal plane, and then lowered slowly together to the table top. This minimizes torsion stress on the lumbar spine that would occur if each leg were lowered independently. It also permits gradual accommodation to the increase in the circulatory capacitance, thereby avoiding sudden hypotension. If pressure on the nerve over the fibula is not prevented by adequate padding or positioning, common peroneal nerve injury is possible. It is manifested as an inability to dorsiflex the foot and a loss of sensation over the dorsum of the foot. Hyperflexion of the hip joint can cause femoral and lateral femoral cutaneous nerve palsy. Obturator and saphenous nerve injury are also complications of the lithotomy position.

Frequently, some degree of head-down tilt is added to a lithotomy position. Depending on the degree of head depression, the addition of tilt to the lithotomy position combines the worst features of both the lithotomy and the Trendelenburg postures. The weight of abdominal viscera on the diaphragm adds to whatever abdominal compression is produced by the flexed thighs of an obese patient or of one placed in an exaggerated lithotomy position. Consequently, the work of spontaneous ventilation is increased for an anesthetized patient in a position that already worsens the ventilation-perfusion ratio by gravitational accumulation of blood in the poorly ventilated lung apices. During controlled ventilation, higher inspiratory pressures are needed to expand the lung (Box 12-3).

COMMON GYNECOLOGIC PROCEDURES

From the anesthesiologist's perspective, gynecologic procedures can be divided into four major categories: transvaginal, perineal, intra-abdominal, and transabdominal (laparoscopic). They are grouped according to the surgical site, position, surgical technique, and equipment used.

Box 12-2   Perioperative Need for Blood

Type and screen
Encourage autologous blood donation
Consider epoetin alfa

Box 12-3   Neuropathies Arising as a Result of Poor Positioning During Gynecologic Surgery

Common peroneal nerve palsy
Lateral femoral cutaneous nerve palsy
Obturator nerve injury
Saphenus nerve injury

Transvaginal Surgery

Dilation and Evacuation

Dilation and evacuation (D&E) is the generic term for curettage abortions at 13 weeks' gestation or later. During the 1970s, D&E emerged as the most frequently used method for second-trimester abortions. Errors in estimating gestational age, especially underestimation, can have serious consequences during a D&E procedure, because the complication rates are directly correlated with the week of gestation and the experience of the surgeon.

Paracervical block with intravenous (IV) sedation and analgesia is the preferred form of anesthesia because the patient is awake and able to report sudden, sharp abdominal pain should uterine perforation occur. In addition, the average blood loss is expected to be less in comparison to general anesthesia because volatile agents increase uterine relaxation and atony. There is, however, an occasional patient who requests general anesthesia. The presence of a full stomach should be assumed in pregnancies older than 12 weeks gestation and where there is a history of emesis or excessive anxiety. Thus, the trachea should be intubated and the cuff inflated to protect the airway from aspiration.

Once the suction curettage is begun, oxytocin is usually given IV, not to exceed 20 U/L, to promote "clamping down" of the uterus and to decrease the bleeding. In cases of bleeding unresponsive to oxytocin, ergonovine maleate 0.2 mg is usually administered intramuscularly (IM) or subcutaneously (SC). It is not recommended for IV use because severe hypertension, dysrhythmia, and even myocardial ischemia may ensue.

Prophylactic antibiotics show a substantial protective effect in women undergoing induced abortion. Doxycycline 100 mg IV is most commonly used to accomplish this goal.

Dilation and Curettage

This procedure is performed to diagnose and treat bleeding from uterine and cervical lesions, to complete an incomplete or missed spontaneous abortion, or to treat cervical stenosis. It is used infrequently as a primary method for pregnancy termination.

Local, regional, or general anesthesia all may be appropriate. If regional anesthesia is chosen, a T10 sensory level is sufficient to provide anesthesia for procedures on the uterus. 0.75% bupivacaine 10 to 15 mg in 7.5% dextrose is used most commonly. Lidocaine, both 2% and 5%, fell out of favor in recent years due to numerous reports of transient neurologic symptoms that can occur in up to one third of patients. If used, general anesthesia is frequently by mask or laryngeal mask airway with O_2/N_2O + volatile anesthetic and spontaneous respiration, as long as there is no indication for endotracheal intubation such as a full stomach, pregnancy 12 weeks and older gesta-

tion, obesity, severe anxiety, nausea, vomiting, or emergent surgery.

As with D&E, oxytocin and occasionally ergonovine are used to promote uterine contraction and decrease bleeding.

Laser Therapy to Vulva, Vagina, or Cervix

Laser therapy is indicated for preinvasive lesions of the vulva, vagina, or cervix. It destroys tissues by the selective application of light energy focused into a beam.

A carbon dioxide (CO_2) laser has a sharply focused beam with a very narrow spot diameter and a high-power density. This is perfect for cutting, and lateral tissue damage is minimized. Yttrium aluminum garnet (YAG) laser is able to penetrate tissue to a much greater depth than CO_2 laser energy. YAG energy scatters in tissue, so thermal damage is greater. Thus, this laser better serves as a coagulator of tissue and for debulking.

Most gynecologic laser procedures are done with local anesthesia and IV sedation, but general anesthesia and regional technique may be used as well. If regional anesthesia is used, T10 sensory level is desirable.

Special attention should be given to protection against eye injury, operating room fires, and aerosolization of viral particles during laser procedure. Goggles should be worn by both the patient and operating room (OR) personnel during laser use to prevent eye injury from the laser. If the patient is asleep, eyes should be covered with saline-soaked gauze. It is always advisable to watch for improper handling of lasers because OR fires can happen rapidly. Vaporization of condyloma may produce aerosolization of viral particles; therefore, appropriate ventilation is suggested to disperse smoke, and a special laser-surgical mask to trap virus-containing particles is recommended.

Perineal Surgery

Radical Vulvectomy

En bloc dissection of the inguinal-femoral region and the vulva is the current treatment for invasive vulvar carcinoma. This surgery involves bilateral excision of lymphatic and areolar tissue in the inguinal and femoral regions, combined with removal of the entire vulva between the labia-crural folds, from the perineal body to the upper margin of the mons pubis. If a large surgical wound is created, skin graft may be necessary.

Patients with vulvar carcinoma are typically elderly and have a high incidence of comorbidity. Careful preoperative assessment is needed to optimize the patient for the surgery. Blood should be available for transfusion, because occasionally femoral vessels may be injured, requiring rapid blood replacement.

Both general and regional anesthesia can be used, alone or in combination. Although vulvectomy is not particularly painful for a prolonged period postoperatively, a continuous epidural technique allows earlier ambulation with less sedation, especially in the elderly.

Operations for Stress Urinary Incontinence

Stress incontinence is a symptom that describes involuntary loss of urine associated with sudden cough or strain. The incidence of genuine stress incontinence is 10% among reproductive-aged women, but may approach 10% to 20% among postmenopausal patients.

There are currently two surgical approaches: suspension by the vaginal route and abdominal suspension procedures. Vaginal approach (Kelly urethral plication) is often the primary surgical treatment, especially when other vaginal surgery needs to be performed. Abdominal approaches (Marshall-Marchetti-Krantz and Burch) are probably more successful in long term.

Patients are usually past childbearing age and need to be assessed for coexisting health problems. Both general and regional anesthesia can be used. A T10 sensory level is sufficient to provide anesthesia for procedures on the uterus and bladder, whereas a T4 level is recommended if the peritoneum is opened.

Intra-abdominal Operations

Hysterectomy (+/− Bilateral Salpingo-Oophorectomy)

After cesarean delivery, hysterectomy is the most commonly performed operation in the United States. Common indications include dysfunctional uterine bleeding, adenomyosis, descent or prolapse of the uterus, uterine leiomyomas, and neoplastic diseases of the uterus or adjacent pelvic organs.

There are two surgical approaches: vaginal and abdominal. Often the approach is decided upon in the OR, where a pelvic examination under anesthesia will determine the true uterine size and the presence of pelvic pathology.

General anesthesia is commonly used; however, regional anesthesia may be also appropriate for simple hysterectomies. A T4–T6 sensory level is sufficient to provide anesthesia for procedures on the uterus.

Heavy blood loss is possible. Blood and evaporative losses are usually greater in patients undergoing abdominal, rather than vaginal hysterectomy. Hysterectomy for gynecologic tumor resection also includes oophorectomy, omentectomy, lymph node dissection, and tumor resection. These resections are often extensive, result in significant blood loss, and require intraoperative fluid replacement. Postoperative pain may also be significant due to the extent of the surgery. These patients may require short-term postoperative ventilation and/or time

in the intensive care unit (ICU). Epidural analgesia for postoperative pain management should be considered.

Tubal Ligation

In the United States, sterilization has become the most commonly used method of contraception among married couples. The procedure can be performed at the time of cesarean delivery, shortly after delivery or induced abortion, or at a time unrelated to pregnancy. The timing of tubal sterilization can influence the choice of anesthetic, the surgical approach, and the method of tubal occlusion. Most tubal sterilizations performed after vaginal delivery are done by minilaparotomy; those not associated with birth are performed by laparoscopy or minilaparotomy.

Complications of general anesthesia are the leading cause of death attributed to sterilization in the United States. The risks inherent in general anesthesia are exacerbated by its use postpartum and during laparoscopy. Sterilization by minilaparotomy can be safely performed under local anesthesia and IV sedation or regional anesthesia. The patient avoids the risks associated with general anesthesia, spends less time sedated or anesthetized, and has a more rapid recovery. Nausea and vomiting are less likely to occur, and the patient is awake to report symptoms that can indicate the occurrence of a complication (Box 12-4).

POSTOPERATIVE CONSIDERATIONS

Good preoperative preparation should decrease the number of issues that might arise in the postanesthesia care unit. Nausea and pain remain the most commonly occurring conditions that require treatment. As discussed, extensive procedures may warrant epidural postoperative analgesia. Otherwise, IV patient-controlled analgesia for

---

Box 12-4 Gynecologic Surgical Procedures

Transvaginal gynecologic surgeries
 Dilation and evacuation
 Dilation and curettage
 Laser therapy to vulva, vagina, or cervix
Perineal gynecologic surgeries
 Radical vulvectomy
 Operations for stress urinary incontinence
Intra-abdominal gynecologic operations
 Hysterectomy
 Tubal ligation
 Abdominal debulking

in-patients or oral opioids +/− NSAIDs or COX-2 inhibitors for out-patients provide good pain control.

SUGGESTED READING

American College of Physicians: Guidelines for assessing and managing the perioperative risk from coronary artery disease associated with major noncardiac surgery. Ann Internal Med 127(4):309–312, 1997.

ASHP: Therapeutic guidelines on antimicrobial prophylaxis in surgery. Am J Health-Syst Pharm 56:1839–1888, 1999.

Bucklin BA, Smith CV: Postpartum tubal ligation: Safety, timing, and other implications for anesthesia. Anesth Analg 89:1269–1274, 1999.

Doyle RL: Assessing and modifying the risk of postoperative pulmonary complications. Chest 115:77S–81S, 1999.

Fahy BG, Barnas GM, Nagle SE, Flowers JL: Effects of Trendelenburg and reverse Trendelenburg postures on lung and chest wall mechanics. J Clin Anesth 8(3):236–244, 1996.

Garfield JM, Muto MG, Bizzari-Schmid M: Anesthesia for Gynecologic Surgery. Principles and Practice of Anesthesiology. New York, Mosby, 1993.

Goldman L: Cardiac risk in noncardiac surgery: An update. Anesth Analg 80(4):810–820, 1995.

Guaschino S, De Santo D, De Seta F: New perspectives in antibiotic prophylaxis for obstetric and gynecologic surgery. J Hospital Infect 50(Suppl A):S13–S16, 2002.

Halliwill JR, Hewitt SA, Joyner MJ, Warner MA: Effect of various lithotomy positions on lower-extremity blood pressure. Anesthesiology 89(6):1373–1376, 1998.

Hampl KF, Heinzman-Wiedmer S, Luginbuehl I, et al: Transient neurologic symptoms after spinal anesthesia: A lower incidence with prilocaine and bupivacaine than with lidocaine. Anesthesiology 88(3):629–633, 1998.

Hampl KF, Schneider MC, Pargger H, et al: A similar incidence of transient neurologic symptoms after spinal anesthesia with 2% and 5% lidocaine. Anesth Analg 83:1051–1054, 1996.

Hampl KF, Schneider MC, Ummenhofer W, Drewe J: Transient neurologic symptoms after spinal anesthesia. Anesth Analg 81:1148–1153, 1995.

Harrison BA, Burkle CM: Cardiorespiratory emergencies associated with pelvic surgery. Clin Obstet Gynecol 45(2):518–536, 2002.

Jaffe RA, Samuels SI: Anesthesiologist's Manual of Surgical Procedures, 2nd edition. Portland, OR, Lippincott, Williams and Wilkins, 1999.

Katz J, Cohen L, Schmid R, et al: Postoperative morphine use and hyperalgesia are reduced by preoperative but not intraoperative epidural analgesia and the prevention of central sensitization. Anesthesiology 98(6):1449–1460, 2003.

Narr BJ, Warner ME, Schroeder DR, Warner MA: Outcomes of patients with no laboratory assessment before anesthesia and a surgical procedure. Mayo Clinic Proc 72(6):505–509, 1997.

Leigh JM, Walker J, Janaganathan P: Effect of preoperative anesthetic visit on anxiety. Br Med J 2:987–989, 1997.

Maranets I, Kain ZN: Preoperative anxiety and intraoperative anesthetic requirements. Anesth Analg 89:1346–1351, 1999.

Martin J: Patient Positioning. In Barash P, Cullen B, Stoelting R (eds): Clinical Anesthesia, 2nd edition. Philadelphia, JB Lippincott, 1992, pp 709–735.

McFarland JG: Perioperative blood transfusions. Chest 115:113S–121S, 1999.

Meyer R: Rofecoxib reduces perioperative morphine consumption for abdominal hysterectomy and laparoscopic gastric binding. Anaesth Inten Care 30(3):389–390, 2002.

Papadimitriou L, Livanios S, Katsaros G, et al: Prevention of postoperative nausea and vomiting after laparoscopic gynecologic surgery. Combined antiemetic treatment with tropisetron and metoclopramide alone. Eur J Anesth 18(9):615–619, 2001.

Parker BM, Tetzlaff JE, Litaker DL, Maurer WG: Redefining the preoperative evaluation process and the role of the anesthesiologist. J Clin Anesth 12(50):350–356, 2000.

Rock JA, Jones HA (eds): Te Linde's Operative Gynecology, 9th edition. Philadelphia, Lippincott, Williams and Wilkins, 2003.

Sawaya GF, Grady D, Kerlikowske K, Grimes DA: Antibiotics at the time of induced abortion: The case for universal prophylaxis based on a metaanalysis. Obstet Gyn 87(5 Pt 2):884–890, 1996.

Smetana GW: Preoperative pulmonary evaluation. N Engl J Med 340(12):937–944, 1999.

Southorn P: Preoperative management of the medically at-risk patient. Clin Obstet Gyn 2002; 45(2): 449–468

Speir BR, Freeman MG: Psychological Aspects of Pelvic Surgery. In Rock JA, Jones HA (eds): Te Linde's Operative Gynecology, 9th edition. Philadelphia, Lippincott, Williams and Wilkins, 2003.

Stone SG, Foex P, Sear JW, et al: Risk of myocardial ischemia during anesthesia in treated and untreated hypertensive patients. Br J Anaesth 61(6):675–679, 1988.

Stovall TG: Clinical experience with epoetin alfa in the management of hemoglobin levels in orthopedic surgery and cancer. Implications for use in gynecologic surgery. J Reprod Med 46(5 Suppl):531–538, 2001.

Thomas R, Jones N: Prospective randomized, double-blind comparative study of dexamethasone, ondansetron, and ondansetron plus dexamethasone as prophylactic antiemetic therapy in patients undergoing day-case gynecological surgery. Br J Anaesth 87(4):588–592, 2001.

Tsui BCH, Stewart B, Fitzmaurice A, Williams R: Cardiac arrest and myocardial infarction induced by postpartum intravenous ergonovine administration. Anesthesiology 94(2):363–364, 2001.

Updike GM, Manolitsas TP, David E, et al: Pre-emptive analgesia in gynecologic surgical procedures: Preoperative wound infiltration with ropivacaine in patients who undergo laparotomy through a midline vertical incision. Am J Obstet Gyn 188(4):901–905, 2003.

Verdolin MH, Toth AS, Schroeder R: Bilateral lower extremity compartment syndromes following prolonged surgery in the low lithotomy position with serial compression stockings. Anesthesiology 92(4):1189-1191, 2000.

Walsh J, Puig MM, Lovitz MA, Turndorf H: Premedication abolishes the increase in plasma beta-endorphin observed in the immediate preoperative period. Anesthesiology 66:402-405, 1987.

Warner MA, Warner DO, Harper CM, et al: Lower extremity neuropathies associated with lithotomy positions. Anesthesiology 93(4):938-942, 2000.

White PF: Pharmacologic and clinical aspects of preoperative medication. Anesth Analg 65:963-974, 1986.

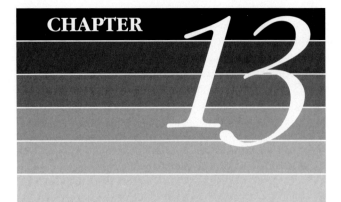

Management of Pelvic Pain

MIRJANA LOVRINCEVIC

ETIOLOGY

Chronic pelvic pain can be classified as the following:
1. Pain arising from the reproductive tract
2. Pain arising from other organ systems
3. Nonorganic disease, but evidence of a psychiatric disease
4. No evidence of organic or psychiatric disease

Chronic pelvic pain arising from the reproductive tract:
- Endometriosis
- Pelvic adhesions
- Pelvic venous congestion
- Cyclic pain
- Cancer pain

Chronic pelvic pain arising from the other organ systems:
- Irritable bowel syndrome
- Recurrent cystitis and interstitial cystitis
- Abdominal myofascial pain

Chronic pelvic pain without evidence of an organic disease, but with evidence of a psychiatric disease:
- Mood disorder
- Anxiety disorders
- Personality disorders
- Psychoses

Chronic pelvic pain with no evidence of organic or psychiatric disease:
- History of physical and /or sexual abuse

HISTORY

History-taking is the first and probably the most important part of the evaluation of a patient with pelvic pain. Patients are usually asked to complete a standardized medical and pain questionnaire that is followed by a structured interview. Particular attention is paid to association of symptoms with menstrual cycle because some of these occur only with menses, others increase with menses, and still others are not related to menses at all. Patients are also asked to point to all areas of pain: it is not uncommon to have patients point to their legs, flank, and upper abdomen. Irritable bowel syndrome, appendicitis, pyelonephritis, cholecystitis, ulcers, and other diseases not originating from the pelvic area may be coincidentally or indirectly related to cyclic hormonal changes. Screening for dysmotility disorders of the bowel should be also included. Associated symptoms are of particular importance because they are dependent on the primary cause of the pain or the involvement of adjacent structures. Special attention should be paid to a sexual history, including history of physical and sexual abuse. Standardized screening psychometric measures, such as West

Haven-Yale Multidimensional Pain Inventory (WHYMPI), a marital adjustment scale (Locke-Wallace), and the Beck Depression Inventory can prove to be very useful as well.

PHYSICAL ASSESSMENT

Physical assessment starts with a standardized exam and narrows down to particular areas of tenderness.

Reproducing trigonal or urethral tenderness usually points toward diagnosis of urethral syndrome or interstitial cystitis.

If the pain is limited to a localized area and is reproduced and exacerbated by direct palpation of these areas of maximal tenderness, myofascial pain is suspected. Injections at abdominal wall and pelvic floor muscle trigger points seem to be very successful if the patient is cooperative in "pinpointing" the painful areas.

In young patients, cyclic pelvic pain and dysmenorrhea are common with endometriosis. Focal tenderness correlates with deep fibrotic endometriosis or other fibrotic pathology. Studies showed that diagnosing deep disease could be facilitated by examination during menses.

DIAGNOSTIC INVESTIGATIONS

In context of a multidisciplinary approach to the patient with chronic pelvic pain, systematic diagnostic methods are used. Laboratory examination should include a complete blood count, sedimentation rate, urinalysis, cervical smear and cultures, cytology, CA-125 level, and radiographic studies, such as ultrasonography, hysterosalpingography, or contrast radiography of the gastrointestinal tract. The results are integrated with the information obtained from the history and physical examination. Additional tests might be performed when specific pathology is suspected: cystoscopy with hydrodistention and bladder biopsy, and intravesical potassium sensitivity for interstitial cystitis; pelvic phlebography to document the presence of venous congestion of the pelvis; microlaparoscopy under local anesthesia and conscious pain mapping for various etiologies of pelvic pain as well as a preoperative assessment for patients with central pelvic pain considering either laparoscopic uterosacral nerve ablation or presacral neurectomy; classic laparoscopy and/or laparotomy as the ultimate diagnostic method.

Chronic Pelvic Pain Arising from the Reproductive Tract

Endometriosis refers to the presence of extrauterine endometrial tissue and the clinical sequelae produced by its normal function in an abnormal site.

Endometriosis-associated pelvic pain commonly persists throughout the reproductive years, and a clinical diagnosis may be made on the basis of a history with the triad of symptoms: dysmenorrhea, dyspareunia, and abnormal uterine bleeding, as well as classic physical findings of uterosacral nodularity. The American Society for Reproductive Medicine is trying to adjust the classification of endometriosis so that it is able to predict outcome with respect to pregnancy, as well as to aid in the management of chronic pelvic pain.

CURRENT CONTROVERSY: CONSERVATIVE VERSUS INVASIVE TREATMENT FOR ENDOMETRIOSIS

- Recent studies have demonstrated that surgical therapy offers no better pain control than medical therapy with gonadotropin-releasing hormone agonist.
- Recurrence of symptoms after surgical intervention occurs in 44% of patients within 1 year of treatment.
- Repeated operations are associated with a progressive reduction in the chance of permanent success.
- Gonadotropin-releasing hormone analogues have been associated with significant pain control. Downside? Significant osteoporosis.
- Various combinations of estrogen and progestin were found to be effective in reducing chronic pain of endometriosis. Contraindications are the same as for oral contraceptives, in general.
- Androgens produce atrophy of the endometriotic implants and control of pain. Virilization, however, is a very undesirable side effect.

Multiple attempts have been made to correlate stage of disease and severity of pain. Important variables include depth of invasion, histology, location, and preoperative physical findings and investigations, and although the endometriosis stage is not directly related to the degree of pain, it is related to the persistence of pelvic pain.

Whereas in the past laparoscopy was commonly used for the diagnosis and treatment of women with endometriosis and pelvic pain, recent studies have demonstrated that surgical therapy offers no better results in terms of pain relief than medical therapy with a gonadotropin-releasing hormone agonist. In fact, from the results of the randomized controlled trials, recurrence of symptoms after surgical intervention occurs in 44% of patients within 1 year of treatment by an experienced surgeon. Repeated operations are associated with a progressive reduction in the chance of permanent success and are not always feasible.

Gonadotropin-releasing hormone analogs (e.g., leuprorelin) are the newest medications used for the treatment of endometriosis and have been associated with significant control of pain. Significant osteoporosis, however, can occur when used for more than 6 months.

Various combinations of added estrogen and progestin have been used to decrease osteoporosis.

Gestagens alone, such as lynestrenol, might be used as second-line drugs for long-term and continuous treatment in the management of endometriosis. A low daily oral dose of cyproterone acetate and a continuous monophasic oral contraceptive containing ethinyl estradiol and desogestrel were found to be similarly effective in reducing chronic pelvic pain in one of the studies. Subcutaneous implantation of buserelin acetate was also found to be effective, although adverse effects were significant.

The observation that hyperandrogenic states induce atrophy of the endometrium has led to the use of androgens (e.g., danazol) in the treatment of endometriosis. The efficacy of danazol is based on its ability to produce a high androgen/low estrogen environment that results in the atrophy of endometriotic implants and control of pain.

CURRENT CONTROVERSY: TREATMENT OF PELVIC ADHESIONS

Laparoscopic adhesiolysis seems to be effective therapeutic measure according to numerous retrospective studies, whereas some prospective studies showed no benefit, except for the small subset of patients with adhesions involving the bowel.

Pelvic adhesions are bands of fibrous tissue that join abdominal organs to each other or the abdominal wall. Adhesions develop rapidly after damage to the peritoneum during surgery, infection, trauma, or irradiation. Until recently, it was thought that the pain secondary to adhesions occurs because of restricted organ mobility and stimulation of stretch receptors. However, it was shown that adhesions contain sensory nerve fibers capable of producing pain stimuli independently.

Laparoscopic adhesiolysis seems to be an effective therapeutic measure to relieve chronic pelvic pain according to numerous retrospective studies, whereas one prospective randomized trial showed no benefit, except for the small subset of patients with dense adhesions involving the bowel.

Pelvic venous congestion in association with chronic pelvic pain was first time described in the late 1950s. The primary problem is retrograde flow in incompetent ovarian and pelvic veins, confirmed by injecting contrast into the ovarian and/or internal iliac veins. Patients usually complain of pain in the pelvic area when standing or in the upright position, during or after intercourse, and in association with varices in the thighs, buttocks, perineum, vulva, or vagina. Although the transuterine venogram supports the diagnosis, the degree of organic disease is minimally related to pain and functional impairment.

Meta-analyses reviewing controlled trials of treatment in patients suffering from pelvic congestion syndrome showed that progestogen was associated with a reduction of pain during treatment. Counseling supported by ultrasound scanning was associated with reduced pain and improvement in mood. Adhesiolysis was not associated with an improved outcome apart from where adhesions were severe.

Embolization of the ovarian veins has emerged as an attractive modality lately: transcatheter embolization of the ovarian veins is a safe and feasible technique leading to complete relief of symptoms in more than half of cases. It should be emphasized, though, that careful selection of patients and use of appropriate angiographic and technical skills by the interventional radiologist are requisite for the success of this therapeutic alternative.

Cyclic pain, or primary dysmenorrhea, is colicky, low abdominal pain during menstruation that occurs predominantly in young women. As a rule, it is not associated with any other diseases, such as endometriosis. Increased uterine tone and high-amplitude contractions during menstruation result in decreased uterine blood flow, all due to increased endometrial prostaglandin production. Considering high prevalence rates (43% to 90% in some studies), dysmenorrhea may not even come to medical attention, although it frequently causes absenteeism and decreased quality of life.

The risk factors for dysmenorrhea are early age at menarche, long menstrual periods, smoking, alcohol intake, and weight above the 90th percentile.

Considering the relation of this condition to hormonal changes during menstrual cycle, and increased prostaglandin production, it is not surprising that nonsteroidal anti-inflammatory drugs and combined oral contraceptives are the most commonly used treatments. Calcium antagonists, glyceryl trinitrate, transcutaneous electric nerve stimulation, acupuncture, and herbal remedies have also been reported to provide pain relief, although their long-term effectiveness is not known.

Cancer pain requires special attention, because it is not only a manifestation of a serious disease with often-poor prognosis, but it is also associated with negative expectations, depressed mood states, and a decrease in a patient's quality of life. Patients with gynecologic malignancies may experience chronic pain as a result of either the disease process itself or cancer treatment.

Pelvic pain has been reported frequently by women with gynecologic cancer. It is usually described as a vague, poorly localized sensation of fullness, pressure, and discomfort, although intermittent shooting pains or a burning sensation deep in the perineum are reported as well.

The Cancer Relief Program of the World Health Organization (WHO) developed the analgesic ladder that has become a widely accepted method of drug selection (Fig. 13-1). Although it is not strictly followed especially

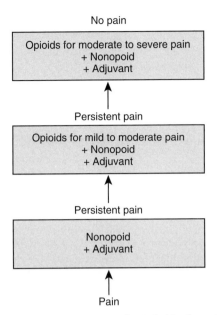

No pain

Opioids for moderate to severe pain
+ Nonopoid
+ Adjuvant

Persistent pain

Opioids for mild to moderate pain
+ Nonopoid
+ Adjuvant

Persistent pain

Nonopoid
+ Adjuvant

Pain

Figure 13-1 WHO three-step analgesic ladder for pain management.

with the development of transdermal and invasive therapies, it forms the basis for an approach to managing all types of pain in the cancer patient. The initial approach for patients with mild to moderate pain is to use a nonopioid analgesic first, with addition of an adjuvant agent if indicated. If this does not provide adequate relief, if the pain increases, or if the pain is severe on presentation, an opioid should be instituted, with or without a nonopioid or adjuvant drug.

CLINICAL CAVEAT: ANALGESIC LADDER

- Nonopioid analgesics: acetaminophen, nonsteroidal anti-inflammatory medications, COX-2 specific inhibitors
- Opioid analgesics: oral (e.g., morphine, hydrocodone, oxycodone) and/or transdermal (fentanyl patch)
- Adjuvant analgesics: for neuropathic pain (tricyclic antidepressants, antiepileptics) and for musculoskeletal (corticosteroids, spasmolytics)

Nonopioid analgesics most commonly used are nonsteroidal anti-inflammatory drugs and acetaminophen. The former group works through the inhibition of enzyme cyclo-oxygenase and decreased tissue production of prostaglandins. The latter has no anti-inflammatory properties. Nonopioid analgesics have a "ceiling effect" for analgesia—they reach a point at which no therapeutic gain is achieved by increasing doses beyond those recommended.

Opioid analgesics are the mainstay of therapy for cancer pain. The pure opioid agonists are used almost exclu-

sively, and it is customary to initially prescribe opioids such as codeine, hydrocodone, or oxycodone that are also available in combination with nonopioids. More potent opioids are chosen when patients do not respond to the initial choice of opioids.

Adjuvant therapy includes different classes of medications that can be combined with analgesics at any level of the WHO ladder to potentiate their effect, to provide inherent analgesic action, and/or to improve mood, sleep, nausea, anxiety, and/or somnolence.

Tricyclic antidepressants have been indicated in the cancer pain population to treat neuropathic pain syndromes. The tertiary amines (amitriptyline, doxepin) are often used as a first line of therapy because of their greater analgesic effect. If excessive sedation is an issue, a secondary amine (desipramine, nortriptyline) would be a more appropriate choice.

Anticonvulsants are particularly useful in treatment of lancinating, shooting, electric shock–like sensations, and paroxysmal dysesthesias. Gabapentin and oxcarbazepine are newer antiseizure medications that have been shown to be effective in neuropathic pain unresponsive to traditionally used carbamazepine, clonazepam, or phenytoin.

Corticosteroids enhance the analgesic effect of other drugs. They also provide excellent anti-inflammatory effects and are especially beneficial in patients with bone pain and in those with pain caused by nerve trunk or spinal cord compression. Dexamethasone has the added benefit of improving mood, appetite, and energy, and it causes less fluid retention than prednisone.

Other adjuvant analgesics are used to manage opioid-refractory malignant pain. These include bisphosphonates, radiopharmaceutical drugs, and calcitonin. The bisphosphonates currently used in clinical practice to treat pain due to bone metastases include pamidronate, zoledronic acid, and clodronate (the former two are approved in the United States for this indication). So far, zoledronic acid has demonstrated clinical superiority. The pain resulting from infiltrated bone with released pain mediators may be effectively alleviated by yet another analgesic method, radiopharmaceuticals. Currently, five artificial isotopes of naturally occurring radioactive elements are in medical use: strontium (89 Sr), phosphorus (32 P), rhenium (186 Rh), samarium (153 Sm), and tin (117 m Sn).

When the pain cannot be controlled with oral medications, the intrathecal route is considered. When opioids alone are used, profound analgesia is achieved at a much lower dose, without the motor, sensory, or sympathetic block associated with intrathecal local anesthetic administration. However, in cancer patients, the presence of neuropathic pain is the most frequent reason to use an intrathecal technique, and the addition of a local anesthetic, clonidine, or both is necessary to achieve adequate pain control. Combinations of low-dose opioids with local anesthetic and/or clonidine act synergistically to produce effective analgesia while decreasing the side effects of individual drugs by allowing lower doses of each. Very infrequently, patients will not achieve adequate pain control with triple intrathecal therapy. In the future, the use of adenosine, aspirin, and ziconotide may become a viable alternative for patients with complex pain problems.

Chronic Pelvic Pain Arising from the Other Organ Systems

Irritable bowel syndrome is characterized by abdominal pain, alteration in bowel habits, and absence of detectable organic disease. Not only is the etiology of this entity unclear, but also it is possible that this syndrome includes a number of disorders for which specific causes may eventually be discovered. Although chronic pelvic pain and irritable bowel syndrome are seen in high rates in patients with psychopathology, demographic data such as age, parity, marital status, race, income, or education were not found to be consistent risk factors. Treatment includes spasmolytics, heating pads, a diet high in bran and fiber, with avoidance of opioids as much as possible.

Interstitial cystitis is a clinical syndrome that is characterized by urinary urgency and frequency and/or pelvic pain in the absence of an apparent cause. It is also known as a chronic urethral syndrome. Trauma, allergies, periurethral inflammation or fibrosis, urethral spasm, urethral stenosis, hypoestrogenism, stress, and psychiatric disorders have all been suggested as a cause, but none has been proven. Risk factors associated with this entity include grand multiparity, two or more abortions, hospital delivery, delivery without episiotomy and pelvic relaxation, and are thought to be so by virtue of traumatization of the pelvic structures and urethra and decreasing urethral blood supply.

A small subset of patients has worsening of symptoms with menstrual cycle variation, and that population seems to do well with hormonal therapy. Is it because of the increase in the perception of pain between ovulation and onset of menses, or because of undetected endometriosis? It is not clear, but hormonal therapy offers substantial pain relief.

Other forms of treatment have been used with relative success: antibiotics, tricyclic antidepressants, manual physical therapy, acupuncture and moxibustion, and sacral nerve stimulation (Medtronic Implantable Pulse Generator sacral nerve implant). Recent studies showed that transforaminal sacral nerve stimulation decreases severity and number of hours and rate of pain in patients with intractable pelvic pain. Some older methods, such as urethral dilation, are not used as often as before. Recently trained practitioners find it less efficacious than those who have been practicing for longer periods.

Abdominal myofascial pain is a common physical sequela to psychological stress as well as muscle tension. This is noteworthy because many patients are being treated for myofascial trigger points or post-traumatic neuromas, which are obviously sensitive to muscle tension.

Chronic Pelvic Pain Without Evidence of Organic Disease but with Evidence of a Psychiatric Disease

Psychological morbidity is commonly seen in association with chronic pain. Numerous studies have consistently shown a relationship between the two, but failed to distinguish the direction of any causality. Recent population-based studies have reported that baseline chronic pain is predictive of future psychological distress, in the presence of other physical and psychosocial factors. At the same time, analysis of 20 observational studies failed to show that chronic pain results from a prior psychiatric disorder. The studies provided limited evidence that chronic depression plays a role in the development of new pain locations; that prior nervousness and past negative life events predict work disability; and that depression, anxiety, and a sense of not being in control may predict slower recovery from pain and disability. These findings do not prove that psychological factors have a role in the development of chronic pain, although psychological impairment may precede the onset of pain. Based on current knowledge, psychological problems may arise as a complication of chronic pain.

Chronic Pelvic Pain with No Evidence of Organic or Psychiatric Disease

Among the many socioenvironmental factors influencing chronic pelvic pain outcomes, abuse history is the most widely studied. Previous data indicate that 20% to 30% of women with chronic pelvic pain have experienced childhood sexual trauma or abuse. Recently, the study was conducted comparing women with chronic pelvic pain, women with chronic low back pain, and healthy women with reference to experience of sexual abuse, physical abuse, physical violence, and emotional neglect in childhood. It was found that women with chronic pelvic pain were exposed more frequently to physical violence and suffered more emotional neglect in their childhoods than women in the control group, and that there is a significant association between sexual victimization before age 15 years and later development of chronic pelvic pain. On a physiologic level, women with chronic pelvic pain demonstrate a dysregulation of the hypothalamic-pituitary-adrenal axis (hypocortisolism) that partly parallels neuroendocrine features of abuse-related post-traumatic stress disorder: a persistent lack of cortisol in traumatized or chronically stressed individuals might promote an increased vulnerability for chronic pain syndromes, as well as for chronic fatigue syndrome, fibromyalgia, rheumatoid arthritis, and asthma.

Psychological treatment modalities are tailored to the individual needs of the patient and begin with the most basic interventions, such as behavioral therapy, and move to the next level, such as cognitive therapy, if initial attempts prove to be insufficient.

CONCLUSION

Complexity of pelvic pain requires a multidisciplinary approach to the problem. History-taking, thorough physical examination, laboratory and other diagnostic investigations, along with psychological assessment of the patient are necessary for the understanding of this common problem that strikes women of all ages much too often.

SUGGESTED READING

Aboseif S, Tamaddon K, Chalfin S, et al: Sacral neuromodulation as an effective treatment for refractory pelvic floor dysfunction. Urology 60(1):52-56, 2002.

Choktanasiri W, Rojanasakul A: Buserelin acetate implants in the treatment of pain in endometriosis. J Med Assoc Thailand 84(5):656-660, 2001.

Chwalisz K, Garg R, Brenner RM, et al: Selective progesterone receptor modulators (SPRMs): A novel therapeutic concept in endometriosis. Ann NY Acad Sci 955:373-388, 2002.

Clemons JL, Arya LA, Myers DL: Diagnosing interstitial cystitis in women with chronic pelvic pain. Obstet Gynecol 100(2): 337-341, 2002.

Elliot ML: Chronic pelvic pain: What are the intervention strategies for psychological factors? Am Pain Society Bulletin 10-16, 1996.

Gurel H, Gurel SA, Atilla MK: Urethral syndrome and associated risk factors related to obstetrics and gynecology. Eur J Obstet Gynecol Reprod Biol 83:5-7, 1999.

Harlow SD, Park M: A longitudinal study of risk factors for the occurrence, duration, and severity of menstrual cramps in a cohort of college women. Br J Obstet Gynaecol 103: 1134-1142, 1996.

Heim C, Ehlert U, Hanker JP, Hellhammer DH: Abuse-related post-traumatic stress disorder and alterations of the hypothalamic-pituitary-adrenal axis in women with chronic pelvic pain. Psychosomatic Med 60(3):309-318, 1998.

Hoeger KM, Guzick DS: An update on the classification of endometriosis. Clin Obstet Gynecol 42(3):611-621, 1999.

Jamieson DJ, Steege JF: The prevalence of dysmenorrhoea, dyspareunia, pelvic pain, and irritable bowel syndrome in primary care practices. Obstet Gynecol 87(1):55-58, 1996.

Kaplan B, Rabinerson D, Lurie S, et al: Clinical evaluation of a new model of a transcutaneous electrical nerve stimulation device for the management of primary dysmenorrhoea. Gynecol Obstet Invest 44(4):255-259, 1997.

Koninckx PR, Meuleman C, Oosterlynck D, Cornillie FJ: Diagnosis of deep endometriosis by clinical examination during menstruation and plasma CA-125 concentrations. Fertil Steril 65:280-287, 1996.

Kotani N, Oyama T, Sakai I, et al: Analgesic effect of a herbal medicine for treatment of primary dysmenorrhoea-a double-blind study. Am J Chinese Med 25(2):205-212, 1997.

Kuch K: Psychological factors and the development of chronic pain. Clin J Pain 17(4):33-38, 2001.

Lampe A, Solder E, Ennemoser A, et al: Chronic pelvic pain and previous sexual abuse. Obstet Gynecol 96(6):929-933, 2000.

Lemack GE, Foster B, Zimmern PE: Urethral dilation in women: A questionnaire-based analysis of practice patterns. Urology 54(1):37-43, 1999.

Lentz G, Bavendam T, Stenchever MA, et al: Hormonal manipulation in women with chronic, cyclic irritable bladder symptoms and pelvic pain. Am J Obstet Gynecol 186(6): 1268-1273, 2002.

Ludwig H: Dysmenorrhea. Therapeutische Umschau 53(6): 431-441, 1996.

Maleux G, Stockx L, Wilms G, Marchal G: Ovarian vein embolization for the treatment of pelvic congestion syndrome: Long-term technical and clinical results. J Vascular Intervent Radiol 11(7):859-864, 2000.

Malik E, Berg C, Meyhofer-Malik A, et al: Subjective evaluation of the therapeutic value of laparoscopic adhesiolysis: A retrospective analysis. Surg Endoscopy 14 (1):79-81, 2000.

McBeth J, Macfarlane GJ, Silman AJ: Does chronic pain predict future psychological distress? Pain 96(3):239-245, 2002.

Morgan PJ, Kung R, Tarshis J: Nitroglycerin as a uterine relaxant: A systematic review. J Obstet Gynecol Canada 24(5):403-409, 2002.

Nezhat FR, Crystal RA, Nezhat CH, Nezhat CR: Laparoscopic adhesiolysis and relief of chronic pelvic pain. J Society Laparoendoscopic Surg 4(4):281-285, 2000.

Palter SF: Microlaparoscopy under local anesthesia and conscious pain mapping for the diagnosis and management of pelvic pain. Curr Opin Obstet Gynecol 11(4):387-393, 1999.

Parsons CL, Zupkas P, Parsons JK: Intravesical potassium sensitivity in patients with interstitial cystitis and urethral syndrome. Urology 57(3):428-432, 2001.

Peters AAW, Trimbos-Kemper GCM, Admiraal C, et al: A randomized clinical trial on the benefit of adhesiolysis in patients with intraperitoneal adhesions and chronic pelvic pain. Br J Obstet Gynaecol 99:59-63, 1992.

Porpora MG, Gomel V: The role of laparoscopy in the management of pelvic pain in women of reproductive age. Fertil Steril 68(5):765-779, 1997.

Proctor ML, Smith CA, Farquhar CM, Stones RW: Transcutaneous electrical nerve stimulation and acupuncture for primary dysmenorrhoea. Cochrane Database Systemic Rev 1: CD002123, 2002.

Rapkin AJ, Kames LD, Darke LL, et al: History of physical and sexual abuse in women with chronic pelvic pain. Obstet Gynecol 76:92–96, 1990.

Regidor PA, Regidor M, Schmidt M, et al: Prospective randomized study comparing the GnRH-agonist leuprorelin acetate and the gestagen lynestrenol in the treatment of severe endometriosis. Gynecol Endocrin 15(3):202–209, 2001.

Reiter RC: Evidence-based management of chronic pelvic pain. Clin Obstet Gynecol 41(2): 422–435, 1998.

Selak V, Farquhar C, Prentice A, Singla A: Danazol for pelvic pain associated with endometriosis. Cochrane Database System Rev 2:CD000063, 2000.

Siegel S, Paszkiewicz E, Kirkpatrick C, et al: Sacral nerve stimulation in patients with chronic intractable pelvic pain. Clin Urology 166(5):1742–1745, 2001.

Stocumb JC: Neurologic factors in chronic pelvic pain: Trigger points and the abdominal pelvic pain syndrome. Am J Obstet Gynecol 149:536–540, 1984.

Stones RW, Mountfield J: Interventions for treating chronic pelvic pain in women. Cochrane Database Systematic Rev 4:CD000387, 2000.

Sulaiman H, Gabella G, Davis C, et al: Presence and distribution of sensory nerve fibers in human peritoneal adhesions. Ann Surg 234(2):256–261, 2001.

Surrey ES, Hornstein MD: Prolonged GnRH agonist and add-back therapy for symptomatic endometriosis: Long-term follow-up. Obstet Gynecol 99:709–719, 2002.

Sutton CJ, Pooley AS, Ewen SP, Haines P: Follow-up report on a randomized controlled trial of laser laparoscopy in the treatment of pelvic pain associated with minimal to moderate endometriosis. Fertil Steril 68:1070–1074, 1997.

Sutton CJG, Ewen SP, Whitelaw N, Haines P: Prospective, randomized, double-blind, controlled trial of laser laparoscopy in the treatment of pelvic pain associated with minimal, mild, and moderate endometriosis. Fertil Steril 62:696–700, 1994.

Svanberg L, Ulmsten U: The incidence of primary dysmenorrhea in teenagers. Arch Gynecol 230:173–177, 1981.

Topolanski-Sierra R: Pelvic phlebography. Am J Obstet Gynecol 76:44–45, 1958.

Venbrux AC, Lambert DL: Embolization of the ovarian veins as a treatment for patients with chronic pelvic pain caused by pelvic venous incompetence (pelvic congestion syndrome). Curr Opin Obstet Gynecol 11(4):395–399, 1999.

Vercellini P, De Giorgi O, Mosconi P, et al: Cyproterone acetate versus a continuous monophasic oral contraceptive in the treatment of recurrent pelvic pain after conservative surgery for symptomatic endometriosis. Fertil Steril 77(1):52–61, 2002.

Vercellini P, De Giorgi O, Pisacreta A, et al: Surgical management of endometriosis. Baillieres Clin Obstet Gynaecol 14:501–523, 2000.

Walker EA, Gelfand AN, Gelfand MD, et al: Chronic pelvic pain and gynecological symptoms in women with irritable bowel syndrome. J Psychosom Obstet Gynecol 17(1): 39–46, 1996.

Walker JJ, Irvine G: How should we approach the management of pelvic pain? Gynecol Obstet Invest 45(suppl 1):6–11, 1998.

Weiss JM: Pelvic floor myofascial trigger points: manual therapy for interstitial cystitis and the urgency-frequency syndrome. J Urology 166(6):2226–2231, 2001.

Winkel CA: A cost-effective approach to the management of endometriosis. Curr Opin Obstet Gynecol 12(4):317–320, 2000.

Zheng H, Wang S, Shang J, et al: Study on acupuncture and moxibustion therapy for female urethral syndrome. J Trad Chinese Med 18(2):122–127, 1998.

Zondervan KT, Yudkin PL, Vessey MP, et al: Chronic pelvic pain in the community-symptoms, investigations, and diagnoses. Am J Obstet Gynecol 184(6):1149–1155, 2001.

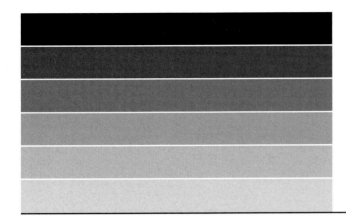

Appendix 1:
Factors That May Place a Woman at Increased Risk from Anesthesia

- Marked obesity
- Severe facial and neck edema
- Extremely short stature
- Difficulty opening her mouth
- Small mandible or protuberant teeth or both
- Arthritis of the neck
- Short neck
- Anatomic abnormalities of the face or mouth
- Large thyroid
- Asthma/other chronic pulmonary disease
- Cardiac disease

- History of problems attributable to anesthetics
- Bleeding disorders
- Severe pre-eclampsia/eclampsia
- Other significant medical or obstetric complications

Adapted from the American Academy of Pediatrics and the American College of Obstetricians and Gynecologists: Guidelines for Perinatal Care, 4th Edition, 1997.

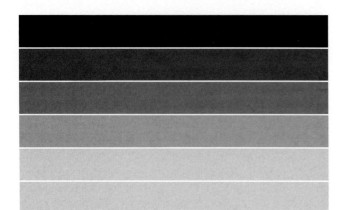

Appendix 2: Guidelines for Regional Anesthesia in Obstetrics

(Approved by House of Delegates on October 12, 1988, and last amended on October 18, 2000. Reprinted from American Society of Anesthesiologists, Park Ridge, Illinois.)

These guidelines apply to the use of regional anesthesia or analgesia in which local anesthetics are administered to the parturient during labor and delivery. They are intended to encourage quality patient care but cannot guarantee any specific patient outcome. Because the availability of anesthesia resources may vary, members are responsible for interpreting and establishing the guidelines for their own institutions and practices. These guidelines are subject to revision from time to time as warranted by the evolution of technology and practice.

GUIDELINE I

REGIONAL ANESTHESIA SHOULD BE INITIATED AND MAINTAINED ONLY IN LOCATIONS IN WHICH APPROPRIATE RESUSCITATION EQUIPMENT AND DRUGS ARE IMMEDIATELY AVAILABLE TO MANAGE PROCEDURALLY RELATED PROBLEMS.

Resuscitation equipment should include, but is not limited to: sources of oxygen and suction, equipment to maintain an airway and perform endotracheal intubation, a means to provide positive pressure ventilation, and drugs and equipment for cardiopulmonary resuscitation.

GUIDELINE II

REGIONAL ANESTHESIA SHOULD BE INITIATED BY A PHYSICIAN WITH APPROPRIATE PRIVILEGES AND MAINTAINED BY OR UNDER THE MEDICAL DIRECTION[1] OF SUCH AN INDIVIDUAL.

Physicians should be approved through the institutional credentialing process to initiate and direct the maintenance of obstetric anesthesia and to manage procedurally related complications.

GUIDELINE III

REGIONAL ANESTHESIA SHOULD NOT BE ADMINISTERED UNTIL: (1) THE PATIENT HAS BEEN EXAMINED BY A QUALIFIED INDIVIDUAL[2] AND (2) A PHYSICIAN WITH OBSTETRIC PRIVILEGES TO PERFORM OPERATIVE VAGINAL OR CESAREAN DELIVERY, WHO HAS KNOWLEDGE OF THE MATERNAL AND FETAL STATUS AND THE PROGRESS OF LABOR AND WHO APPROVES THE INITIATION OF LABOR ANESTHESIA, IS READILY AVAILABLE TO SUPERVISE THE LABOR AND MANAGE ANY OBSTETRIC COMPLICATIONS THAT MAY ARISE.

Under circumstances defined by department protocol, qualified personnel may perform the initial pelvic examination. The physician responsible for the patient's obstetric care should be informed of her status so that a decision can be made regarding present risk and further management.[2]

GUIDELINE IV

AN INTRAVENOUS INFUSION SHOULD BE ESTABLISHED BEFORE THE INITIATION OF REGIONAL ANESTHESIA AND MAINTAINED THROUGHOUT THE DURATION OF THE REGIONAL ANESTHETIC.

GUIDELINE V

REGIONAL ANESTHESIA FOR LABOR AND/OR VAGINAL DELIVERY REQUIRES THAT THE PARTURIENT'S VITAL SIGNS AND THE FETAL HEART RATE BE MONITORED AND DOCUMENTED BY A QUALIFIED INDIVID-

UAL. ADDITIONAL MONITORING APPROPRIATE TO THE CLINICAL CONDITION OF THE PARTURIENT AND THE FETUS SHOULD BE EMPLOYED WHEN INDICATED. WHEN EXTENSIVE REGIONAL BLOCKADE IS ADMINISTERED FOR COMPLICATED VAGINAL DELIVERY, THE STANDARDS FOR BASIC ANESTHETIC MONITORING[3] SHOULD BE APPLIED.

GUIDELINE VI

REGIONAL ANESTHESIA FOR CESAREAN DELIVERY REQUIRES THAT THE STANDARDS FOR BASIC ANESTHETIC MONITORING[3] BE APPLIED AND THAT A PHYSICIAN WITH PRIVILEGES IN OBSTETRICS BE IMMEDIATELY AVAILABLE.

GUIDELINE VII

QUALIFIED PERSONNEL, OTHER THAN THE ANESTHESIOLOGIST ATTENDING THE MOTHER, SHOULD BE IMMEDIATELY AVAILABLE TO ASSUME RESPONSIBILITY FOR RESUSCITATION OF THE NEWBORN.[3]

The primary responsibility of the anesthesiologist is to provide care to the mother. If the anesthesiologist is also requested to provide brief assistance in the care of the newborn, the benefit to the child must be compared to the risk to the mother.

GUIDELINE VIII

A PHYSICIAN WITH APPROPRIATE PRIVILEGES SHOULD REMAIN READILY AVAILABLE DURING THE REGIONAL ANESTHETIA TO MANAGE ANESTHETIC COMPLICATIONS UNTIL THE PATIENT'S POSTANESTHESIA CONDITION IS SATISFACTORY AND STABLE.

GUIDELINE IX

ALL PATIENTS RECOVERING FROM REGIONAL ANESTHESIA SHOULD RECEIVE APPROPRIATE POSTANESTHESIA CARE. FOLLOWING CESAREAN DELIVERY AND/OR EXTENSIVE REGIONAL BLOCKADE, THE STANDARDS FOR POSTANESTHESIA CARE[4] SHOULD BE APPLIED.

- A postanesthesia care unit (PACU) should be available to receive patients. The design, equipment, and staffing should meet requirements of the facility's accrediting and licensing bodies.
- When a site other than the PACU is used, equivalent postanesthesia care should be provided.

GUIDELINE X

THERE SHOULD BE A POLICY TO ASSURE THE AVAILABILITY IN THE FACILITY OF A PHYSICIAN TO MANAGE COMPLICATIONS AND TO PROVIDE CARDIOPULMONARY RESUSCITATION FOR PATIENTS RECEIVING POSTANESTHESIA CARE.

REFERENCES

1. The Anesthesia Care Team (Approved by ASA House of Delegates 10/26/82 and last amended 10/17/01).
2. Standards for Perinatal Care (American Academy of Pediatrics and American College of Obstetricians and Gynecologists, 1988).
3. Standards for Basic Anesthetic Monitoring (Approved by ASA House of Delegates 10/21/86 and last amended 10/21/98).
4. Standards for Postanesthesia Care (Approved by ASA House of Delegates 10/12/88 and last amended 10/19/94).

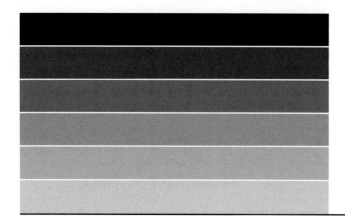

Appendix 3: Optimal Goals for Anesthesia Care in Obstetrics

(Approved by the ASA House of Delegates on October 18, 2000. Reprinted from American Society of Anesthesiologists, Park Ridge, Illinois.)

This joint statement from the American Society of Anesthesiologists (ASA) and the American College of Obstetricians and Gynecologists (ACOG) has been designed to address issues of concern to both specialties. Good obstetric care requires the availability of qualified personnel and equipment to administer general or regional anesthesia, both electively and emergently. The extent and degree to which anesthesia services are available vary widely among hospitals. However, for any hospital providing obstetric care, certain optimal anesthesia goals should be sought. These include:

I. Availability of a licensed practitioner who is credentialed to administer an appropriate anesthetic whenever necessary. For many women, regional anesthesia (epidural, spinal, or combined spinal-epidural) will be the most appropriate anesthetic.

II. Availability of a licensed practitioner who is credentialed to maintain support of vital functions in any obstetric emergency.

III. Availability of anesthesia and surgical personnel to permit the start of a cesarean delivery within 30 minutes of the decision to perform the procedure; in cases of VBAC, appropriate facilities and personnel, including obstetric anesthesia, nursing personnel, and a physician capable of monitoring labor and performing cesarean delivery, immediately available during active labor to perform emergency cesarean delivery.[1] The definition of immediate availability of personnel and facilities remains a local decision, based on each institution's available resources and geographic location.

IV. Appointment of a qualified anesthesiologist to be responsible for all anesthetics administered. There are obstetric units where obstetricians or obstetrician-supervised nurse anesthetists administer anesthetics. The administration of general or regional anesthesia requires both medical judgment and technical skills. Thus, a physician with privileges in anesthesiology should be readily available.

Persons administering or supervising obstetric anesthesia should be qualified to manage the infrequent but occasionally life-threatening complications of major regional anesthesia such as respiratory and cardiovascular failure, toxic local anesthetic convulsions, or vomiting and aspiration. Mastering and retaining the skills and knowledge necessary to manage these complications require adequate training and frequent application.

To ensure the safest and most effective anesthesia for obstetric patients, the director of anesthesia services, with the approval of the medical staff, should develop and enforce written policies regarding provision of obstetric anesthesia. These include:

I. Availability of a qualified physician with obstetric privileges to perform operative vaginal or cesarean delivery during administration of anesthesia. Regional and/or general anesthesia should not be administered until the patient has been examined and the fetal status and progress of labor evaluated by a qualified individual. A physician with obstetric privileges who has knowledge of the maternal and fetal status and the progress of labor, and who approves the initiation of labor anesthesia, should be readily available to deal with any obstetric complications that may arise.

II. Availability of equipment, facilities, and support personnel equal to that provided in the surgical suite. This should include the availability of a properly equipped and staffed recovery room capable of receiving and caring for all patients recovering from major regional or general anesthesia. Birthing facilities, when used for analgesia or anesthesia, must be appropriately equipped to provide safe anesthetic care during labor and delivery or postanesthesia recovery care.

Personnel other than the surgical team should be immediately available to assume responsibility for resuscitation of the depressed newborn. The surgeon and anesthesiologist are responsible for the mother and may not be able to leave her care for the newborn, even when a regional anesthetic is functioning adequately. Individuals qualified to perform neonatal resuscitation should demonstrate:

A. Proficiency in rapid and accurate evaluation of the newborn condition including Apgar scoring.
B. Knowledge of the pathogenesis of a depressed newborn (acidosis, drugs, hypovolemia, trauma, anomalies, and infection), as well as specific indications for resuscitation.
C. Proficiency in newborn airway management, laryngoscopy, endotracheal intubations, suctioning of airways, artificial ventilation, cardiac massage, and maintenance of thermal stability.

In larger maternity units and those functioning as high-risk centers, 24-hour in-house anesthesia, obstetric, and neonatal specialists are usually necessary. Preferably, the obstetric anesthesia services should be directed by an anesthesiologist with special training or experience in obstetric anesthesia. These units will also frequently require the availability of more sophisticated monitoring equipment and specially trained nursing personnel.

A survey jointly sponsored by the ASA and ACOG found that many hospitals in the United States have not yet achieved the above goals. Deficiencies were most evident in smaller delivery units. Some small delivery units are necessary because of geographic considerations. Currently, approximately 50% of hospitals providing obstetric care have fewer than 500 deliveries per year. Providing comprehensive care for obstetric patients in these small units is extremely inefficient, not cost-effective, and frequently impossible. Thus, the following recommendations are made:

1. Whenever possible, small units should consolidate.
2. When geographic factors require the existence of smaller units, these units should be part of a well-established regional perinatal system.

The availability of the appropriate personnel to assist in the management of a variety of obstetric problems is a necessary feature of good obstetric care. The presence of a pediatrician or other trained physician at a high-risk cesarean delivery to care for the newborn or the availability of an anesthesiologist during active labor and delivery when vaginal birth after cesarean delivery (VBAC) is attempted, and at a breech or twin delivery are examples. Frequently, these professionals spend a considerable amount of time standing by for the possibility that their services may be needed emergently but may ultimately not be required to perform the tasks for which they are present. Reasonable compensation for these standby services is justifiable and necessary.

A variety of other mechanisms have been suggested to increase the availability and quality of anesthesia services in obstetrics. Improved hospital design to place labor and delivery suites closer to the operating rooms would allow for more efficient supervision of nurse anesthetists. Anesthesia equipment in the labor and delivery area must be comparable to that in the operating room.

Finally, good interpersonal relations between obstetricians and anesthesiologists are important. Joint meetings between the two departments should be encouraged. Anesthesiologists should recognize the special needs and concerns of the obstetrician, and obstetricians should recognize the anesthesiologist as a consultant in the management of pain and life-support measures. Both should recognize the need to provide high-quality care for all patients.

REFERENCE

1. American College of Obstetricians and Gynecologists. Vaginal birth after previous cesarean delivery. ACOG Practice Bulletin. Washington, DC, ACOG, 1999.

SUGGESTED READING

Committee on Perinatal Health, Toward Improving the Outcome of Pregnancy: The 90s and Beyond. White Plains, NY, March of Dimes Birth Defects Foundation, 1993.

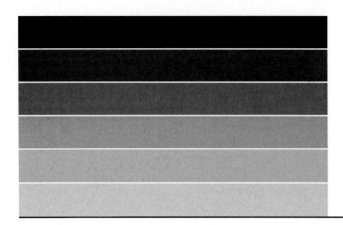

Appendix 4: Standards for Postanesthesia Care

(Approved by House of Delegates on October 12, 1988, and last amended on October 27, 2004. Reprinted from American Society of Anesthesiologists, Park Ridge, Illinois.)

These standards apply to postanesthesia care in all locations. These standards may be exceeded based on the judgment of the responsible anesthesiologist. They are intended to encourage quality patient care but cannot guarantee any specific patient outcome. They are subject to revision from time to time as warranted by the evolution of technology and practice. *Under extenuating circumstances, the responsible anesthesiologist may waive the requirements marked with an asterisk (*); it is recommended that when this is done, it should be so stated (including the reasons) in a note in the patient's medical record.*

STANDARD I

ALL PATIENTS WHO HAVE RECEIVED GENERAL ANESTHESIA, REGIONAL ANESTHESIA, OR MONITORED ANESTHESIA CARE SHALL RECEIVE APPROPRIATE POSTANESTHESIA MANAGEMENT.[1]

1. A Postanesthesia Care Unit (PACU) or an area which provides equivalent postanesthesia care (for example, a Surgical Intensive Care Unit) shall be available to receive patients after anesthesia care. All patients who receive anesthesia care shall be admitted to the PACU or its equivalent **except** by specific order of the anesthesiologist responsible for the patient's care.
2. The medical aspects of care in the PACU (or equivalent area) shall be governed by policies and procedures that have been reviewed and approved by the Department of Anesthesiology.

3. The design, equipment, and staffing of the PACU shall meet requirements of the facility's accrediting and licensing bodies.

STANDARD II

A PATIENT TRANSPORTED TO THE PACU SHALL BE ACCOMPANIED BY A MEMBER OF THE ANESTHESIA CARE TEAM WHO IS KNOWLEDGEABLE ABOUT THE PATIENT'S CONDITION. THE PATIENT SHALL BE CONTINUALLY EVALUATED AND TREATED DURING TRANSPORT WITH MONITORING AND SUPPORT APPROPRIATE TO THE PATIENT'S CONDITION.

STANDARD III

UPON ARRIVAL IN THE PACU, THE PATIENT SHALL BE RE-EVALUATED AND A VERBAL REPORT PROVIDED TO THE RESPONSIBLE PACU NURSE BY THE MEMBER OF THE ANESTHESIA CARE TEAM WHO ACCOMPANIES THE PATIENT.

1. The patient's status on arrival in the PACU shall be documented.
2. Information concerning the preoperative condition and the surgical/anesthetic course shall be transmitted to the PACU nurse.
3. The member of the Anesthesia Care Team shall remain in the PACU until the PACU nurse accepts responsibility for the nursing care of the patient.

STANDARD IV

THE PATIENT'S CONDITION SHALL BE EVALUATED CONTINUALLY IN THE PACU.

1. The patient shall be observed and monitored by methods appropriate to the patient's medical condition. Particular attention should be given to monitoring oxygenation, ventilation, circulation, level of consciousness, and temperature. During recovery from all anesthetics, a quantitative method of assessing oxygenation such as pulse oximetry shall be employed in the initial phase of recovery.[1] This is not intended for application during the recovery of the obstetric patient in whom regional anesthesia was used for labor and vaginal delivery.

2. An accurate written report of the PACU period shall be maintained. Use of an appropriate PACU scoring system is encouraged for each patient on admission, at appropriate intervals prior to discharge, and at the time of discharge.

3. General medical supervision and coordination of patient care in the PACU should be the responsibility of an anesthesiologist.

4. There shall be a policy to assure the availability in the facility of a physician capable of managing complications and providing cardiopulmonary resuscitation for patients in the PACU.

STANDARD V

A PHYSICIAN IS RESPONSIBLE FOR THE DISCHARGE OF THE PATIENT FROM THE POSTANESTHESIA CARE UNIT.

1. When discharge criteria are used, they must be approved by the Department of Anesthesiology and the medical staff. They may vary depending upon whether the patient is discharged to a hospital room, to the Intensive Care Unit, to a short-stay unit or home.

2. In the absence of the physician responsible for the discharge, the PACU nurse shall determine that the patient meets the discharge criteria. The name of the physician accepting responsibility for discharge shall be noted on the record.

REFERENCE

1. ASPAN: Standards of post anesthesia nursing practice, 1992.

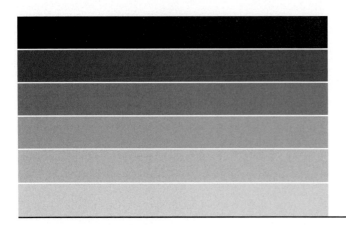

Appendix 5:
Statement on Regional Anesthesia

(Approved by House of Delegates on October 12, 1983, and last amended on October 16, 2002. Reprinted from American Society of Anesthesiologists, Park Ridge, Illinois.)

While scope of practice is a matter to be decided by appropriate licensing and credentialing authorities, the American Society of Anesthesiologists, as an organization of physicians dedicated to enhancing the safety and quality of anesthesia care, believes it is appropriate to state its views concerning the provision of regional anesthesia. These views are founded on the premise that patient safety is the most important goal in the provision of anesthesia care.

Anesthesiology, in all of its forms, including regional anesthesia, is the practice of medicine. Regional anesthesia involves diagnostic assessment, the consideration of indications and contraindications, the prescription of drugs, and the institution of corrective measures and treatment in response to complications. Therefore, the successful performance of regional anesthesia requires medical as well as technical expertise. The medical component generally comprises the elements of medical direction and includes the following:

1. Preanesthetic evaluation of the patient
2. Prescription of the anesthetic plan
3. Personal participation in the technical aspects of the regional anesthetic when appropriate
4. Following the course of the anesthetic
5. Remaining physically available for the immediate diagnosis and treatment of emergencies
6. Providing indicated postanesthesia care

The technical requirements for regional anesthesia will vary with the procedure to be performed.

The decision as to the most appropriate anesthetic technique for a particular patient is a judgment of medical practice that must consider all patient factors, procedure requirements, risks and benefits, consent issues, surgeon preferences, and competencies of the practitioners involved. The decision to perform a specific regional anesthetic technique is best made by a physician trained in the medical specialty of anesthesiology. The decision to interrupt or abort a technically difficult procedure, recognition of complications and changing medical conditions, and provision of appropriate postprocedure care are the duties of a physician. Regional anesthetic techniques are best performed by an anesthesiologist who possesses the competence and skills necessary for safe and effective performance.

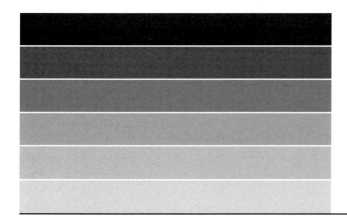

Appendix 6:
Summary of Practice Guidelines for Obstetric Anesthesia

Guidelines are meant to provide basic recommendations for clinical care to assist the anesthesiologist in making patient care decisions. The Guidelines summarized below are intended for peripartum patients.[1]

Preanesthetic Assessment

1. A *focused history and physical* should be performed by the anesthesiologist prior to providing anesthesia care. This should include a history, which reviews issues related to the pregnancy and a limited physical exam including blood pressure, airway assessment, and back exam if regional anesthesia is considered.
2. An intrapartum *platelet count* may be beneficial in reducing complications in patients with pregnancy-induced hypertension or signs of coagulopathy.
3. A *blood type and screen* or cross match should be individualized based on assessment of risk complications.
4. *FHR* should be monitored and documented before and after placement of regional analgesia for labor.

Oral Intake

1. *Clear liquids* may be allowed for uncomplicated laboring patients.
2. *Solid food* should be avoided in labor.
3. Fasting in patients for elective cesarean delivery should be consistent with policies for nonobstetric elective surgery patients.

Intrapartum Care

Choice of *analgesic techniques* should consider patient preference and practitioner preferences. Resources for treatment of complications should be available.

1. *Epidural analgesia* is best with low concentrations of local anesthetic and opioid. Continuous infusion techniques may allow lower analgesia/opioid concentrations while still providing effective analgesia without motor block.
2. *Spinal opioids* may be used for time-limited labor analgesia.
3. *Combined spinal-epidural techniques* may be used to provide rapid, effective analgesia.
4. *MAC* for complicated vaginal delivery may reduce complications and should be available upon request.

Retained Placenta

1. Regional or general *anesthesia* or *sedation/analgesia* may be used for removal of retained placenta.
2. Low-dose *nitroglycerine* is an effective alternative for uterine relaxation during removal of retained placenta.

Cesarean Delivery

1. Choice of anesthetic should be individualized. Regional anesthesia is associated with fewer maternal and neonatal complications when compared with general anesthesia.

Postpartum Tubal Ligation (PPTL)

Timing and anesthetic choice for PPTL should be individualized after evaluation of the patient. PPTL may be safely performed within 8 hours of delivery in many patients.

Management of Complications

1. The institution should have resources available to manage *hemorrhage*. These included large-bore IV catheters, fluid warmers, forced-air body warming, blood bank resources, and rapid IV infusion devices.
2. Resources for *airway emergencies* should include *basic airway equipment* (laryngoscope, ETT, LMA, oxygen, suction, bag and mask) as well as a portable *difficult airway cart*.

The difficult airway cart should contain:

- Various laryngoscope blades and handles
- ETTs
- LMAs
- A device for emergency airway ventilation (e.g., combitube, jet ventilator stylet, crycothyrotomy kit)
- Equipment to establish surgical airway

3. The decision to perform *invasive hemodynamic monitoring* should be individualized.

4. Basic and advanced life support equipment should be immediately available in the Labor and Delivery OR area for *cardiopulmonary resuscitation*.

REFERENCE

1. American Society of Anesthesiologists Task Force on Obstetrical Anesthesia: Practice guidelines for obstetrical anesthesia: A report by the American Society of Anesthesiologists Task Force on Obstetrical Anesthesia. Anesthesiology 90(2):600–611, 1999.

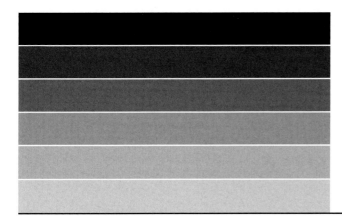

Appendix 7: Statement of Pain Relief During Labor

(Approved by the House of Delegates on October 13, 1999. Reprinted from American Society of Anesthesiologists, Park Ridge, Illinois.)

Labor results in severe pain for many women. There is no circumstance where it is considered acceptable for a person to experience untreated severe pain, amenable to safe intervention, while under a physician's care. In the absence of a medical contraindication, maternal request is a sufficient medical indication for pain relief during labor. Pain management should be provided whenever medically indicated.

Nonetheless, ASA and ACOG have received reports that some third-party payers have denied reimbursement for regional analgesia/anesthesia during labor unless a physician has documented the presence of a "medical indication" for regional analgesia/anesthesia. Of the various pharmacologic methods used for pain relief during labor and delivery, regional analgesia techniques, epidural, spinal, and combined spinal-epidural are the most flexible, effective, and least depressing to the central nervous system, allowing for an alert, participating mother and alert neonate. It is the position of ACOG and ASA that third-party payers who provide reimbursement for obstetric services should not deny reimbursement for regional analgesia/anesthesia because of an absence of other "medical indications."

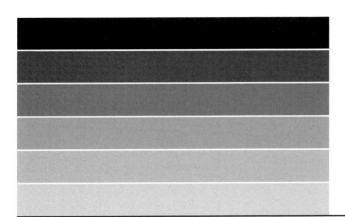

Index

Note: Page numbers followed by f refer to figures; those followed by t refer to tables, and those followed by b refer to boxes.